Advanced Airway Management

Advanced Airway Management

Charles Stewart, M.D., F.A.C.E.P

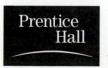
Prentice Hall

Upper Saddle River, New Jersey 07458

Library of Congress Cataloging-in-Publication Data

Stewart, Charles E. (Charles Edward)
     Advanced airway management / Charles Stewart.
        p.; cm.
     Includes bibliographical references and index.
     ISBN 0-13-088191-0 (alk. paper)
        1. Respiratory emergencies.   2. Airway (Medicine).   3. Airway (Medicine)—Intubation.
     4. Respiratory organs—Obstructions.   I. Title.
     [DNLM: 1. Airway Obstruction—therapy. 2. Emergencies. 3. Respiratory
     Therapy—methods. WF 140 S849 2002]
     RC735.R48 S74   2002
     616.2'00425—dc21   2001032191

It is the intent of the authors and publishers that this textbook be used as part of a formal paramedic education program taught by a qualified instructor and supervised by a licensed physician. The care procedures presented here represent accepted practices in the United States. They are not offered as a standard of care. Paramedic-level emergency care is to be performed only under the authority and guidance of a licensed physician. It is the reader's responsibility to know and follow local care protocols as provided by medical advisors directing the system to which he or she belongs. Also, it is the reader's responsibility to stay informed of emergency care procedure changes.

Publisher: Julie Levin Alexader
Acquisitions Editor: Katrin Beacom
Assistant Editor: Kierra Kashickey
Director of Production and Manufacturing: Bruce Johnson
Managing Production Editor: Patrick Walsh
Manufacturing Buyer: Pat Brown
Marketing Manager: Tiffany Price
Production Information Manager: Rachele Triano
Creative Director: Cheryl Asherman
Cover Designer: Gary J. Sella
Compositor: BookMasters, Inc.
Printer/Binder: Banta Harrisonburg

Pearson Education LTD.
Pearson Education Australia PTY, Limited
Pearson Education Singapore, Pte. Ltd.
Pearson Education North Asia Ltd.
Pearson Education Canada, Ltd.
Pearson Educación de Mexico, S.A. de C.V.
Pearson Education—Japan
Pearson Education Malaysia, Pte. Ltd.
Pearson Education, Upper Saddle River, New Jersey

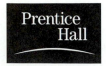

10 9 8 7 6 5 4 3 2 1
ISBN 0-13-088191-0

Brief Contents

Contents

Preface

There is no more important task in emergency medicine than airway control. Whatever the method, it must be effective, for the problem airway does not allow the luxury of waiting until "the consultant" arrives or until the problem cures itself.

To illustrate how important airway control is, merely try holding your breath for one minute. Go ahead—try. Consider how uncomfortable this feels. Now consider a patient who does not have adequate ventilation or who cannot breathe. This patient may be in the acute phase of dying unless you control the situation immediately. This is exactly how important airway control is in emergency care—especially in the field.

If you are not skilled in airway control or attuned to the importance of proactive airway management, then the other fine emergency skills that you possess won't matter much. More of your patients will die from inadequate airway control than hemorrhage or trauma. At normal body temperature, irreversible brain damage begins after 4 to 6 minutes of anoxia. There are few survivable gunshot wounds or other mechanisms of trauma that will cause death in this time. When airway control is achieved early in the management of severe trauma, survival of these trauma victims is improved.[1]

Appropriate control of the airway is the single most important skill that you will ever possess in the management of the acutely ill and injured patient. Indeed, this is the single most important task of the emergency physician, emergency nurse, emergency physician's assistant, emergency medical technician, or paramedic and first responder.

Although the need for better airway control is critical, the means to accomplish this task is anything but clear. The ideal airway maintenance technique would be simple to use, adaptable to every patient, protect the airway from aspiration, and easily provide adequate ventilation. However, this technique does not yet exist!

[1] Regal, G., Stalp, M., Lehmann, U., and Seekamp, A. "Prehospital care, importance of early intervention on outcome." *Acta Anes Scand*, 1997;71–75.

Acknowledgments

I would like to express my appreciation to several people who encouraged and supported me throughout the process of writing this book.

First, I would like to thank my family, the most important people in my life. My heartfelt gratitude is extended to my wife, Kathleen for her love, encouragement, and support. She read every word of this text, offered many comments, and shared the miseries and the mysteries of the author's craft. Her organizational skills helped make deadlines happen and her management of the Red Pencil Brigade brought vibrant field experience into the written word. My mother Kitty and father Sherman put a love for the English language into my life and taught me that anything in life worth having is worth working for—two indispensable tools that helped me get to where I am today. I also thank my mother-in-law Bernice who has shared her family with me. Thanks, also, to my daughters, Kaylan and Tracy, for their love and affection.

I would like to express my gratitude to Judy Streger, Greg Vis, Kierra Bloom, and Katrin Beacom from the Brady group of Prentice Hall, who recruited me to write this text and encouraged me through the ups and downs of the effort. Pat Walsh headed production and Jennifer Welsch organized the BookMasters' side of production.

My close friends and sharp-tongued critics in the "Krasneeya Karendash Brigade" (Russian for Red Pencil Brigade) reviewed every chapter and suffered through the many revisions, late night phone calls, and pleas for a "reference for that thought." Their years of field experience has contributed much to this text. They include:

Tracy Evans, RN, APRN, MS, MPH, EMT-P
Trauma Coordinator
Norwalk Hospital
A fresh view with field experience, teaching, and critical analysis of the work. I was happy to find a new friend and contributor in Tracy.

Dr. James Frisk
Ear, Nose, and Throat Surgery
Dakota Heartland Hospital
Perhaps the most gentle and understanding surgeon I have ever met.

Jacquline Harris, EMT-P
911 Coordinator for Fort Carson
Field experience, an outstanding teacher for the troops, and a long time friend.

Colleen Hayes, MBA, RN, EMT-P
CEO, Vertical Villages, Inc.
Founder/Editor EMSvillage.com
Senior Faculty, The Stamford Hospital EMS Institute
Associate Professor, Norwalk Community College Paramedic Program
Insightful comments, cogent thoughts, outstanding teacher, and both field and hospital experience. I was delighted to make a friend and find a critic in Colleen.

Dexter W. Hunt, MEd, EMT-P
The Hunt Group
Rural transports, air medicine, tactical medicine, and outstanding author, teacher, and a damn good friend. Dexter was constantly getting me to simplify, cut and pare the text.

Jo Ann Hanks, EMT-P
Boise, Idaho
Rural transports, medium-sized city medicine, and Dexter's constant, Jo Ann reviewed and probably toned down Dexter's polemic.

Robert G. Nixon, BA, EMT-P
Life Care Medical Training
The West Coast view, part I; and superb educator, author, and a damn good friend.

Paul M. Maniscalco, MPA, PhD(c), EMT-P
The New York City streets, part I; disaster medicine, scholarly analysis, and the long view mark Paul's contributions. I am happy to count him as both a friend and critic.

Mike Poynter, EMT-P
Flight Paramedic
University of Kentucky Air Medical Service
Mike looked at the text from both the aeromedical and the tactical approaches. A friend of more than 10 years, I was happy to have his input.

Norm Rooker EMT-P/FF
San Francisco, California, Fire Dept.
The West Coast view, part II

David Spiro EMT-P
Organ Recovery/Placement Coordinator
Finger Lakes Donor Recovery Network
The New York City streets, part II; teaching, and street applications.
David literally read every word of this text at least twice. A long time
friend, author and educator in his own, and A Patron of the Arts.

M. Kathleen Stewart, EMT
Colorado Springs, Colorado
As she said, you really do intubate the bubbles!

The author and publisher would like to thank the following reviewers for
their helpful feedback at the various stages of development of this book:

Brenda M. Beasley, RN, BS, EMT-P
EMS Education Director
Calhoun College

David Becker
Chief Medical Officer
Castle Rock Fire and Rescue Department

John L. Beckman
Firefighter/Paramedic
Addison Fire Protection District; Ems Instructor
Highland Park Hospital

Mary Bell, MICP
Assistant Director/EMS Educator
Trinitas Hospital MICU

Christopher Black
Director, EMS and Fire Science
Arizona Western College

Lee Burns, BS, EMT-P
Saratoga Emergency Medical Services

Donna M. Galganski-Pabst
York County Fire and Life Safety

Scott Tomek
Paramedic
Lakeview Hospital EMS
EMS Instructor
Century College

The author would like to express appreciation to the unnamed Brady staff who guided this text through the publication process. These people aren't often recognized, but without them, books simply wouldn't exist.

Charles Stewart, MD, FACEP
February, 2001

Advanced Airway Management

Chapter **One**

Introduction

Philosophy

Intubation of the larynx and trachea is taught in every ACLS course and is required of almost every emergency provider. This does not mean that every patient is easy to intubate or that the technique is simple. In some trauma patients, intubation is literally impossible to accomplish—even in the well-lighted and controlled environment of an emergency department that routinely manages such trauma.

In a patient with a medical illness, deciding exactly when to intubate the patient may be one of the most challenging judgment calls in clinical practice or it may be quite easy. The patient may be frankly moribund on arrival or may simply be "running out of steam." The minimal morbidity associated with short-term intubation justifies the procedure in marginal cases in most patients. When the patient has risk factors for a difficult intubation, the clinician may choose to delay rather than risk a failed intubation. This delay may be to the patient's detriment. Conversely, attempting to intubate an unwilling awake patient is fraught with hazards.

This book is a compendium of techniques that may be used when routine intubation is either not possible, is laden with risk, or has failed after multiple attempts. Much of it is *not* designed to be a sequential approach—if this fails, then do that—but rather a review of techniques that have been used successfully in similar situations. Difficult intubations require the ability to use a variety of techniques, depending on the patient's condition, habitus, and urgency.

Primum Non Nocere

The Latin means "Above all, do no harm." A multitude of therapeutic options are available for airway management, including oxygen delivery systems, various tubes and tools, and a variety of techniques for placing these tubes and using these tools. The techniques that the operator (every caregiver that intubates, from EMT through physician) uses to protect the airway and provide oxygen and ventilation to the patient should not damage the patient. In emergency medicine, we have often tried new devices and techniques designed to be more effective or to simplify the clinician's job. Many of these techniques, such as the esophageal obturator airway, have not withstood careful scrutiny. A wise clinician seeks neither the newest technique and fashion nor blindly follows outdated trends. The same astute clinician carefully follows and reads the literature about airway management because it is a singularly important task in emergency medicine.

> *The military puts it very simply:*
> *When the idiot-proof device is built, Mr. Murphy will find a more ingenious idiot. By careful evaluation of risks, benefits, and hazards of the technique or tool, you can avoid being Mr. Murphy's idiot!*

Proper Preparation—The Right Stuff

When the operator is an expert, an observer may note that "every intubation is easy" (Figure 1-1). What the observer does not see is the continuous evaluation and preparation performed by the true expert prior to the intubation. The

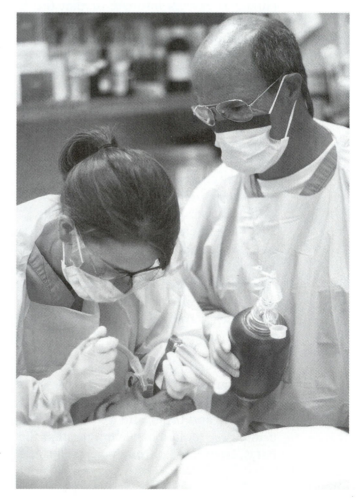

Figure 1-1 EMS airway management in the ED. *Source:* Courtesy of Mark C. Ide.

expert will anticipate the problems and subtly alter his or her behavior so that no difficulties are ever encountered. From the moment that the expert clinician decides that intubation might be needed, the behavior and activities will be directed to patient safety and operator competency. The laryngoscope will be fitted with the desired blade and the light checked. The patient will be correctly positioned in the sniffing position as described by Magill over 70 years ago.[1] Additional padding will be provided for the obese patient if it is required. An operating suction device fitted with either a tonsil or similar suction tip will be put under the patient's left shoulder. An assistant will be directed to the right of the patient with no other duties but to help the operator. A spare blade will be easily at hand. The tube will be checked, lubricated, and a stylet inserted. The patient's monitors will be attached and checked prior to the intubation attempt. The operator will assess the ability to ventilate the patient with a face mask. The patient will be oxygenated to the greatest extent possible, depending on the illness that requires emergent intubation. An intravenous dose of sedative agent will be sufficient to ensure rapid and deep loss of consciousness. This will be followed by a dose of rapidly acting paralytic sufficient to provide complete neuromuscular blockade. The operator will make no attempt at laryngoscopy until complete paralysis has been achieved. The assistant will provide Sellick's maneuver. The pre-prepared tube will be placed on the first attempt . . . the operator will put aside the laryngoscope and note "easy intubation—first shot!"

The intent of this book is to provide every physician, every nurse-clinician, every paramedic, and every EMT who intubates with the ability to have the "right stuff" every time.

Protection

Protection of the Cervical Spine

Protection of the cervical spine is a high priority in emergency medicine. This means avoidance of motion, particularly flexion of the neck. There is no question that all airway maneuvers cause some motion of the neck. The methods with the least motion, or the least harmful motion, are still controversial. They included in-line traction, immobilization with gentle orotracheal intubation, nasotracheal intubation with immobilization, and performance of a surgical airway. A complete discussion of this topic, together with the rationale for each, is presented in the chapter on difficult intubations (Figure 1-2).

Protection from Aspiration

Aspiration is another avoidable complication that can be exacerbated by the clinician. Many of our patients have a full stomach, often have either head trauma or intoxication (and frequently both), and are at grave risk of vomiting. If vomiting occurs without protection of the airway by either the patient or the clinician, then we have not helped our patient. When the patient aspirates stomach contents, the subsequent mortality can be as high as 70 percent. The paramedic or emergency physician is often not aware of this death because the patient dies some days later of pneumonia.

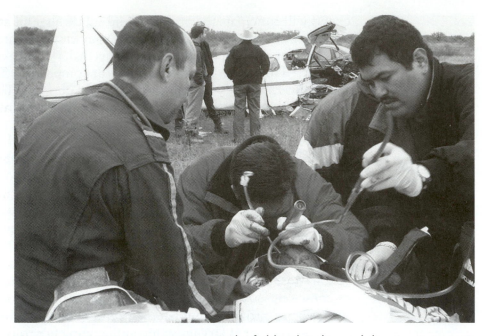

Figure 1-2 Airway management in the field with in line stabilization. *Source:* Courtesy of Mark C. Ide.

Signs and Symptoms of an Inadequate Airway

- **Apnea.** Obviously, if the patient is not breathing, there is something wrong with either the mechanics, the airway plumbing, or the drive to breathe. All of these must be evaluated rapidly.
- **Rate and depth of respiration.** In an adult, the normal respiratory rate is between 10 and 20. An increase in respiratory rate is often the first clue to the patient's ability to ventilate and needs evaluation by the clinician. Likewise, a slowed rate of respiration may be caused by hypothermia, narcotic overdose, or hypothyroidism. Of course, in order to know the rate of respirations, the operator must actually count the respirations and not just guesstimate.

  Shallow respirations may be seen with trauma to the chest wall, pleuritic chest pain from any reason, narcotic overdoses, or abdominal trauma and pathology.
- **Aphonia or hoarseness.** Often an early clue to the patient's ability to maintain the airway.
- **Cyanosis.** A rapidly noted and important physical sign is the bluish color to the skin, called cyanosis. Unfortunately, this is often a late finding in hypoxia. Visual identification of cyanosis generally means that the patient has 5 grams of desaturated hemoglobin per 100 cc of blood. If the patient has too many red blood cells (polycythemia), this 5 grams of desaturated hemoglobin is reached easily, and the patient has adequate saturated hemoglobin to supply all bodily needs. Likewise, if the patient is profoundly anemic, they may not have enough red blood cells to produce the color of cyanosis. Methemoglobinemia and sulfhemoglobinemia may mimic cyanosis.
- **Diaphoresis.** When the patient is working too hard at the mechanics of breathing, diaphoresis is quite common.

- **Drooling.** When the patient is drooling, suspect that either the airway or the esophagus is obstructed and that the patient can no longer handle his or her own secretions.
- **Abnormal respiratory effort.** The signs of increased work of breathing and abnormal respiratory efforts allow the wary clinician to spot the patient in respiratory distress from a distance. A patient with abnormal respiratory effort must be treated rapidly.
  - **Tracheal tug.** This characteristic sign of respiratory distress is a retraction over the trachea in the angle bounded by the sternocleido-mastoid muscles and the sternal notch.
  - **Nasal flaring.** An early sign of distress, particularly in children, is nasal flare or widening of the nostrils as the patient inspires.
  - **Retractions and use of accessory muscles.** The patient with increased work of breathing for any reason will recruit additional muscles to help with the movement of air. As these muscles contract and relax during respiration, they produce retractions. Retractions may be seen in the intercostal, supraclavicular, infraclavicular, and neck areas.
  - **Diaphragmatic breathing.** As the patient increases the breathing effort, abdominal muscles are recruited to help.
- **Tripod position.** As work of breathing continues to increase, the patient will start to lean forward, place both hands on the thighs, and support the upper body with the upper extremities. This tripod position should be recognized immediately, as the patient is in imminent danger of respiratory arrest.
- **Paradoxical chest motion.** There are two types of paradoxical chest motion.
  - **Upper airway obstruction.** When the patient has a partial or complete upper airway obstruction, the patient's attempts to depress the diaphragm will cause the chest and abdomen to have a rocking motion. This is often seen together with retractions and tracheal tug.
  - **Flail chest.** In a patient with multiple fractured ribs in a segment of the chest wall—a flail chest—the patient will pull this isolated segment of chest wall in as they try to inspire.
- **Neck vein distention.** The patient with cardiac tamponade, tension pneumothorax, right heart failure, or volume overload may have engorged neck veins. Although absence of jugular venous distention does not preclude any of these potential disasters, presence of jugular venous distention in the patient who is struggling to breathe should be evaluated.

Abnormal Respiratory Sounds

- **Rales.** Crackles or rales, also called the Rice Krispies™ sound, represent alveolar filling, pulmonary fibrosis, pneumonia, COPD, or pulmonary edema. In general, rales indicate an abnormal lung compliance. Although the patient may require intubation for the underlying disease, rales mandate treatment but not necessarily intubation.
- **Rhonchi.** The coarse sounds produced by mucus or other secretions as air flows past or through the secretions. The presence of rhonchi argues

for cough and suctioning of the patient. A bronchodilator may be indicated in this patient.

- **Grunting respirations.** Grunting is an ominous sign of impending respiratory failure. It is produced by partial closure of the glottis on the end of expiration. Grunting seems to provide an increased end-expiratory pressure and keeps the terminal airways open.[2] Grunting localizes the respiratory disease to the lower respiratory tract. That is, patients who grunt have pneumonia, asthma, or bronchiolitis and not upper respiratory obstruction.

- **Stridor.** The word *stridor* comes from the Latin word "stridulus," meaning creaking, whistling, or grating. Inspiratory stridor is often associated with obstruction at or above the vocal cords. This may be by tumor, epiglottitis, foreign body, or swelling from trauma or allergic reaction. Expiratory stridor is most often seen with obstruction below the cords, as in allergic reaction or croup.

  Stridor will resolve with endotracheal intubation. The clinician should be very wary, as the patient with stridor has a high risk for a failed intubation. This may well leave the clinician in the "can't intubate, can't ventilate" situation.

- **Gurgling.** Gurgling respirations imply pooled secretions that must be removed because the patient is not able to adequately handle these secretions.

- **Wheezing.** The high-pitched whistles usually associated with bronchospasm can be caused by asthma, reactive airway disease, inhalation of noxious gases, pulmonary edema, and mechanical obstruction of the airway. The astute clinician knows that "all that wheezes is not asthma." Higher-pitched wheezes usually occur during expiration when the airways shrink as they lose the support of the distended lung around them.

  Asymptomatic small-airway obstruction may have wheezes only during forced expiration. With mild small-airway obstruction, the wheezes may be heard only at end-expiration.

  Unilateral wheezing is common with an aspirated foreign body. Unilateral wheezing may also be found with pulmonary emboli.

  The patient with wheezing from asthma may benefit from inhaled bronchodilators. The emergency provider must be very wary of the other causes for wheezing while administering the bronchodilator.

Abnormal Mental Status

- Agitation
- Anxiety
- Tachypnea

An old adage says:
Good judgment is the result of experience.
Bad judgment will build a lot of experience quickly!

NORMAL VITAL SIGNS

Group	Age	Resp	Respiratory Danger Window	Pulse	Pulse Danger Window
Newborn	Birth–6 Weeks	30–50	<30, >50	120–160	<100, >160
Infant	7 Weeks–1 year	20–30	<20, >30	80–140	<80, >120
Toddler	1–2 years	20–30	<20, >30	80–130	<80, >110
Preschool	2–6 years	20–30	<20, >30	80–120	<80, >110
School Age	6–13 years	(12–20)–30	<20, >30	(60–80)–100*	<80, >100
Adolescent	13–16 years	12–20	<12, >20	60–100*	<60, >100
Adult	16+ years	12–20	<12, >20	60–100*	<60, >100

*Well-conditioned athletes may have pulses that are as low as 40 without any disease process.

END NOTES

[1] Magill, I. W. "Technique in endotracheal anesthesia." *Br Med J* 1930; 2:817.

[2] American Heart Association. *Textbook of Pediatric Advanced Life Support.* Dallas, TX: The American Heart Association, 1994.

Chapter **Two**

Anatomy

Normal breathing involves the exchange of inspired and expired air through the intact passage from mouth and/or nose to the alveoli of the lung. The emergency provider at all levels must understand the anatomy of the airway in order to master any of the techniques used to maintain or re-establish an airway.

Components of the Upper Airway

The upper airway extends from the nasal or oral opening to the larynx. It includes the nose, mouth, pharynx, and larynx.

Nose

The external nose is formed by the nasal bones, the upper and lower nasal cartilages, and the cartilaginous nasal septum (Figure 2-1). The nose is bony in its upper portion and cartilaginous in the lower portion.

The maxillary, frontal, nasal, ethmoid, and sphenoid bones make up the lateral and superior walls of the nasal cavity. The hard and soft palate form the floor of the nasal cavity (Figure 2-2).

The nasal cavity is divided into two passages by the nasal septum. Each nasal passage has a roof, a floor, a medial wall formed by the nasal septum, and a lateral cartilaginous wall. The anterior opening is the nostril, and the posterior opening is the nasopharynx. The nasal septum is made up of the anterior nasal septal cartilage and the perpendicular plate of the ethmoid bone and vomer.

The lateral walls of the nose are composed of irregular bony projections covered by soft tissue and mucous membranes. These irregular projections are called the turbinates. The lacrimal ducts, the anterior ethmoid sinus, the maxillary sinus, and the sphenoid sinus open into the lateral wall of the nose. The eustachian tubes connect the ear with the nasal cavity.

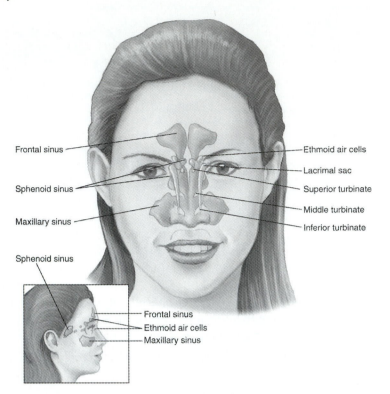

Frontal sinus

Sphenoid sinus

Maxillary sinus

Sphenoid sinus

Ethmoid air cells

Lacrimal sac

Superior turbinate

Middle turbinate

Inferior turbinate

Frontal sinus
Ethmoid air cells
Maxillary sinus

Figure 2-1   Surface anatomy of the face.

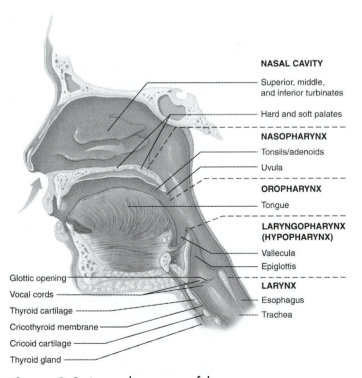

NASAL CAVITY

Superior, middle, and inferior turbinates

Hard and soft palates

NASOPHARYNX

Tonsils/adenoids

Uvula

OROPHARYNX

Tongue

LARYNGOPHARYNX (HYPOPHARYNX)

Vallecula

Epiglottis

LARYNX

Esophagus

Trachea

Glottic opening
Vocal cords
Thyroid cartilage
Cricothyroid membrane
Cricoid cartilage
Thyroid gland

Figure 2-2   Internal anatomy of the nose.

The tissue of the nasal cavity is delicate, endowed with abundant nerves, and extremely vascular. Trauma to this area can be both bloody and very painful. Improper or aggressive placement of airway devices can cause significant bleeding or destroy mucosal surfaces.

The sinuses are mucous membrane-lined cavities in the bone. These cavities connect with the nasal cavity. The sinuses are thought to assist in moistening and heating the air inhaled through the nose.

When sinus openings are plugged by swelling, foreign bodies or material, or trauma, they can become infected. These infections are intensely painful. Nasal airway devices such as nasopharyngeal airways and nasal intubation can cause this extremely painful infection. Indeed, if the patient has been intubated for more than 24 hours and develops a fever, the astute clinician will include sinusitis in the diagnostic evaluation.

The nose has several functions in addition to being the main conduit for incoming air. Inspired air is warmed, humidified, and filtered during flow over the turbinates. The nose acts as a resonant chamber for phonation. The nose is also the organ of smell.

Mouth

The cheeks, lips, floor of the mouth, and hard and soft palate form the oral cavity or mouth. The mandible, tongue, and associated soft tissues form the floor of the mouth.

Behind the lips are the gums and teeth. There are 32 teeth in the adult, all permanent. There are 20 deciduous or "baby" teeth in the child, although this varies by age. All deciduous teeth are present by about three years of age and start to shed by about 6 years of age. From 6 to 10 years of age, the mouth has a mixture of both deciduous and permanent teeth.

It takes significant force to dislodge a normal permanent tooth. This is not true for teeth with periodontal disease, cavities, or for deciduous teeth. Relatively minor trauma can destroy, break, or dislodge diseased teeth. This may be quite important for the field or emergency department provider who breaks, or dislodges a tooth during intubation.

Dislodged teeth can cause significant and long-lasting pulmonary infections if aspirated. A dislodged tooth or broken tooth fragment simply must be located either by direct inspection or x-ray. For the field provider, this means that when the patient report is given to the emergency physician, any tooth trauma noted must be reported so that the emergency physician will look for a tooth on chest x-ray. Failure to include this trauma in a report would be considered malpractice.

Pharynx

The pharynx is a muscular tube that connects the oral and nasal cavities with the larynx and esophagus (Figure 2-3). It is divided into three sections: the nasopharynx, the oropharynx, and the hypopharynx (also called the laryngopharynx).

The nasopharynx is directly behind the nasal cavity. The lower boundary is the level of the soft palate. Within the nasopharynx are five passages: the two nasal passages, the two eustachian tubes, and the outlet to the oropharynx.

The roof of the nasopharynx is formed by the sphenoid and the occipital bones of the skull. The posterior wall of the nasopharynx is separated

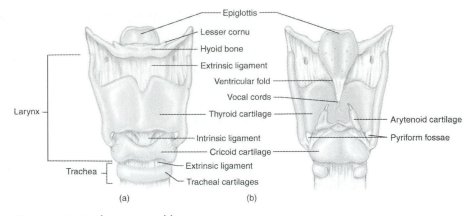

Figure 2-3 Pharynx and larynx.

from the spinal column by the arch of the first cervical vertebra, the deep muscles of the neck, and the prevertebral fascia.

The mucous membranes of the roof and posterior walls of the nasopharynx contain the adenoid lymphatic tissue. When enlarged, the adenoid tissue can cause chronic nasal airway obstruction. Normally, during puberty, the adenoid tissue shrinks. Large adenoids make nasal intubation quite difficult.

The oropharynx is directly posterior to the opening of the mouth and extends from the soft palate to the epiglottis. The posterior wall of the oropharynx is formed by the prevertebral fascia and the second and third cervical vertebral bodies. The lateral walls of the oropharynx contain the tonsils. The tonsillar fossae are formed by the anterior pillars (the palatoglossal folds) and the posterior pillars (the palatopharyngeal folds).

In some children, the tonsils may reach considerable size and may obstruct the view of the larynx during intubation. The tonsils, like the adenoids, normally shrink during puberty.

The uvula is located at the posterior of the soft palate. The uvula can become so edematous that oral intubation is quite difficult. It is important to remember that if the uvula is swollen, nasal intubation will be equally difficult.

Directly medial to the tonsils is the posterior part of the tongue (base of the tongue.) The top surface of the posterior part of the tongue is rough with taste buds.

Because the mouth and nose can be used for both breathing and swallowing food and liquids, there are a number of mechanisms that prevent mixing the two functions. These include coughing to remove particulate and liquid matter from the airway and the gag reflex to prevent liquids from entering the airway.

Just beyond the posterior part of the tongue is one of the most important airway landmarks—the epiglottis. The emergency practitioner must be able to rapidly identify the epiglottis during laryngoscopy. It is a landmark that points the way to the glottic opening where an endotracheal tube is placed. The epiglottis is a small flap-like structure made of cartilage and covered with mucosa. The epiglottic cartilage forms the anterior border of the laryngeal inlet and is attached to the hyoid bone and the thyroid cartilage. The bulk of the epiglottis projects posteriorly to the tongue and into the pharynx. The anterior surface of the epiglottis is concave. Its particular function is not certain—it is tempting to think it is a flap valve that falls over the cords to protect against aspiration, but patients without this structure rarely aspirate.

The arytenoid cartilages are pyramidal structures that articulate with the posterior portion of the cricoid cartilage. The muscles of voice control are attached to the arytenoid and the vocal cords. They then extend posteriorly to the arytenoids from the thyroid cartilage. The action of the laryngeal muscles will change the size of the opening between the vocal cords.

Just anterior and superior to the epiglottis is the vallecula. The vallecula is a fold of tissue formed at the base of the tongue and the epiglottis. The vallecula is an important landmark for intubation. The curved series of laryngoscope blades are designed to lift the epiglottis when placed in the vallecula.

The hypopharynx extends from the epiglottis to the cricoid cartilage. It communicates with three structures: the oropharynx, the inlet of the larynx, and the esophagus. On each side of the larynx are the piriform sinuses. The piriform sinuses act to divert food away from the larynx during swallowing.

Larynx

The larynx is a box formed with the thyroid cartilage on the front. The arytenoid, corniculate, and the cuneiform cartilages form the back of the box. The epiglottal cartilage caps the top of the box. The cricoid cartilage is shaped like a backward signet ring and forms part of the back and the bottom of the box. The box opens into the oropharynx and the trachea. The thyroid cartilage forms the anterior prominence called the Adam's apple. The thyroid cartilage is larger in males.

The larynx serves to protect the airway from aspiration and to form the sounds of the voice. The oldest function of the larynx is protection of the airway from aspiration. This function is found in our amphibian ancestors. The constrictor mechanisms result in effective and rapid closure of the airway that prevents food and liquid from entering the lower airway.

The nerve supply to the larynx is through the superior laryngeal nerve and the recurrent laryngeal nerve. These are both branches of the vagus nerve. The superior laryngeal nerve divides into the internal and external laryngeal nerves. The internal laryngeal nerve supplies the sensory fibers to the mucosa above the level of the vocal cords. The external laryngeal nerve supplies motor function to the cricothyroid muscle. The remainder of the laryngeal muscles are supplied by the recurrent laryngeal nerve, which comes from the area of the aortic arch.

Cricoid The cricoid (from Greek *cricos,* meaning "ring") cartilage is the only cartilaginous structure in the larynx that has no ligaments. The cricoid cartilage is located below the thyroid cartilage. Some authors consider the cricoid cartilage to be the first ring of the tracheal cartilage. The narrow portion of the cricoid cartilage provides room for the cricoid membrane and is the space where the cricoid membrane is punctured in an emergent surgical intubation.

Since the cricoid cartilage is a complete ring, pressure on the anterior cricoid cartilage will push on the esophagus. This is the basis of Sellick's maneuver or cricoid pressure in occluding the esophagus and preventing aspiration.[1] In children, the narrowest portion of the upper airway is the cricoid cartilage.

The cricoid cartilage has two surfaces that articulate with the thyroid cartilage. The thyroid cartilage is attached above to the hyoid bone by the thyrohyoid membrane and below to the cricothyroid membrane.

The larynx is lined with mucous membranes. These membranes are richly enervated and have abundant blood vessels. The nerve supply is from the vagus nerve. The nerve endings are quite sensitive so that liquid or particulate matter in the airway will trigger gag or cough reflexes.

Since the nerve supply is from the vagus nerve, stimulation by endotracheal intubation or other devices can trigger bradycardia, hypotension, or decreased respiratory rates. This is particularly true in younger patients.

Vocal Cords The vocal cords are located just behind the prominence of the thyroid cartilage (Adam's apple). The cords are located just above the cricoid cartilage. They are composed of the thickened upper edges of the cricothyroid ligament and extend to the paired and mobile arytenoid cartilages. Because they are subject to repeated trauma during speaking, they are covered with a layer of epithelium (Figure 2-4).

The motor nerve supply to the larynx originates from the recurrent laryngeal branch and the superior laryngeal branch of the vagus nerve. The recurrent laryngeal nerve runs alongside the thyroid on both sides of the trachea and is susceptible to trauma during a tracheostomy. The superior laryngeal nerve supplies the cricothyroid muscle, which tenses the vocal cords. Damage to the recurrent laryngeal nerve may cause vocal cord dysfunction if one side is damaged or catastrophic respiratory obstruction if both nerves are damaged.

The Lower Airway

The lower airway extends from the larynx to the parenchyma of the lung. The lower airway progressively narrows until the alveoli are entered. Exchange of oxygen and carbon dioxide occur in the alveoli.

Components of the Lower Airway

- Trachea
- Bronchi
- Alveoli
- Chest wall

The lung parenchyma is arranged into two lungs with three lobes each. In the left lung, the middle lobe is atrophied to allow for the mass of the heart. The remnant of the left middle lobe is often called the lingular lobe.

Trachea

The trachea descends to the level of the fifth or sixth thoracic vertebra and then splits into the right and left mainstem bronchi (Figure 2-5). The adult trachea is about 10 to 15 centimeters long. There are between 16 and 20 c-shaped cartilages that form the trachea. The first tracheal ring attaches to the cricoid cartilage by the cricotracheal ligament. The open ends of the c-shaped cartilages face posteriorly. The posterior trachea is membranous tissue and is in contact with the anterior wall of the esophagus.

The trachea is lined with both mucus-producing cells and cilia. The mucus traps particulate matter. The cilia sweep the mucus towards the larynx where it is coughed up or swallowed.

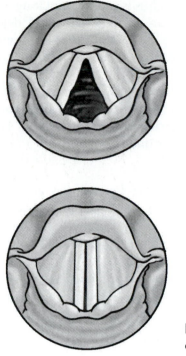

Figure 2-4 Glottis and vocal cords.

In adults, the right mainstem bronchus is shorter and straighter than the left. The position and shape of the heart decreases the size of the left lung and moves it more laterally. The right bronchus is a direct continuation of the trachea, so most foreign bodies and aspirations are likely to enter the right mainstem bronchus. The right mainstem bronchus is anterior to the pulmonary artery.

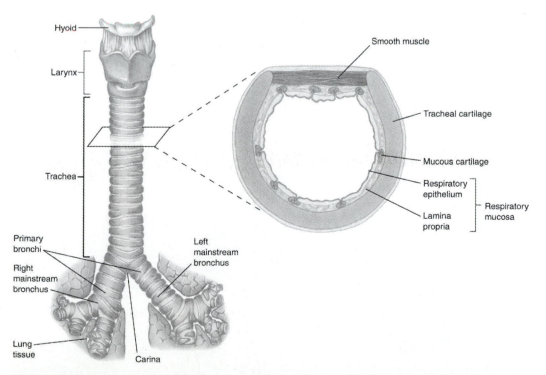

Figure 2-5 Components of the lower airway (trachea and both mainstem bronchi).

The left mainstem bronchus is smaller and longer than the right. The left mainstem bronchus makes an angle of about 35 degrees with the trachea, while the right makes an angle of about 25 degrees with the trachea. The left bronchus is anterior to both the esophagus and the aorta.

The mainstem bronchi enter the lung at the hilum. They rapidly divide into progressively smaller tubes—the bronchioles. After about 22 divisions, the bronchioles lose cartilage and become respiratory bronchioles. These structures have a limited capacity for gas exchange. The respiratory bronchioles terminate in the alveolar ducts.

The Alveoli

The ends of the respiratory bronchioles are the alveolar ducts which end in the balloon-like clusters of alveoli, or air sacs. The membranes of the alveoli are about two cell layers thick and are the chief functional unit for respiratory gas exchange. Only limited gas exchange can occur in the larger respiratory bronchioles and alveolar ducts.

There is a massive surface area to the alveoli—almost 40 square meters. This facilitates gaseous diffusion of oxygen and carbon dioxide into the respiratory capillaries (Figure 2-6).

The Pleura

The pleura is a membranous connective tissue that covers the inner surface of the chest, the mediastinal structures, and the lungs. The chest wall layer

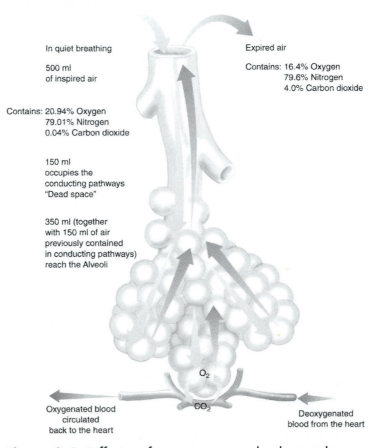

In quiet breathing

500 ml
of inspired air

Expired air

Contains: 16.4% Oxygen
79.6% Nitrogen
4.0% Carbon dioxide

Contains: 20.94% Oxygen
79.01% Nitrogen
0.04% Carbon dioxide

150 ml
occupies the
conducting pathways
"Dead space"

350 ml (together
with 150 ml of air
previously contained
in conducting pathways)
reach the Alveoli

O_2

CO_2

Oxygenated blood
circulated
back to the heart

Deoxygenated
blood from the heart

Figure 2-6 Diffusion of gases across an alveolar membrane.

is called the parietal pleura. The parietal pleura has many nerve fibers. The visceral pleura lines the mediastinal structures and the lungs. It has no nerve fibers.

The space between the parietal pleura and the visceral pleura usually has no fluid and no gas. When it contains fluid, the patient has a pleural effusion or hemothorax. When it contains gas, the patient has a pneumothorax.

Airway

The anatomy of the airway has three axes: the oral axis, the pharangeal axis, and the tracheal axis. Successful visualization of the vocal cords and subsequent intubation are dependent on the alignment of these three axes. The best way to align all three axes is to place the head in the flexed neck occiput raised 5–10 cm position, also called the sniffing position.

Respiratory Physiology

Respiration and Ventilation

Ventilation is the mechanical process that moves the gases in and out of the lungs so that respiration can occur. Respiration is defined as the exchange of gases. Respiration may be further divided into the respiration that occurs within the lungs, or pulmonary respiration, and respiration that occurs within the cell, or cellular respiration. Pulmonary respiration occurs as gases are exchanged with the outside environment through the airway and into the alveoli. Oxygen is coupled to hemoglobin in the pulmonary capillaries. During cellular respiration, oxygen is liberated from oxygenated hemoglobin and enters the cells. Carbon dioxide is picked up by the blood stream, transported as bicarbonate, and then liberated into the alveoli.

Pulmonary Circulation

The circulatory system is essential for ventilation and respiration to occur. In the pulmonary capillaries, the oxygen within the alveoli is picked up by hemoglobin in the red blood cells. The oxygenated blood is transported to the left heart by the pulmonary veins. From the left heart, the blood is swept into the peripheral tissues by the arterial circulation. Progressively smaller arteries lead to arterioles, which become capillaries. Within the tissue capillaries, the oxygen is released for cellular respiration. Carbon dioxide is picked up, and the capillaries become venules and finally veins. The venous circulation sweeps into the right heart and is pumped into the lung through the pulmonary artery.

The lung tissue itself receives its blood supply from the bronchial arteries as a subdivision of the aorta. Bronchial veins return the blood from the lungs into the venous system and the right heart.

Regulation of Respiration

The respiratory rate does not usually fall under conscious control. Physical and chemical mechanisms will signal the respiratory centers to provide an involuntary impulse to breathe. We can voluntarily override the existing controls and either hold our breath or hyperventilate.

Respiratory Drives

The main respiratory center is in the medulla oblongata, located in the brainstem. The medulla is connected to the respiratory muscles by the vagus nerve. As noted, the urge to breathe is involuntary.

When the medulla fails to initiate ventilation properly, a secondary control system located in the pons will assume the task. This apneustic center will ensure continual ventilation. A third back-up system, called the pneumotaxic center and also located in the pons, will drive expiration.

Other involuntary ventilation controls are the chemical receptors in the medulla and secondary chemoreceptors in the carotid bodies and the arch of the aorta. The chemoreceptors sense decrease in the arterial oxygen (PaO_2), increase in the arterial carbon dioxide ($PaCO_2$), and decreases in the arterial pH.

The most sensitive of the chemoreceptors is located in the medulla and responds to cerebral spinal fluid pH. A decreased CSF pH will rapidly trigger increased respiratory rate. Since the CSF pH responds quite quickly to a change in the arterial $PaCO_2$, any increase in $PaCO_2$ will cause an increase in respiratory rate.

This can lead to a serious problem when the patient hyperventilates and then tries to hold the breath. An example of this is the youngster who tries to swim farther by hyperventilating. The $PaCO_2$ will be driven far down by the hyperventilation. The child will furiously swim and exhaust the oxygen carried in the lungs and bloodstream before the CO_2 rises enough to trigger an involuntary ventilation. This may lead to a hypoxic seizure and subsequent aspiration of water.

Hypoxia is a profound stimulus of respiration, but the hypoxic drive is far slower in effect. The carotid body and the arch of the aorta contain chemoreceptors that monitor the oxygen content of the arterial blood. The hypoxic drive is stronger than the carbon dioxide chemoreceptors.

When a patient has a chronically elevated $PaCO_2$, the carbon dioxide receptors become less sensitive. This occurs when the patient has lung damage from COPD or other chronic lung diseases. As the $PaCO_2$ rises in these patients, the central nervous system will rely less on $PaCO_2$ to initiate ventilation.

It has been widely quoted in emergency literature that giving high-flow oxygen to patients with chronic obstructive pulmonary disease and hypoxic drive will shut down the hypoxic respiratory center and cause them to stop breathing. This appears to be a myth that is not substantiated by data. In good studies that have followed arterial blood gases and respiratory parameters in these patients, administration of oxygen does not cause apnea or even substantial slowing of respiratory drive.[2][3][4] There appears to be a transient rise in the patient's $PaCO_2$, but by 30 minutes after initiation of oxygen therapy, the carbon dioxide and oxygen levels stabilize.[5] As Dr. Crossley and his colleagues discussed in their cogent study of the problem, the problem with administration of oxygen to the COPD patient is not apnea, but inadequate respiratory reserves and subsequent difficulty in elimination of carbon dioxide. Indeed, they administered 70 percent FIO_2 with no significant effect on any respiratory parameter.

The basic issue in this problem is oxygen. The human body, particularly the heart and brain, are not at all forgiving of hypoxia. Medical decision-making based on the mythology that administration of oxygen causes apnea and cardiorespiratory arrest in patients by shutting off the hypoxic drive may cause the field provider or even the emergency physician to withhold or deliver inadequate oxygen to the patient in respiratory failure. This will often be fatal for the patient and is a practice that should be condemned by informed medical providers. The solution for inadequate respiratory reserves and subsequent respiratory failure is to provide ventilation for the patient.

Causes of Upper Airway Compromise

Declining Consciousness

If the patient is in a supine position, an alteration of consciousness from any cause will compromise oropharyngeal muscle tone and allow the tongue to fall posteriorly onto the posterior pharynx. This is the leading cause of airway obstruction. This can often be recognized by the presence of stridor or snoring respirations. When the patient is apneic or is moving little or no air, then there are no sound clues to airway obstruction.

If the patient is unconscious, normal airway protection may also be lost. The potential for aspiration of secretions and vomitus is significantly increased. If risk of trauma to the neck is minimal, this problem is best handled by putting the patient in a lateral position, so that the tongue cannot move posteriorly, which allows secretions and vomitus to drain out of the airway.

Trauma

Trauma may result in direct injury to the airway or may cause swelling around the airway. The trauma may also cause an altered mental state, rendering the patient unable to protect his or her airway. Trauma can also produce foreign bodies (such as teeth, pieces of dental work, bone, vomitus, or food being consumed at the time of the injury), or hemorrhage that can further destroy the patient's ability to protect his or her own airway.

Soft Tissue Swelling

Soft tissue swelling may be caused by allergic reactions, idiopathic angioedema, infection, inhalation injuries, or trauma. Any soft tissue swelling may compromise the airway and the ability to move air to the lungs.

Infections

Infections, such as Ludwig's angina, croup, retropharyngeal abscess, peritonsillar abscess, or epiglottitis, can directly obstruct the airway with swelling. Pneumonia and bronchitis can clog the airway with purulent secretions.

Neoplasms

Growth of tumors can impinge on the airway. Neoplasms also cause remote damage that affects the airway, including diaphragmatic paralysis and recurrent laryngeal nerve damage that affects the vocal cords.

Aspirated Foreign Bodies

Aspirated foreign bodies can cause both complete and partial obstruction of the airway. Aspirated materials may also damage airway structures with resultant pneumonia, bronchial destruction, laryngospasm, or inflammation.

Vocal Cord Dysfunction

Vocal cord dysfunction can result from damage to the recurrent laryngeal nerve by trauma or tumor. Direct damage to the cords may cause laryngospasm. Tumors of the vocal cords may cause hoarseness or even obstruction of the cords.

End Notes

[1] Sellick, B. A. "Cricoid pressure to control regurgitation of stomach contents during induction of anaesthesia." *Lancet* 1961;2:404–406.

[2] Hoyt, J. W. "Debunking myths of chronic obstructive lung disease." *Crit Care Med* 1997;25:1451.

[3] Aubier, M., Murciano, D., Fournier, M., et al. "Central respiratory drive in acute respiratory failure of patients with chronic obstructive pulmonary disease." *Am Rev Resp Dis* 1980;122:191–199.

[4] Aubier, M., Murciano, D., and Milic-Emili, J. "Effects of administration of O_2 on ventilation and blood gases in patients with chronic obstructive pulmonary disease during acute failure." *Am Rev Respir Dis* 1980;122:747–754.

[5] Crossley, D. J., McGuire, G. P., Barrow, P. M., and Houston, P. L. "Influence of inspired oxygen concentration on deadspace, respiratory drive, and $PaCO_2$ in intubated patients with chronic obstructive pulmonary disease." *Crit Care Med* 1997;25:1522–1526.

Chapter **Three**

Airway Maneuvers

*Special thanks to Tracy Evans, RN,
for her help with the section on suctioning.*

There are four main aspects of proper airway positioning. First, positioning improves opening of the upper airway. The head-tilt–jaw-thrust, and chin-lift maneuvers accomplish this airway opening.

Second, positioning can improve visualization for endotracheal intubation. This is best accomplished by the "sniffing" or open airway position which lines up the axes of the mouth, soft palate, and trachea. The technique for this positioning will be further discussed in the section on intubation.

Third, the patient's position on the bed influences the mechanics of ventilation. A supine position is not necessarily the best position for the patient to breathe, even if it is the best position for the operator to work. The supine position decreases the functional residual capacity, increases a ventilation-perfusion inequality, and increases pulmonary shunting. All of these cause decreased oxygenation. If the patient's cardiovascular status will tolerate some degree of the sitting position, respiratory function will be improved. This is particularly true in the morbidly obese patient and the patient with congestive heart failure.

An interesting problem of positioning is in the patient with possibility of cervical spine injury who also has either morbid obesity or congestive heart failure. Although recommendations to elevate the head of the bed will help the problem somewhat, spinal immobilization may not be tolerable in some patients.

A final aspect of positioning is the prevention and management of aspiration. Passive regurgitation can occur when the patient is supine. The sitting position markedly decreases the possibility of vomiting. Vomiting in this position requires active regurgitation with at least a pressure difference of the distance between the glottis and the gastro-esophageal sphincter. At the very least, the patient should be placed in the "coma" position, so that aspiration is less likely. (The coma position is in lateral decubitus position with legs positioned so that the patient stays on the side.)

If vomiting does occur, then the unconscious patient should be placed in the Trendelenburg, or head down, position for suctioning. The unconscious vomiting patient should be rapidly intubated to protect the airway and to allow suctioning of the secretions.

Head-Tilt–Chin-Lift Maneuver

The head-tilt–chin-lift maneuver is recommended for adults and children over the age of 8 years (Figure 3-1).

Indications

*   Initial management of the compromised airway
*   Relief of mild anatomic airway obstruction
*   Stimulus to respiratory drive in altered levels of consciousness
*   Recommended for the patient who has no neck trauma

Contraindications

*   Possible (suspected) cervical spine injury
*   Down's syndrome

Patients with Down's syndrome have a significant incidence of incomplete ossification of C1 and C2 and cervical vertebral subluxation.

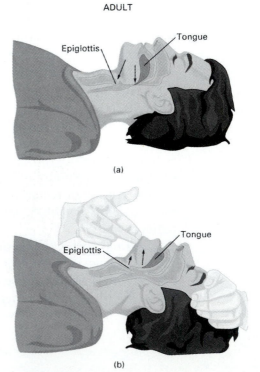

Figure 3-1 Head tilt maneuver.

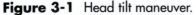

- Prior spinal fusion
- Known cervical spine pathology

Examples of this may include ankylosing spondylitis and rheumatoid arthritis, as well as trauma to the neck. Mobility of the neck in these two diseases is markedly limited.

- Advanced age due to decreasing mobility of the aging neck and increasing osteoarthritis.

Technique
- Place the patient in supine position.
- Position yourself at the side of the patient's head.
- Using one hand on the forehead, tilt the patient's head back while keeping mouth closed.
- Use the other hand under the bony part of the chin to lift the jaw anteriorly to open the airway.

The chin is lifted with the fingers of one hand while the forehead is pushed down with the palm of the other (Figure 3-2).

- Head remains in neutral position.

If neck injury is suspected, then lift the chin without the head tilt.

- Lift chin to move the hyoid bone away from posterior pharyngeal wall.

Complications
In children under the age of 5, the cervical spine can flex substantially. The head tilt maneuver can worsen the obstruction by pushing the posterior pharynx towards the tongue and epiglottis. The airway is best maintained in children by leaving the head in a neutral, or "sniffing," position.

In the adult, avoid extensive hyperextension of the neck or pressure on the patient's soft tissues below the chin. Either can actually worsen the airway.

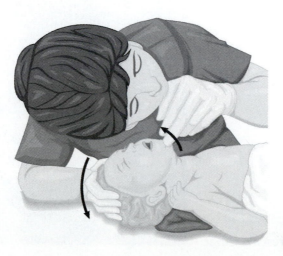

Figure 3-2 Chin lift maneuver.

Jaw-Thrust Maneuver

Technique

• Place the patient in the supine position.
• Assume a position at the patient's head.
• Open mouth slightly.
• Put one hand on each side of the jaw at the angle of the mandible.
• Lift the jaw forward and gently tilt the patient's head to open the airway.

A two-handed techniques works best (Figures 3-3, 3-4). The elasticity of the mandibular joint capsule and the strength of the masseter muscle will tend to pull the mandible back if the grip is relaxed.

Jaw-Lift Technique Maneuver

• Grip the ramus of the mandible with the fingers of each hand and lift the mandibular teeth over and in front of the maxilla.
• Don't tilt the patient's head.

Use caution . . . the patient can bite you when this technique is used.

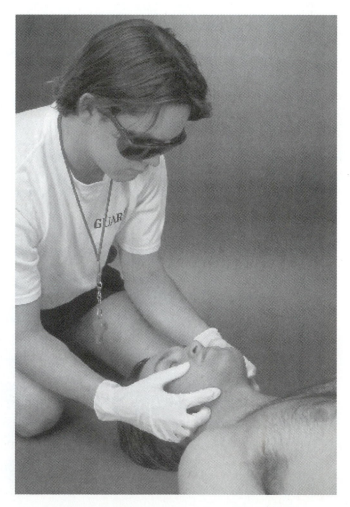

Figure 3-3 Jaw thrust maneuver.

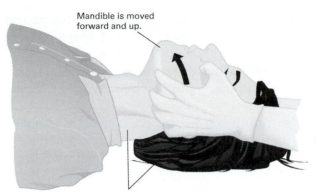

Mandible is moved forward and up.

Head and neck are kept in neutral in-line position.

Figure 3-4 Jaw thrust maneuver.

Sniffing Position

During laryngoscopy, there must be an unobstructed line of view from the operator's eye through the mouth and into the larynx for endotracheal intubation to proceed without difficulty. The space anterior to the larynx determines the ease with which the laryngeal axis can be brought in line with the pharyngeal axis during laryngoscopy. Difficulty may occur if the cords, the upper teeth, or the tongue are displaced (Figures 3-5, 3-6).

The term anterior larynx imples that the larynx lies anteriorly to the line of sight of the operator when the patient is supine. The tongue or the epiglottis may obstruct the view of the larynx.

The sniffing position has the neck flexed slightly and the head extended slightly. This position optimizes the alignment of the oral-pharyngeal axis and the pharyngeal-laryngeal axis. A small towel may be placed behind the adult's occiput to help maintain this relationship.

Suctioning

Indications

Ongoing hemorrhage, vomiting, or particulate debris in the airway will require suction to clear the airway. Any of these substances can occlude or partially obstruct the airway and impede the flow of air, the insertion of an airway adjunct, or a definitive airway.

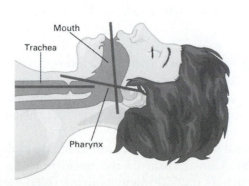

Mouth

Trachea

Pharynx

Figure 3-5 The neutral position.

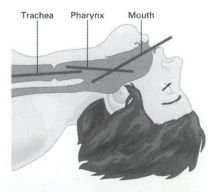

Trachea   Pharynx   Mouth

Figure 3-6 Open airway or sniffing position.

Suctioning equipment must be available for every patient. If the patient is allowed to aspirate vomit, blood, or debris, there will be a sharp increase in possible morbidity and mortality for this patient. This increase in morbidity will not be seen by the EMS or emergency department providers. The patient will not develop aspiration pneumonia until much later in the hospital course.

Eighty to 120 mmHg of suction is needed for orotracheal suctioning. Higher pressures are needed for tracheobronchial suctioning. Equipment should generate a flow rate of at least 30 liters per minute during suctioning.

Contraindications

The only relative contraindication to suctioning is cardiac arrhythmia, which may be exacerbated by tracheal suctioning. There are no absolute contraindications to suctioning. If the airway is obstructed, it must be cleared.

Methods and Techniques
Oral Suctioning

Steps:

1. Don the appropriate personal protective equipment. Gloves and eye protection are a minimum.
2. Check the suction equipment. (Ideally, suction should be checked prior to every shift and after every mission.)
3. Pre-oxygenate the patient if at all possible.
4. Insert the suction tip into the mouth. A dental or specialized suction tip is appropriate. A tonsil sucker is adequate, but definitely not ideal. A whistle tip catheter should be used only for suctioning the trachea and bronchi in the intubated patient.
5. Withdraw the suction slowly, occluding the finger port to begin suctioning. Suction for no more than 5–15 seconds in adults and 5 seconds in children.
6. In many cases, the secretions will be thick or viscous and can obstruct the flow through the suction tubing. If necessary, clean out the catheter between attempts by placing the tip into a container of sterile water or saline and covering the finger port to create suction. Observe until the tubing is clear.
7. After suctioning, allow the patient to breathe supplemental oxygen or ventilate with a bag-valve mask for 15–30 seconds between suction attempts.

Nasal Suctioning Because airway obstruction occurs most often in the mouth and oropharynx, nasal suction is seldom required. Infants have obligate nasal breathing, so the airway can be obstructed by mucus, vomitus, or blood. If nasal suction is needed, the emergency provider should use either a bulb syringe or a catheter suction tip.

Vigorous nasal suctioning can cause epistaxis and futher complicate airway management. Constriction of the nasal mucosa with vasoconstrictor drops or spray such as 0.25% phenylephrine (Neo-Synephrine) may reduce the potential for injury.

Steps:

1. Don the appropriate personal protective equipment. Again, gloves and eye protection are the minimum required equipment.
2. Check the suction equipment. Check for suction by occluding the whistle-stop port. Check to ensure that the bulb syringe tip is not occluded.
3. Pre-oxygenate the patient if at all possible.
4. Ensure adequate catheter length to suction the nasopharyngeal and oropharyngeal cavities by measuring the length from the patient's nose to the tip of the ear. This will allow for adequate insertion depth.
5. Lubricate the end of the catheter with a water-soluble jelly or Lidocaine jelly (optional).
6. Insert the catheter with the whistle-stop open, avoiding suctioning while rotating the catheter as it is inserted. If resistance is encountered, stop the insertion, withdraw slightly, and reinsert. If the second attempt is still unsuccessful, remove the catheter and make an attempt using the other nostril.

or

7. Squeeze the bulb of a bulb syringe. Insert it into the nostril and release the bulb, allowing it to expand and suction the debris out of the nose.
8. Once the catheter has been inserted to the appropriate depth as measured before the catheter was inserted, cover the whistle-stop with your thumb or finger, and suction while withdrawing the catheter. Watch for fluids moving up the inside of the catheter toward the collection container. Each attempt should be limited to 5 to 15 seconds in an adult and 5 seconds in a child.
9. If necessary, clean out the catheter between attempts by placing the tip into a container of sterile water or saline and covering the whistle-stop to create suction and observe until the tubing is clear. The bulb syringe is cleaned by holding it with the tip downward and vigorously squeezing the bulb to force the debris out of the tip.
10. After suctioning, allow the patient to breathe supplemental oxygen or ventilate with a bag-valve mask for 15–30 seconds between suction attempts.

Tracheobronchial Suctioning Tracheobronchial suctioning clears secretions and aspirated material from the trachea and bronchi of patients who have no cough reflex or who have an artificial airway. Ideally, tracheal suctioning should be performed under sterile conditions. When that is not an option, tracheal suction should be done in as clean a manner as possible (Figure 3-7).

Open Systems

In an open system, the endotracheal tube is separated from the bag-valve mask. Almost all field and emergency department suctioning is conducted through an open system. The provider will remove the ventilation device, whether a bag-valve mask or a ventilator. The suction catheter is then inserted into the open endotracheal tube. Because the endotracheal tube is open and separated, the patient is at an increased risk for a dislodged tube, infection, and trauma.

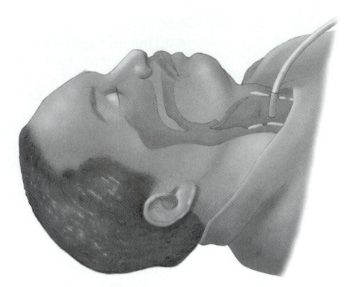

Figure 3-7 Tracheal stoma suctioning.

Steps:

1. Don the appropriate personal protective equipment. As always, gloves and eye protection are minimum required equipment.
2. Pre-oxygenate the patient.
3. Check the suction equipment. Check for suction by occluding the whistle-stop port.
4. Choose an appropriate catheter size. The catheter diameter should be one-half the diameter of the endotracheal tube and can be estimated by multiplying the endotracheal tube diameter in millimeters by two. For example, an 8.0 ET would require a 16 Fr catheter. This catheter diameter is critical when suctioning the pediatric patient.
5. Estimate the catheter depth that will be needed to reach the carina of the patient's trachea. This can be estimated externally by measuring from the xiphoid process of the sternum around the ear and then to the corner of the mouth.
6. The bag-valve mask is removed from the endotracheal tube and the soft-tip catheter is introduced into the endotracheal tube and advanced to the level of the carina. Insert the catheter to the correct depth as measured. The whistle-stop is not covered until the catheter is placed at the correct level and is occluded for suctioning as the catheter is withdrawn.
7. Withdraw the suction slowly, occluding the whistle-stop to begin suctioning. Suction for no more than 5–15 seconds in adults and 5 seconds in children.
8. In many cases, the secretions will be thick or viscous and can obstruct the flow through the suction tubing. If necessary, clean out the catheter between attempts by placing the tip into a container of sterile water or saline and covering the whistle-stop to create suction. Observe until the tubing is clear.
9. The secretions may be thinned by injecting 3–5 ml of sterile water down the endotracheal tube.
10. After suctioning, allow the patient to breathe supplemental oxygen or ventilate with a bag-valve mask for 15–30 seconds between suction attempts.

Closed systems

In a closed system there is a port to allow suctioning without separating the bag-valve-mask or ventilator from the endotracheal tube. Closed systems are more commonly used in patients who are on a mechanical ventilator. The field operator may see the closed suctioning systems during transport of the patient from hospital to hospital. These systems, while more expensive, allow for concomitant oxygenation and reduce the risk of infection.

Most of the models available have a port for medication instillation, allowing the system to remain closed. This reduces the risk of dislodging the ET tube while detaching and re-attaching the bag-valve mask for suctioning or for medication administration via syringe and aerosolization.

The steps to use this system are essentially the same as those listed for the open system.

Complications

- Difficulty in passing a tracheal catheter.

    Never force a tracheal catheter. Use a lubricant to ease the passage of the catheter. Remove the catheter and then re-attempt the procedure using a rotating motion for the tracheal catheter.

- Tissue damage and bleeding

    Carefully select the catheter. Use caution with a dental tip or open tubing. When using wall suction and high suction pressures, the operator can literally amputate the uvula or perform a partial tonsillectomy. Do not suction aggressively.

    Consider a vasoconstrictor when nasal suctioning with a catheter tip.

- Hypoxia

    Hypoxia during suctioning is real. If the patient is receiving supplemental oxygen, that oxygen-rich atmosphere is literally sucked out of the oral cavity and replaced by room air. Limit suctioning time to 5–15 seconds and ventilate for 15–30 seconds after each attempt. This should be true for all suction techniques.

    If possible, hyperventilate the patient with 100 percent oxygen before and after each effort. Do not apply suction while you are inserting the catheter.

- Dysrhythmias

    Vagal stimulation can produce bradycardia and possible hypotension. During tracheal suctioning, suction gently.

    Sympathetic stimulation can also occur during tracheal suctioning, causing tachydysrhythmias and ventricular fibrillation. Suction gently.

- Increased intracranial pressure

    This may be transient. In patients with already elevated intracranial pressure, this can exacerbate the condition.

- Bronchoconstriction

    Bronchoconstriction may result from mechanical irritation of the bronchi by a suction tip catheter. This may resolve with the cessation of suction or may require a bronchodilator.

Precautions

There are no specific contraindications to suctioning, only guidelines for appropriate suctioning. Do not use a damaged, kinked, or defective catheter.

Equipment

There are numerous tools available for suctioning that include both portable and nonportable equipment.

Manual

Manually Operated (V-Vac) (Res-D-Vac) At first consideration, the manually operated unit may seem the least desirable suction for either field or hospital (Figure 3-8).

The units operate by squeezing or pumping manually and are limited by the technician's hand strength. The manually operated units deliver the least amount of vacuum and have the smallest collection container of all manufactured suction machines.

The major advantages are the inherent simplicity and cost. Because of this, they function as a formidable back-up unit.

There are no batteries to fail. The unit does not require any electrical power at all. Deep in the field, in rescue efforts in disasters, or even in an elevator with no power outlets, these units will continue to operate. This may be the difference between a clear patent-open airway and aspiration of blood and vomitus.

These units are substantially less expensive than an electrically powered suction unit. They are lighter weight, making them usable for a portable equipment bag and for rescue operations.

Bulb Syringe The bulb syringe is most often used to clear the mouth and nose of the newborn, but could be used to clear the airway of a child or adult. Another manually powered tool, this unit requires less strength from the operator, but has substantially less vacuum. The capacity is limited to the bulb, and the unit must be manually cleared after each use.

Suction is achieved by manually compressing the bulb, inserting the tip into the mouth or nose, and releasing the bulb. The bulb acts as the vacuum and the collection device. This unit is quite limited, but inexpensive and a *pinch* can clear secretions. (No pun intended.)

A larger version of the bulb syringe is the "turkey baster." This large syringe may be useful as a field expedient for suctioning. It has limited ability to remove large volumes, is easily clogged by large chunks of vomitus, and does not fit into the nasopharynx. It simply can't be used to suction an endo-

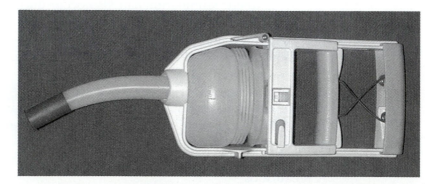

Figure 3-8 Manual powered portable suction unit. *Source:* Big Yank Suction System, courtesy of CONMED, Corp. and Dr. Vandenburg.

tracheal tube. The turkey baster is useful in mass casualty situations or where the power is out for long periods of time.

Battery-Powered Portable Equipment Portability is the attractive feature in these units. They are smaller and as such have a smaller collection container, shorter tubing, and less power. The batteries are rechargeable. Most units may be charged with either AC or DC (12v).

The portable unit should be able to provide an air intake of at least 20 L/min to operate effectively. Like the fixed suction unit, if the power supply is lost, the unit cannot function (Figure 3-9).

On-Board Ambulance Equipment These units are mounted in ambulances and powered by the vacuum produced by the vehicle's manifold.

Wall-Mounted Hospital Equipment These suction units are wall-mounted in hospitals and electrically powered by vacuum pumps. Both types of fixed suction provide an air intake of 30 L/min and provide vacuum of more than 300 mm Hg when the tube is clamped. These devices have an on/off control and more sophisticated units have a dial control to adjust the amount of vacuum used (Figure 3-10).

In addition to their higher power-suctioning capabilities, these units have larger collection units than portable suction devices. Because they are mounted to the wall, they are immobile and, as such, require longer connective tubing. If the power supply fails, so does the suction unit.

Disposables

Dental Suction A dental tip suction is the most useful tip for removing particulate debris from the mouth and upper airway. This tip is less likely to become plugged with vomitus than any other type of suction tip.

The dental suction tip can damage soft oropharyngeal tissues if used vigorously.

When a dental suction tip is not available, then the open suction line may be used, but if this becomes clogged, the whole tubing must be replaced.

The dental tip should be available during resuscitation and should be available on the crash cart or in the ambulance gear.

Catheter Tip Suction This device has many names: French catheter, soft suction, catheter-tip, and whistle tip. The catheter tip is designed for suctioning the trachea and bronchi through a tracheal tube.

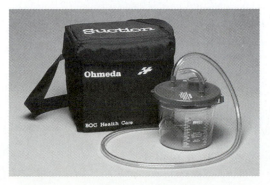

Figure 3-9 Battery-powered portable suction device. *Source:* Ohmeda suction system, courtesy of Ohmeda Medical.

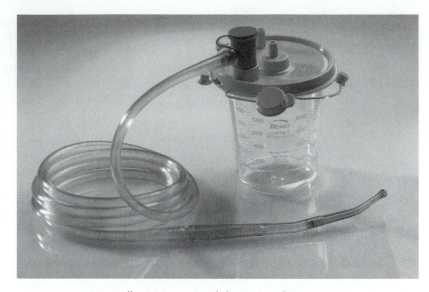

Figure 3-10 Wall suction unit with large tonsil-type suction. *Source:* Big Yank Suction System, courtesy of CONMED, Corp. and Dr. Vandenburg.

The catheter tip suction is the least likely suction to be successful in resuscitation of a patient. This device has a small diameter, making it ineffective for large particulate matter, such as clots of blood, pieces of tissue, or vomitus. The smaller diameter limits the flow of fluid as it is removed, so the catheter can't remove large volumes of fluid rapidly.

The catheter tip is virtually useless until the patient has been intubated. After intubation, this device is effective for suctioning the trachea and bronchi through the endotracheal tube. It can be used in the oropharynx or nasopharynx as well, but with the previously described limitations.

It should be available, but generally can be considered second line equipment, rather than primary gear to be carried to the patient.

Tonsil Tip Suction (Yankauer Suction) This tip is designed to prevent obstruction of the tip by tissue and clot. It is very effective at clearing hemorrhage and secretions. The blunted end causes less damage to airway structures.

Although the tonsil suction tip is well built for suctioning blood and clots, it is not designed for vomitus. It is easily clogged by soft large particles, such as pizza and similar vomitus.

Specialized versions of this suction tip device such as the "Big Yank" are depicted in Figure 3-11.

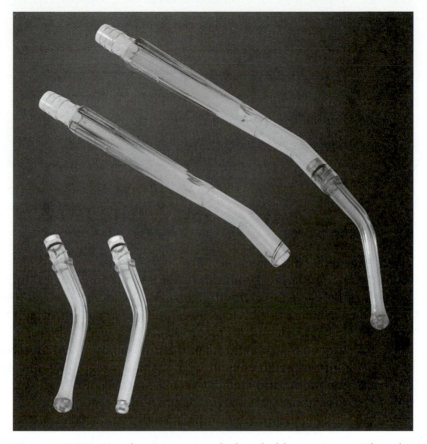

Figure 3-11 Tonsil suction unit with detachable tip. *Source:* Photo by Charles Stewart and Associates; www.storysmith.net.

Chapter **Four**

Airway Aids

The simplest artificial airways are the oropharyngeal and the nasopharyngeal airways. Both of these airways will prevent the tongue from falling back against the posterior pharynx and obstructing the airway.

More complex airway aids include the esophageal obturator airway, the Combitube, Pharyngotracheal lumen airway, the cuffed oropharyngeal airway, and the laryngeal mask airway. None of these devices are equivalent to endotracheal intubation for either ventilation or airway control. In selected patients, however, they may be acceptable and even helpful.

Oropharyngeal Airway

Indications and Contraindications

Oral airways are indispensable adjuncts to airway management. They facilitate ventilation in patients who have lost the gag reflex and have obstruction of the airway from relaxation of the tongue and soft palate. The toothless patient is particularly prone to this problem, and ventilation is improved when an oral airway is used.

A second use of these airways is as a bite block for the intubated patient. If the intubated patient is inadequately sedated, they may bite down and obstruct the endotracheal tube. On rare occasions, the patient may even cut the tube by biting it.

Indications for Oropharyngeal Airway

- Complete or partial upper airway obstruction
- Adjunct for suctioning the oral cavity
- Bite block in the unconscious, seizing, or intubated patient

This procedure should not be attempted while the patient is actively seizing.

Contraindications for Oropharyngeal Airway

- An intact gag reflex is an absolute contraindication
- Dental or mandibular fracture (relative contraindication)
- Acute episode of reactive airway disease, such as asthma (relative contraindication)

Equipment

The oropharangeal airway comes in two styles and in sizes from 000 for neonates to size 4 for large adults (see Figure 4-1). The Guedel oral airway has a central suctioning chamber, while the Berman airway is a curved strut shaped liked an I-beam, on cross section. Both types are semicircular in shape and curved to fit behind the tongue in the lower portion of the posterior pharynx. The rigid proximal end of the Guedel airway is reinforced to prevent collapse if the patient bites.

The oropharyngeal airway may be made of plastic, hard rubber, or metal. The metal oropharangeal airway is reusable, but rarely seen in modern emergency practice. Although infant and newborn sizes of the oral airway are manufactured, they are not particularly useful in these children.

Other Equipment Needed

- Anesthesia 10% lidocaine or Cetacaine spray (This is not needed in the patient who has no gag reflex)
- Plastic or nylon flanged oral airways of proper size
- Tongue depressor
- Suction apparatus

Positioning of Patient

- Supine or lateral

Technique

There are two techniques to insert an oral airway (Figures 4-2 - 4-5). Either one is appropriate. The most important part of the technique is to choose the proper size for the patient (Figure 4-6).

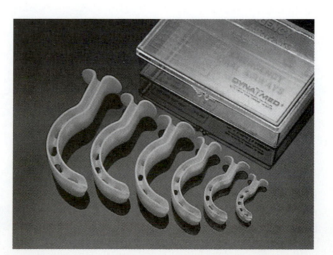

Figure 4-1 Oropharyngeal airway.

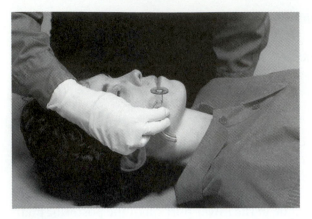

Figure 4-2 Measuring for oropharyngeal airway.

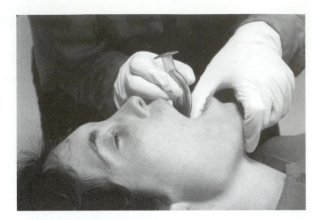

Figure 4-3 Insertion of oropharyngeal airway.

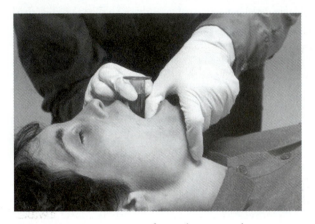

Figure 4-4 Insertion of oropharyngeal airway—rotation step.

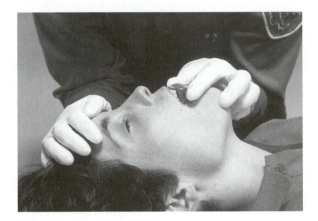

Figure 4-5 Oropharyngeal airway proper position.

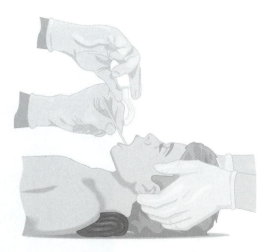

Figure 4-6 Insertion of oropharyngeal airway in child, tongue blade technique.

Tongue Blade Technique

- Open mouth
- Place tongue blade at the base of the tongue
- Push the tongue anteriorly (if the tongue is pushed down, it may obstruct the airway)
- Place the airway in the mouth with concave *facing the tongue*

Place the distal end at the posterior wall of the orpharynx. Use the jaw thrust maneuver or the chin lift maneuver to lift the tongue forward off of the posterior pharyngeal wall. Tap the airway down to place it so that the curve lies beyond the base of the tongue.

Rotation Technique

- Insert the airway with concave side *facing the palate.* (The convexity should be pointed towards the patient's feet.)
- Insert in mouth until the tip is past the uvula.
  - No tongue blade is needed for this technique.
- Rotate the airway 180 degrees to sweep behind the tongue from the side.
  - Do not use this method if the patient has had oral trauma or poor dentition.
  - This technique may increase bleeding or dislodge teeth.
- When the airway is in proper position, the concavity points toward the feet. The airway is then pushed until the hub is on the teeth.

Complications

- Exacerabation of reactive airway disease
- Retching or vomiting
- Increased airway obstruction if not properly placed

This airway is very uncomfortable and should not be used in the awake or awakening patient. It will activate the gag reflex. Treatment is to remove the airway and suction the oropharynx. Do not ever tape the airway in place because it must be easily removed if the patient starts to retch or vomit.

If an oral airway is not properly placed, it can increase the obstruction by pushing the tongue back against the posterior oropharynx. The patient will become more difficult to ventilate after insertion of the airway. The treatment is to remove the device and reinsert it appropriately.

If the oral airway is too long, it may press the epiglottis against the glottic opening and obstruct the airway.[1] The treatment is to remove the device and reinsert an appropriate size.

Other complications during oral airway insertion include precipitation of laryngospasm; tooth breakage; soft tissue ulceration; pressure necrosis of the lips, palate, tongue, or posterior pharyngeal wall; and tongue trauma. Never trap the tongue between the airway and the teeth or endotracheal tube.

Nasopharyngeal Airway

The nasopharyngeal airway is made of rubber or soft plastic (Figure 4-7). It is available in several sizes and is about 6 inches in length. In some texts, the nasopharyngeal airway is also called a nasal trumpet or NPA.

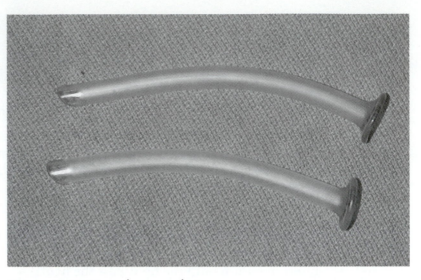

Figure 4-7 Nasopharyngeal airway.

Indications

This airway is better tolerated in an awake patient and is easier to insert in the seizing patient and the patient with trismus.

- Upper airway obstruction in awake or comatose patients
- Dental or oral trauma
- Failure of an oral airway or inability to insert an oral airway
- Seizing patient
- Trismus

Contraindications

- Nasal occlusion
  Nasal jewelry may occlude the nares. These ornaments should be removed, if possible, before using a nasopharyngeal airway.
- Nasal fracture (relative contraindication depending on the severity of the nasal fracture) (known or suspected)
- Basal skull fracture (known or suspected)
- Deviated septum
- Coagulopathy
- CSF rhinorrhea
- Prior transsphenodial surgery
- Prior posterior pharyngeal surgery

Equipment

- Cotton swabs
- Nasal airways of the proper sizes
- Suction apparatus
- Surgical lubricant or 4% lidocaine jelly

Positioning of the Patient-Supine, Lateral, or Sitting

Technique
- Select size of airway desired.

Measure from the tip of the nose to the bottom of the ear. Do not choose an airway that is longer than this distance as it will cause the patient to gag. Then look for the largest size that will fit into the patient's nostril. Look in both nostrils for septal deviation, nasal trauma, polyps, and so on. Select the nostril that appears to be most open (Figures 4-8 - 4-11).

- Anesthetize the area with lidocaine jelly prior to the procedure. Although this is not strictly necessary for use of this device, it will make the patient more comfortable.
  – Alternatively apply Cetacaine spray to the nares
  – Alternatively use surgical lubricant for insertion
- Neo-Synephrine or similar topical vasoconstrictor such as Afrin™ may be useful to help pass the tube.
- Pass the airway gently into the nose with the concave side facing the trunk and the bevel side facing the nasal septum. (If required, the tube *can* be inserted with the bevel side away from the nasal septum.)

The airway will follow a path that is parallel to the hard palate. This path is also perpendicular to the facial place and does not follow the curve of the nose. The proper pathway has little resistance. If there is substantial resistance, then tube position is probably wrong or the tube is too big. If resistance is felt, try a smaller tube or try the other side of the nose.

Ensure that the patient has proper airway positioning after the nasopharyngeal airway is inserted. The tube should lie in the hypopharynx.

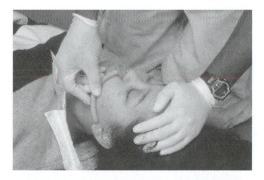

Figure 4-8 Insertion of nasopharyngeal airway.

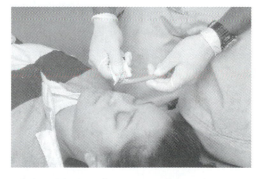

Figure 4-9 Lubrication of nasopharyngeal airway.

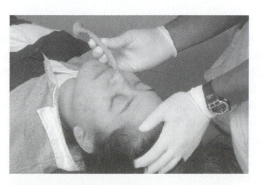

Figure 4-10 Insertion of nasopharyngeal airway.

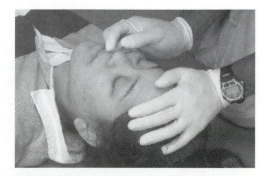

Figure 4-11 Insertion of nasopharyngeal airway.

Complications

- A nasal airway that is too long may provoke gagging or may enter the esophagus and cause gastric distention.
- A nasal airway that is too short is useless.
- The nasal airway may precipitate laryngospasm in some patients.
- Epistaxis

    This is not a welcome complication in the patient who already has a compromised airway!
- Submucosal tunneling

    This complication only occurs when a stiff nasal airway is forced despite resistance. Unfortunately, the more pliable, less traumatic nasal airways are less effective at keeping the upper airway open.

Nasal airways should not be used for more than two days. Longer may cause mucosal injury, sinusitis, or otitis. The nasal airway becomes uncomfortable and can cause pressure necrosis of the nasal mucosa. Never use a nasal airway in one nostril and an NG tube in the other nostril. This can cause compression injury to the nasal septum.

Esophageal Airways

The esophageal airway is an intermediate device that goes beyond the maintenance of a patent airway. The devices described in this section allow ventilation, but also occlude the esophagus. The EOA should be considered an obsolete airway. It is important to review the functioning of this device in order to appreciate the advantages of later, similar devices.

As early as 1903, Kausch proposed the use of a double lumen gastric tube with an inflatable balloon designed to block the esophagus at the cardio-esophageal junction.[2] The first practical device was invented by Don Michael, with details published in *Lancet* in 1968.[3] The original esophageal obturator airway had a pointed end and a face mask that only covered the mouth. The operator had to block the nose with a pinch clamp! This device was adapted by Gordon and developed into a clinically usable apparatus.[4]

These airways should be regarded at best as a temporary adjunct until a more secure airway can be established. They should not ever be used as a replacement for endotracheal intubation, unless the provider either isn't credentialed to intubate or simply can't intubate the patient.

Esophageal obturator airway

The esophageal obturator airway (EOA) is a nondefinitive airway used in the prehospital phase of resuscitation by emergency medical technicians when trachael intubation is either not feasible or not allowed by state or local rules. (Figure 4-12).

The esophageal obturator airway was approved for use in cardiopulmonary resuscitation in 1973 by the American National Conference of Standards for cardiopulmonary resuscitation.[5]* The original endorsement of the

---

*Interestingly, the chairman of the steering committee for this conference was A. S. Gordon, the person who took Don Michael's tube and developed it further.

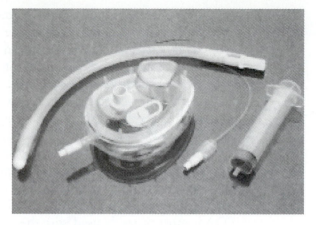

Figure 4-12 Esophageal obturator airway (EOA).

EOA stated, "It appears to be a very useful airway adjunct, but its future role remains to be determined." It has remained controversial since its introduction.

Use of the EOA has been taught to thousands of physicians, nurses, paramedics, and emergency medical technicians through the ACLS programs. Despite this widespread teaching in every ACLS course, the EOA is no longer used. This decline is due both to significant intrinsic problems with the EOA and to increased training and experience of emergency providers in performing endotracheal intubation. With the decline in the use of the EOA, most physicians and many new field providers have had little experience with this device yet it is the prototype for other devices.

The EOA is a tube 33 cm long with a closed end and a 30 cc balloon at the distal end. It resembles an endotracheal tube with the distal end occluded and contains sixteen 3 mm holes in the mid-proximal end. These holes are located in the area of the hypopharynx when the tube is properly positioned. The tube comes with a hard plastic mask fitted with a large low-pressure compliant cuff. A key and slot ensures that the mask will lock onto the tube in the proper position.

The face mask must be held tightly over the nose and mouth and make an acceptable seal in order to ventilate the patient. The inflated esophageal balloon blocks the esophagus and prevents both vomiting and air from entering the stomach. When the face mask is properly sealed, the air must enter the trachea—the only unobstructed orifice.

Proper positioning of the tube in the esophagus means that there is no air passing into the stomach because of the obturator and balloon. If the trachea is intubated inadvertently, then there should be no breath sounds in the lungs. The tube must be removed and reinserted.

A newer modification of the EOA is the esophageal gastric tube airway (EGTA). This device is similar to the EOA with the addition of a port for nasogastric suctioning and removal of air from the stomach. Ventilation from the EGTA is identical to mask ventilation with the addition of esophageal occlusion.

Purported advantages of the EOA include the ability to position the esophageal obturator blindly and rapidly and the ability to insert the tube without neck movement. Much less training is required for proficiency in inserting the airway and no laryngoscope is required for visualization during insertion. The EOA may also be quicker to insert than the endotracheal tube.

Disadvantages include inadvertent tracheal intubation, a failure to adequately ventilate the patient with the EOA, increased gastric distention, and esophageal trauma. The EOA should be considered a temporary airway and should be replaced within 2 hours of insertion.

Of these disadvantages, the most clinically important is ventilation. Inadequate ventilation is common because when the tube is inserted, a mask with seal is needed to ventilate the patient. This has all of the problems associated with bag-mask-valve ventilation that were previously described. Inadequate ventilation has been recognized as a complication early in the deployment of this airway adjunct.[6] In this study, measurements of exhaled tidal volumes were all inferior with the EOA and inadequate for survival in two patients. The face mask seal with the EOA was considered difficult. A later paper stated that ". . . the EOA is most properly used with the patient who will not be moved and ventilatory assistance need occur only for short periods of time."[7] Subsequent papers have confirmed that the EOA fails to provide adequate ventilation and has a lower PaO_2 and higher $PaCO_2$ in the prehospital setting.[8 9 10 11]

A major problem with ventilation is the construction of the device. The inadequately trained individual sees the long tube inserted into the patient, attaches the bag-valve to the device, and starts to "ventilate" the patient. [Unless exceptional care is used to seal the mask—the same care required for BVM—then the device simply does not function properly and the patient is not ventilated.] Any "second generative device" must address this problem.

Indications For many years, the American Heart Association proposed use of the EOA in apneic or deeply unconscious patients. Gordon, a co-developer of the tube, restricted its use to the apneic, areflexic patient. The EOA was thought to be faster to insert, capable of being inserted in patients with neck trauma, and appropriate for use by EMS providers with minimal training. The EOA and EGTA have been abandoned with the 2000 ACLS standards.

Likewise, the American College of Surgeons felt that the EOA requires less neck motion than with the standard tracheal intubation. It has been advocated for airway management in the unconscious injured patient who requires airway support.

Contraindications

Conscious patient The EOA is contraindicated in conscious or semiconscious patients because it would induce vomiting. An EOA could be contraindicated in the patient with an altered level of consciousness where the coma can be rapidly reversed, such as a narcotic overdose, a benzodiazepine overdose, or hypoglycemic coma.

Ability to insert any more effective airway If the patient can be intubated, then they should be intubated rather than use an EOA.

Age less than 16 or small-size adult The EOA and all of its look-alikes were designed for the adult body. There is no pediatric version available. If the adult size is used on a small adult or child, it will be inserted too deeply and the balloon may be in the stomach and not occluding the esophagus. Some authors specify a minimum age of 15–16 years, and others point out that the size of the patient is more important than the age.

Large adult If the patient is over 6 feet, 7 inches in height, then the balloon will not be below the carina when it is inflated. If the balloon is inflated while it is above the carina, it may actually occlude the trachea by pressure from behind.

Upper airway secretions The airway is not protected with the EOA and its relatives. The presence of active bleeding in the mouth, oropharynx, and nose or excessive secretions represents a relative contraindication to the use of these devices.

Known esophageal disease It is also contraindicated in known incidences of esophageal trauma, pathology, and ingestion of corrosive poison. In these patients it is thought to cause further esophageal damage. In patients with esophageal varices, it may provoke uncontrolled hemorrhage.

The inventor of the device, Dr. T. A. Don Michael felt that this device should not be used in any extensive facial or head trauma.[12]

Method The proper steps for insertion of the EOA are the following:
- Check the balloon and lubricate the tip with water-soluble lubricant.
- Attach mask and lock in place.
- Prepare suction and have available for immediate use should the patient vomit when the EOA is inserted.
- Place head in neutral position.
- Grasp jaw with thumb along tongue and lift up and forward.
- Insert the tube along the right side of the pharynx. Advance the tube along the posterior pharynx with gentle steady pressure.
- Seal the mask on the face and blow (watching for the rise of the chest wall).
- Auscultate the chest for equal breath sounds and epigastrium for air passage through water. If water sounds are heard, then the tube is probably not in the appropriate place.
- Inflate the balloon with about 20–30 cc of air. Don't attempt to adjust the position of the balloon while the tube is inflated.
- Continue to monitor chest wall motion with each ventilation.
- For effective ventilation, breath sounds must be audible bilaterally.

Complications The author cannot recommend the use of the EOA or EGTA under any circumstances. This recommendation has been affirmed by the 2000 ACLS standards by the American Heart Association. There is no data that shows that the EOA performs better than mouth to mask ventilation. There are abundant studies and case reports that show significant, including lethal, complications of the EOA and similar devices. If the operator cannot intubate the patient due to lack of equipment or skill, then mouth to mask ventilation offers a safer, less expensive, and more effective alternative. There is simply no question that the time spent on training for the use of the EOA is more effectively used in training for endotracheal intubation or continued training in basic airway management techniques such as mouth to mask ventilation.

Tracheal insertion Unrecognized tracheal intubation is devastating, because the tube is designed to completely occlude the esophagus. Placing the tube in the trachea and inflating the balloon means that the patient now has a completely obstructed trachea and will die unless this is rapidly recognized and corrected. In experience with 29,000 placements of the EOA, inadvertent tracheal intubation occurred in 5 percent of the patients.[13] In another study, only 2.9 percent incidence was reported, but the mortality of this complication was 100 percent.[14] A third series in the Canadian literature cited an incidence of this mortal complication of between 5 percent and 10 percent.[15]

Vomiting The 1996 ACLS course taught that if an EOA is inserted, then the patient should be intubated with an endotracheal tube before removal of the EOA because vomiting often occurs after the EOA is removed or the balloon is deflated. Although this warning is appropriate, from the author's personal experience, the obstruction and distortion of the oropharynx by the large diameter of the EOA makes this more difficult. Often it is appropriate to disregard the ACLS warnings, remove the EOA, and trust Sellick's maneuver to inhibit vomiting and aspiration.

Regaining consciousness Again, this is not an airway to use in the conscious patient because of profound vomiting.

Rupture of esophagus and laceration of esophagus Rupture of the esophagus or laceration of the esophagus is an extremely grave condition with a very high morbidity and mortality, particularly when it is not promptly recognized. The location of the perforation is an important factor in the outcome, as well as determinant of the appropriate therapy. Esophageal perforation can occur following emergency who has bloody nasogastric drainage, a pneumothorax, an increasingly pleural effusion, a pneumomediastinum, or a widening mediastinum and who has been resuscitated with this tube.[16][17]

This is not a "rare" occurrence. Esophageal lacerations were found in 8.5 percent of patients in whom the EOA was used.[18]

As a precaution against pressure-related complications in the esophagus, the EOA should not be left in place for longer than 2 hours.

Combined Esophageal and Tracheal Airways

These airways provide for the possibility of intubation of either the esophagus or the trachea. They appear to be safer, although each has some of the complications of the EOA.

Pharyngotracheal Lumen Airway

The pharyngeal-tracheal lumen airway is a two-tube modification of the EOA. The PtL was designed specifically to avoid two major problems associated with the EOA: inadequate mask seal and inadvertent tracheal intubation. This tube potentially solves the problem of accidental tracheal intubation seen with the EOA. It is easier to ventilate the patient with a PtL than with the EOA. The pharyngotracheal lumen airway has two cuffed tubes. The first tube is short with a large diameter. This tube is color-coded green. A large cuff surrounds the tube's lower third. This cuff will be used to occlude the oropharynx.

If the longer tube is passed into the trachea, it is simply used as an endotracheal tube. If the longer tube goes into the esophagus, then the shorter tube is used to ventilate the patient. The longer tube then is used to occlude the esophagus.

Each of the PtL's tubes is equipped with a standard 15/22 mm connector. The distal cuff on the longer tube resembles the cuff of an endotracheal tube. Both cuffs are inflated simultaneously with the same port. There is a separate clamp on each cuff.

To ensure appropriate placement, the operator must auscultate during ventilation through both tubes. If the distal lumen is in the esophagus, then ventilation should be through the proximal lumen. If the distal lumen is in the trachea, then the tube is used like an endotracheal tube. The balloon in the hypopharynx eliminates the need for a mask, so that the operator can concentrate on ventilation rather than mask seal.

The pharyngotracheal lumen airway appears to provide adequate oxygenation and ventilation. Although the PtL may perform marginally better than mouth-to-mask ventilation, there is little rational justification for use of a more expensive and more dangerous device. The time spent on training for use of the PtL may well be more effectively used in training for endotracheal intubation.

Intubation around this device is quite difficult. In most cases, the tube should be removed from the patient prior to intubation.

Complications

Migration of this tube is a potential hazard. The tube can potentially migrate from tracheal placement to esophageal placement. If the operator does not recognize the proper lumen to use, the patient will not be ventilated appropriately—with disastrous results. Frequent reassessment of tube position is essential when using this device.

Pharyngeal or laryngeal trauma may occur with poor technique. The tube must be removed if the patient awakens or if the gag reflex returns.

Contraindications

The PtL should not be used in a patient under 5 feet in height (there is no pediatric model). Although the literature cites an arbitrary age of 16 as a contraindication, its use depends more on the patient's size. Again, if the patient has a known esophageal disorder, then this tube should not be used. Finally, these tubes should not be used in the conscious patient or when the patient has a gag reflex.

Although it is not documented in the literature, if the distal cuff is inflated in the esophagus of a very tall patient, it would be possible to occlude the trachea, as described in the section on EOA. The emergency provider should be wary of this possibility when using the PtL.

Insertion of the Pharyngotracheal Lumen Airway

1. Place the patient's head in a neutral position.
2. Prepare and check all equipment.

3. Stabilize the cervical spine, as appropriate. Hyperextend the neck if there is no risk of cervical spine injury. Use the neutral position if the patient has had possible cervical spine trauma.
4. Insert the pharyngotracheal lumen airway in the midline through the oral pharynx. Use a jaw lift maneuver to open the airway.
5. Inflate both distal cuffs of the pharyngotracheal lumen airway.
6. Using the bag-valve device, deliver a breath into the green lumen. Auscultate the chest as you do so. If the patient's chest rises and you can hear breath sounds in the chest, then the long tube has passed into the esophagus. Continue to ventilate the patient with the green tube. Inflate the pharyngeal balloon completely.
7. If the chest does not rise and you do not hear breath sounds in the chest, then the long tube has passed into the trachea. Remove the stylet from the clear tube and ventilate the patient with the bag-valve device from the clear tube.
8. Confirm placement of either tube with a capnometer and/or pulse oximeter.
9. Continue ventilatory support with 100 percent oxygen.

Esophageal Tracheal Combitube

The Combitube (Sheridan, Argyle, New York) (EtC) (Figure 4-13 and 4-14) is another two-lumen tube that permits nonvisualized placement in either the trachea or the esophagus (see Figures 4-15 and 4-16). It is designed for oral insertion without visualization of the vocal cords.[19][20] It is functionally and structurally similar to the PtL.

The longer, blue port is the distal port; the shorter, clear port is the proximal port and terminates in the hypopharynx. The proximal lumen ends in numerous holes in the tube at the level of the hypopharynx. The distal part of the tube is again designed like the cuff of an endotracheal tube. There is a large balloon designed to occlude the oropharynx surrounding both tubes.

The Combitube is inserted blindly through the mouth and into the posterior oropharynx. It is then advanced until the distal tube is either in

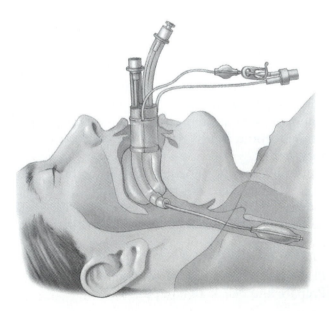

Figure 4-13 Combitube.

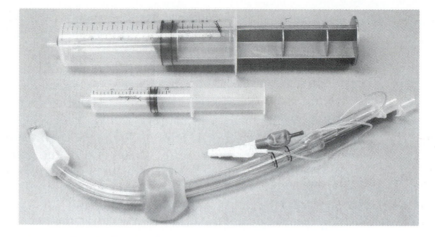

Figure 4-14 Combitube.

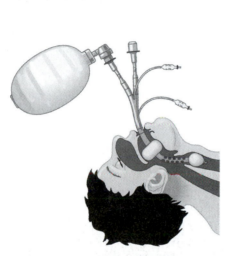

Figure 4-15 Combitube in esophagus.

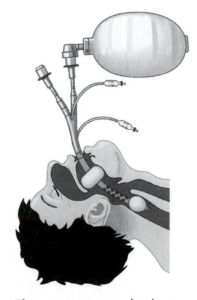

Figure 4-16 Combitube in trachea.

esophagus or trachea. The operator can determine which port ventilates which orifice by ventilating the patient. The operator should first ventilate the longer, distal blue port. Esophageal intubation with this port is quite likely. If breath sounds are heard and stomach sounds are not, then the longer port should be used for ventilation. If gurgles are heard in the stomach and no breath sounds are heard, then attach the bag-valve-mask to the distal port.

The latex pharyngeal balloon is filled with 100 cc of air, and the distal plastic cuff is inflated with 10 cc to 15 cc of air. There is no need for any type of external mask to be sealed around the mouth or lips.

When the Combitube was used in hospitalized comatose or cardiac arrest patients, the "rescuers" were able to achieve arterial blood gas parameters and tidal volumes that were comparable to endotracheal intubation.[21] In another large study, the Combitube appeared to be more effective in ventilation and airway control than the EGTA or the LMA.[22] The Combitube had the best overall insertion and ventilation rates in this study and was associated with the least problems in ventilation.

Only one prospective study has examined the prehospital use of Combitube.[23] In this study, the success rate was only 71 percent compared to intubation rates of 85 percent to 95 percent for visualized endotracheal intubation by paramedics. The authors of this study attributed the lower success rate to poor technique and inadequate skill retention (the very problems cited as reasons not to teach endotracheal intubation!). The authors also noted that Combitube insertion was successful 64 percent of the time after a failed endotracheal intubation.

One case report describes the use of the Combitube in two patients with rapidly enlarging cervical hematomas.[24]

Available data shows that oxygenation is comparable to that achieved by endotracheal intubation. $PaCO_2$ has been elevated when the Combitube is used. Although this device may be useful in prehospital airway support and possibly useful as a rescue airway in failed endotracheal intubation, effective employment depends on continued training and frequent use. The time spent on training for use of the Combitube may well be more effectively used in training for endotracheal intubation.

Advantages[25]

Blind Intubation

Blind intubation can be performed by those medical providers who have not been trained in endotracheal intubation. The skill level requires minimal training.

Suited for Difficult Conditions

The tube's airway is suitable for difficult intubations. Little space and no view of the cords is needed to intubate the patient. This has led to the inclusion of the Combitube in the ASA failed intubation algorithm.[26] The Combitube is considered an appropriate short-term airway by the American Heart Association ACLS 2000 program.

No Mask Needed

This means that the operator can concentrate on ventilation rather than mask positioning.

No Movement of Head or Neck Needed

The insertion technique can be performed with the head and neck in the neutral position. Movement of the head and neck for insertion is not needed.

Gastric Fluid Can Be Aspirated (in some cases)

When the tube is inserted in the esophageal position, the stomach fluids can be aspirated via the "distal" channel.

Complications

Since this tube can be inserted into the esophagus, all of the complications associated with the blind esophageal insertion are possible. Again, ventilation of the wrong lumen will be disastrous. There are significant disadvantages to use of the Combitube:

Maintaining adequate seal of the pharyngeal balloon is difficult. The same pharyngeal balloon makes endotracheal intubation impossible. This device simply must be removed to adequately visualize the cords and intubate the patient.

The Combitube does not isolate or protect the airway. Indeed, suctioning secretions through the tube is impossible when the tube has been placed in the esophagus.

The Combitube has been associated with a significantly higher and longer lasting increase in catecholamine concentrations after insertion than either intubation or insertion of an LMA. This implies that the Combitube is more stressful than either of these airway devices and may be deleterious in the patient who has increased intracranial pressure, cardiovascular disease, or aortic dissection.

Contraindications

The regular Combitube should not be used in a patient under 5 feet in height. There is a Combitube SA for patients 4 to 5 feet tall. (There is no pediatric model.) An arbitrary age of 16 is set, but the height restriction would be more appropriate. Again, if the patient has a known esophageal disorder, then this tube should not be used. Finally, these tubes should not be used when the patient has a gag reflex or is conscious.

Inserting the Esophageal Tracheal Combitube

1. Place the patient's head in a neutral position.
2. Prepare and check all equipment.
3. Stabilize the cervical spine, as appropriate.
4. Insert the esophageal tracheal Combitube in the midline through the oral pharynx. Use a jaw lift maneuver to open the airway. Advance the tube through the hypopharynx to the depth indicated by the markings on the tube. There are black rings on the tube that should be at the level of the teeth.
5. Inflate the pharyngeal cuff with about 10 ml of air.
6. Inflate the distal cuff with about 10–15 ml of air.
7. Ventilate through the blue port first. Auscultate over the chest and stomach. If breath sounds are heard in the chest, continue to ventilate with a bag-valve device and 100 percent oxygen.
8. If breath sounds are heard in the stomach, change the bag-valve device to the clear connector.
9. Reconfirm placement and appropriate ventilation port with end tidal CO_2 detector and/or pulse oximeter.
10. Secure the tube.

Oral-Pharyngeal Airway Devices
Laryngeal Mask Airway (LMA)

The LMA was first introduced in 1983 by A. I. J. Brain at the London Hospital.[27] The FDA approved the LMA for use in the United States in August

1991. The LMA is commonly used for anesthesia in Europe, but is not widely available in the United States. The LMA is currently used in some (but certainly not all) U.S. operating rooms by anesthesiologists for failed intubation and is mentioned in their failed intubation algorithm (Figure 4-17).[28]

There are few U.S. emergency departments that advocate or use the LMA and fewer prehospital organizations. (Less than 1 percent surveyed academic emergency departments had this device available.[29]) The author knows of no prehospital organizations that employ the LMA.

Despite the lack of notoriety in the United States, the LMA is a safe alternative for use in all age groups and should be considered for an airway after failed intubation attempts. The LMA has been extensively used in the field, but not in the United States.[30] This field experience with the LMA reveals no significant problems when proper training was provided (Figures 4-18 - 4-23).

Five sizes of the LMA are now available. Size 1 is designed for a patient who weighs less than 6.5 kilograms and size 2 is designed for the 6.5 kilogram to 20 kilogram patients.[31] Size 1 has been successfully used on a 1.2-kg child.[32]

Each LMA costs about $200 and is guaranteed for at least 10 sterilizations by the manufacturer. This high initial cost further decreases the popularity of this device in most prehospital organizations. Most anesthesia groups use the LMA for up to 50 sterilizations without significant deterioration of the airway.

The laryngeal mask (LMA) consists of a large bore tube with a distal inflatable molded mask (Figure 4-24). The mask is placed above the laryngeal inlet to direct gases into the lungs. The apparatus was also designed to improve the flow of gas through the trachea, since the cuff does not constrict the airway at any point.

The mask portion is triangular and can be easily inserted into the hypopharynx. The mask is constructed to inflate, fill the hypopharynx, and cover

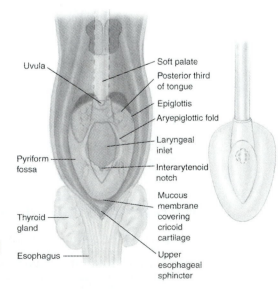

Figure 4-17 LMA position and anatomy. *Source:* Courtesy of LMA America

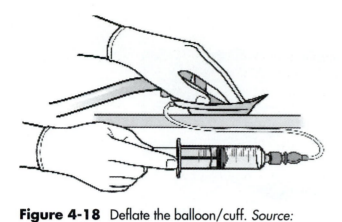

Figure 4-18 Deflate the balloon/cuff. *Source:* Courtesy of LMA America.

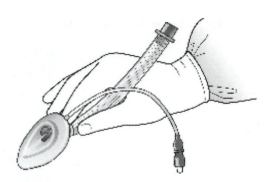

Figure 4-19 Proper position to hold LMA. *Source:* Courtesy of LMA America.

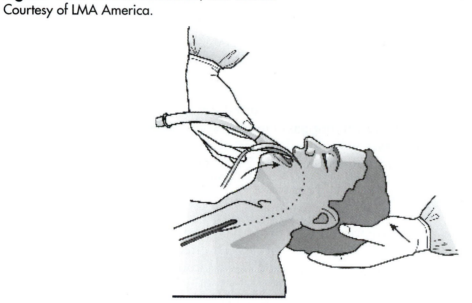

Figure 4-20 Insert LMA with cuff anteriorly. *Source:* Courtesy of LMA America.

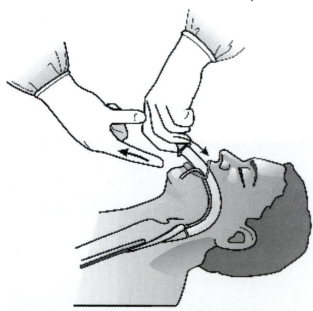

Figure 4-22 Slide LMA into position. *Source:* Courtesy of LMA America.

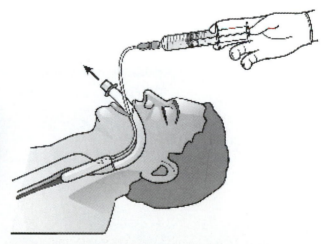

Figure 4-23 Inflate the cuff. *Source:* Courtesy of LMA America.

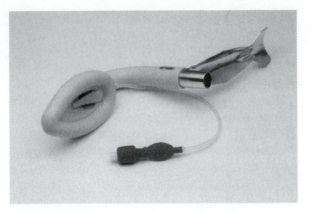

Figure 4-24 A variant of the LMA that is designed for intubation. *Source:* Courtesy of LMA America.

the laryngeal opening. The distal tip of the triangle rests in the esophagus. The device will not pass into the esophagus because of its size. An open slit in the mask will allow direct inspection of the larynx with a flexible bronchoscope or passage of a tube for high-pressure jet ventilation.[33]

Incorrect placement of the LMA is an infrequent problem. Exact placement is not crucial for a clinically patent airway, and only 44 percent of airways that are evaluated by fiberoptic examination will be found perfectly placed. Approximately correct placement of this device has occurred in nearly 90 percent of the cases on the first attempt, even by untrained operators.[34] There appears to be a smaller margin of error in positioning the device in children. When the infant's body position is altered with an LMA in place, the patency may be compromised. The LMA position should always be rechecked when body movement of a child is required.

Occasionally, the child's epiglottis may be kinked or folded by the LMA. This may lead to later edema or latent airway compromise.[35]

Advantages
Advantages of this device over an endotracheal tube include increased ease and speed of placement, lower incidence of coughing and sore throat after the procedure, and insertion of the device requires no laryngoscope.[36] Compared

TABLE 4-1 LMA SIZES	
Mask Size	**Patient Weight**
1	Neo-6 kilograms
2	6.5–25 kilograms
3	25 kilograms–Adult
4	Normal Adult
5	Large Adult

with a face mask, the LMA is easier to use, produces less hand fatigue, and improves oxygen saturation.

The LMA appears to be a good alternative to use of the face mask in the adult patient. Indeed, even with inexperienced operators, the LMA appears to provide better ventilation of patients than bag-valve ventilation.[37] (The students using the LMA actually did better than anesthesiologists using face masks.) It also requires less hand pressure to hold in proper position.[38] Face masks require repositioning more frequently than the LMA in order to adequately ventilate the patient. The LMA lets the operator perform other functions while ventilation continues.

This has led to the inclusion of the LMA in the ASA failed intubation algorithm.[39] The LMA is considered an appropriate short-term airway by the American Heart Association ACLS 2000 program.

Since the LMA does not require use of a laryngoscope and does not pass through the vocal cords, it limits trauma to this area. With this decrease in complications, better ventilation than bag-valve mask, and a high success rate of insertion by inexperienced personnel, this airway may represent a significant improvement in EMS and first responder airway skills.

Insertion of the LMA is only a moderate stimulus that causes little hemodynamic changes. The LMA may induce minor changes in blood pressure and heart rate, which usually return to normal within one minute. Spontaneous ventilation is possible with the LMA.[40]

Contraindications to the Use of the LMA

- Inability to extend the neck or open the mouth greater than 1.5 cm
- Abdominal surgery
- Airway obstruction at or below the pharynx
- Low pulmonary compliance
- Full stomach or increased risk of regurgitation
- The patient has a suspected foreign body in the trachea or the bronchial system.

Complications

In over 2,300 patients, problems with LMA use were recorded in about 11.5 percent of the cases.[41] The most common problem was air leakage around the LMA. Leakage was usually resolved by insertion of a fresh, new LMA. This suggested that the LMA should be replaced at least as frequently as recommended by the manufacturer, or at least after about 50 uses.

Although the LMA appears to provide better oxygenation than the face mask, it provides little protection for the airway from aspiration of vomitus. Although aspiration is repeatedly implicated as a complication of the LMA, no studies reveal a significant incidence of aspiration. This may be because these studies are in the anesthesia literature and the proper screening of patients has decreased the risk of aspiration. This screening in not always possible in emergency medicine.

Some patients can be screened easily. The trauma patient, the obese patient, and the patient who has recently eaten or consumed quantities of alcoholic beverages are not good candidates for LMA for use because of known increased risks for aspiration.

The anesthesia literature recommends H^2 blockers, such as cimetidine (Tagamet™) or ranitidine (Zantac™) and metoclopramide (Reglan™) for the obese patient when employing the LMA. This is simply not an option for emergency patients.

Other complications of the LMA include laryngospasm (1.6%), oropharyngeal or uvular bruising, and hypoxemia (PO < 90%) on insertion. The LMA may be difficult to insert when tonsillar hypertrophy is present.

The cuff of the LMA should be kept inflated until the gag reflex returns. This will prevent aspiration of secretions. The LMA may be removed when the patient opens his mouth on command.

Technique for Insertion of the Laryngeal Mask Airway

1. The patient is placed in the sniffing position, and the jaw is allowed to fall open.
2. Organize the equipment for the procedure. Always have a backup method, such as bag-valve-mask available. Determine the size of the tube. See Table 4-1.
3. Fully deflate the cuff.
4. Position the tube for insertion.
   a. Lubricate the dorsal surface of the cuff.
   b. Flatten mask tip against the hard palate before sliding downward into position. The curved portion of the LMA points toward the patient and away from the operator.
   c. Avoid accidental aspiration of lubricant by using no lubrication on the ventral surface of the cuff.
   d. The tube and cuff are advanced until the tip is in the esophagus. Use the index finger to push at the junction of the tube and the mask and advance the airway. Stop when resistance is encountered. Note that a black line is located on the posterior surface of the LMA to aid in confirming correct position of the tube. If this line is twisted to the anterior or on the side, then the LMA is in the wrong position.
   e. Avoid the epiglottis by pressing downwards and backwards against the posterior wall of the pharynx during insertion.
5. Verify position with direct visualization or by using a laryngoscope.
6. Inflate cuff with about 20cc of air. The soft tissues over the larynx should rise. If there is substantial resistance to inflation, then the position of the LMA should be reassessed.
7. Attach the bag and begin ventilation. Look for chest expansion with ventilation.
8. Secure the tube in place similarly to an endotracheal tube.

Cuffed Oropharyngeal Airway (COPA)

The cuffed oropharyngeal airway (COPA) is a modified Guedel airway with an inflatable distal cuff that is broad and flattened posteriorly, and narrow and more pointed anteriorly (see Figure 4-6a). It was engineered to form a seal in the proximal laryngopharynx with the pointed anterior cuff elevating the epiglottis from the posterior pharyngeal wall to provide a clear airway.[42][43] The proximal end of the device has a standard 15/22 mm connector, an integrated bite block (tooth lip guard), and two posts for attaching an elastic strap that holds the device in place (see Figure 4-6b).

The COPA is 1 cm longer than the corresponding Guedel airway. The COPA is available in sizes 8, 9, 10, and 11. The size is the distance in centimeters between the tooth lip guard and the distal tip of the COPA.

The proper COPA size is selected by placing the distal tip of the COPA at the angle of the jaw. The device is then held perpendicularly to the jaw. In the correct position the guard should be 1 cm above the lips of the patient. The fixation strap posts are centered over the corners of the mouth.

The insertion technique for COPA is similar to that of the standard Guedel oropharyngeal airway, with the patient's head placed in "sniffing" position. Although the COPA device can be inserted more easily by inexperienced users, it is more difficult to obtain an adequate airway seal for positive-pressure ventilation, and additional manipulations may be necessary after insertion.

Comparative studies between the COPA and LMA have shown that the LMA forms a better seal in apneic, paralyzed, and spontaneously breathing nonparalyzed patients.[44] The LMA allows for ventilation with greater peak inspiratory pressures.

The COPA and the LMA have essentially the same complications and contraindications.[45] The ease of insertion of the COPA device may make it an attractive alternative to the LMA for use by inexperienced medical personnel in emergency situations.

End Notes

[1] Spoerel, W. E. "The unprotected airway," in Spoerel, W. E., ed., *Problems of the upper airway.* Boston, MA: Little, Brown, and Company, 1972;10: 1–36.

[2] Benson, D. M. "The esophageal obturator airway: Things are seldom what they seem" in *JACEP* 1976;5:43.

[3] Don Michael, T. A., Lambert, and E. H., Mehran, A. "Mouth to lung airway for cardiac resuscitation," in *Lancet* 1968;12:1329.

[4] Don Michael, T. A., and Gordon A. S. "Esophageal obturator airway: A new adjunct for artificial respiration," in *Proceedings of the National Conference on Standards for CPR and ECC.* Washington, DC: American Heart Association, 1973.

[5] "Standards for cardiopulmonary resuscitation (CPR) and emergency cardiac care (ECC)" in *JAMA* 1974;227(suppl):833–868.

[6] Bryson, T., Benumof, J. L., and Ward, C. F. "The esophageal obturator airway. A clinical comparison to ventilation with a mask and oropharangeal airway," *Chest* 1978;74:57–539.

[7] Meislin, H. W. "The esophageal obturator airway: A study of respiratory effectiveness," in *Ann Emerg Med* 1980;9:171.

8 Johannigman, J. A., Branson, R. D., Johnson, D. J., et al. "Out of hospital ventilation: Bag-valve device vs. transport ventilator," *ACAD Emerg Med* 1995;2:719–724.

9 Auerbach, P. S., and Geehr, E. C. "Inadequate oxygenation and ventilation using the esophageal gastric tube airway in the prehospital setting," in *JAMA* 1983;250:3067–3071.

10 Smith, J. P., Bodai, B. I., and Auborg, R., et al. "A field evaluation of the esophageal obturator airway," in *J Trauma* 1983;23:317–321.

11 Smith, J. P., Bodai, B. I., Seifkin, A., et al. "The esophageal obturator airway: A review," in *JAMA* 1983;250:1081–1084.

12 Don Michael, T. A. "The esophageal obturator airway (letter)," in *JAMA* 1982;247:754.

13 Don Michael, T. A. "Esophageal obturator airway," *Med Instrum* 1977; 11:231.

14 Gertler, J. P., Cameron, D. E., Shea, K., et al. "The esophageal obturator airway: Obturator or obtundator?" in *J Trauma* 1985;25:424.

15 Donen, N., Tweed, W. A., and Dashfsky, S. "The esophageal obturator airway: An appraisal," in *Can Anes Soc J* 1983;30:194–200.

16 Carlson, W. J., Hunter, S. W., and Bonneabeau, R. C. "Esophageal perforation with obturator airway," in *JAMA* 1979;241:1154–1155.

17 Fluck, R. R., Wagner, I. J., and Wiezalis, C. P. "The esophageal obturator airway—A review," in *Resp Care* 1982;27:1373–1379.

18 Goldenburg, I. F., Campion, B. C., Siebold, C. M., et al. "Morbidity and mortality in patients receiving the esophageal obturator airway and endotracheal tube in prehospital cardiopulmonary arrest," in *Minn Med* 1986; 69:707.

19 Blostein, P. A., Koestner, A. J., and Hoak S. "Failed rapid sequence intubation in trauma patients: Esophageal tracheal Combitube is a useful adjunct," in *J Trauma* 1998;44:534–537.

20 Bigensahn, W., Pesau, B., and Frass, M. "Emergency ventilation using the Combitube in cases of difficult intubation," in *Eur Arch Otorhinolaryngol* 1991;248:129–131.

21 Pepe, P. E., Zacharia, B. S., and Chadra, N. C. "Invasive airway techniques in resuscitation," in *Ann Emerg Med* 1993;22:393–403.

22 Tanigawa, K., and Shigematsu, A. "Choice of airway devices for 12,020 cases of nontraumatic cardiac arrest in Japan," in *Prehosp Emerg Care* 1998;2:96–100.

23 Atherton, G. L., and Johnson, J. C. "Ability of paramedics to use the Combitube in prehospital cardiac arrest," in *Ann Emerg Med* 1993;22: 1263–1268.

24 Bigenzahn, W., Pesau, B., and Frass, M. "Emergency ventilation using the Combitube in cases of difficult intubation," in *Eur Arch Otorhino* 1991; 248:129–131.

25 Ibid.

26 Benumof, J. L. "Laryngeal mask airway and the ASA difficult airway algorthim," in *Anes* 1996;84:686–699.

27 Brain, A. I. J. "The Laryngeal mask: A new concept in airway management," *Br J Anesth* 1983;55:801–804.

28 Sofferman, R. A., Johnson, D. L., and Spencer, R. F. "Lost airway during anesthesia induction: Alternatives for management," *Laryngoscope* 1997; 107:1476–1482.

29 Nayyar, P., and Lisbon, A. "Non-operating room emergency airway management and endotracheal intubation practices: A survey of anesthesiology program directors," in *Anesth Analg* 1997;85:62–68.

30 Tanigawa, K., and Shigematsu, A. "Choice of airway devices for 12,020 cases of nontraumatic cardiac arrest in Japan," in *Prehosp Emerg Care* 1998;2:96–100.

31 Pinkowsy, M. "Laryngeal mask airway: Uses in anesthesiology," in *South Med J* 1996;89:551–555.

32 Brimacombe, J., and Gandini, D. "Pediatric airway management," in *Br J Hosp Med* 1995;53:175.

33 Heard, C. M. B., Caldicott, L. D., Fletcher, J. E., and Selsby, D. S. "Fiberoptic guided endotracheal intubation via the laryngeal mask airway in pediatric patients: A report of a series of cases," in *Anesth Analg* 1996;82:1287–1289.

34 Leach, A. B., and Alexander, C. A. "The laryngeal mask: An overview," in *Eur J Anesthesia Suppl* 1991;4:19–31.

35 Mizushima, A., Wardall, G. J., and Simpson, D. L. "The laryngeal mask airway in infants," in *Anesthesia* 1992;47:849–851.

36 Tait, A. R., Pandit, U. A., Voepel-Lewis, T., et al. "Use of the laryngeal mask airway in children with upper respiratory tract infections: A comparison with endotracheal intubation," in *Anesth Analg* 1998;86: 706–711.

37 Martin, P. D., Cyna, A. M., Hunter, W. A. H., et al. "Training nursing staff in airway management for resuscitation," in *Anesthesia* 1993;48:33–37.

38 Benumof, J. L. "Laryngeal mask airway: Indications and contraindications," in *Anesthesiology* 1992;77:843–846.

39 Benumof, J. L. "Laryngeal mask airway and the ASA difficult airway algorithm," in *Anes* 1996;84:686–699.

40 Bahk, J. H., Han, S. M., and Kim S. D. "Management of difficult airways with a laryngeal mask airway under propofol anesthesia," in *Pediatric Anesthesia* 1999;9:163–166.

41 Verghese, C., Smith, T. G. C., and Young, E. "Prospective survey of the use of the laryngeal mask airway in 2359 patients," in *Anesthesiology* 1993; 48:58–60.

42 Greenberg, R. S., and Toung, T. "The cuffed oropharyngeal airway: A pilot study," in *Anesthesiology* 1992,77:A558 (Abstract)

43 Greenberg, R. S., Brimacombe, J., Berry, A., and Gouze, V., et al. "A randomized controlled trial comparing the cuffed oropharyngeal airway and the laryngeal mask airway in spontaneously breathing anesthetized adults," in *Anesthesiology* 1998;88:970–977.

[44] Brimacombe, J., and Keller, C. "The cuffed oropharyngeal airway vs. the laryngeal mask airway: A randomized cross-over study of oropharyngeal leak pressure and fiberoptic view in paralyzed patients," in *Anes* 1999;54: 683–702.

[45] Ezri, T. Ady, N., Szmuk, P., et al. "Use of cuffed oropharyngeal airway versus laryngeal mask airway in elderly patients," in *Can J Anes* 1999;44: 363–367.

Chapter **Five**

Oxygenation and Ventilation Aids

After a patient airway has been established, adequate oxygenation and ventilation must be provided. If the patient cannot ventilate adequately, then the emergency provider must ventilate the patient.

Oxygen Delivery Systems

Oxygen therapy is generally indicated when hypoxia is present. Clinical situations where hypoxia is common include pulmonary diseases, such as COPD, asthma, and pneumonia; cardiac disease; shock; cerebral vascular disease; burns; bleeding; trauma; and shock from any cause. High altitude also causes hypoxia (aviators and climbers require supplemental oxygen), but these delivery systems are beyond the scope of this book.

Oxygen is indicated as a primary treatment for carbon monoxide poisoning. One hundred percent oxygen will reduce the half-life of carboxyhemoglobin from 4 hours to 1 hour.

Oxygen can be supplied by either portable bottles or wall outlets connected to a central reservoir, whether in an ambulance or in a hospital. Portable oxygen tanks are found in ambulances, hospitals, physician's offices, airlines, and many patients' homes. Although airline oxygen can be used for patient care, medical oxygen contains too much moisture to be used as supplemental oxygen in an aircraft. Industrial oxygen should not be used for patient care, as it may contain poisonous contaminants.

Oxygen can also be supplied as a liquid. This is the usual method with a hospital's oxygen supply. The final delivery to the patient is always oxygen gas. Liquid oxygen has several hazards associated with transport, including enhancing flammability of surrounding materials and the extreme cold temperatures required to liquefy oxygen. It is not usually found at a patient's home or in EMS due to the hazards associated with transport.

By international treaty, oxygen tanks are color coded green. In the United States they are pin indexed to prevent attachment of a regulator designed for another gas. The most common cylinders available in the United States are listed in Table 5-1.

To calculate how long the oxygen will last in a cylinder:

$$\text{Tank life in minutes} = (\text{tank pressure in psi} \times 0.28) / \text{liters per minute flow}$$

Regulators for oxygen tanks can be either high-pressure regulators or low-pressure regulators. The standard low pressure regulator is 50 psi. This pressure is used to deliver oxygen to patients and allows low-flow oxygen devices to be used. High-pressure regulators are used to transfer gas at high pressure from one tank (usually a storage tank) to another.

Respiratory Drives

In the normal patient, variations in the CO_2 level in the bloodstream provide the major stimulus for breathing. As the CO_2 builds up, the desire to take another breath becomes profound. Patients with chronic obstructive pulmonary disease may develop a decreased sensitivity to elevated CO_2 levels because of their continuous exposure to these higher CO_2 levels. These patients will typically function with hypoxia driving the stimulus to breathe.

If the COPD patient is given oxygen in sufficient amounts, the remaining stimulus to breathe may theoretically be destroyed and the patient may stop breathing. This factoid is often cited in EMS literature as an admonition not to use high flow oxygen for patients. This admonition is not substantiated by any controlled studies and should be ignored. Indeed, in at least one study, administration of 100 percent oxygen to patients with known COPD resulted in only a transient drop of the patient's ventilation. Within 15 minutes the tidal volume and respiratory rate had returned to baseline levels for the patient.[1]

Methods of oxygen delivery used in the spontaneously breathing patient are summarized in Table 5-2.

TABLE 5-1 AVAILABLE OXYGEN CYLINDERS

Tank (Cylinder) Type	Volume in Liters	Cylinder Factor	Hours of Oxygen at 2 liters/min	Hours of Oxygen at 10 liters/min
D	450	0.20	3.5	.7
E	650	0.28	5.0	1.0
G	5600	2.41	44.0	8.8
H, K	6900	3.14	58.	10.4

Larger tanks are available and may be used in hospitals, clinics, and residences. Oxygen concentrating systems capable of delivering about 90 percent oxygen have been developed and may be used in some residences and hospitals.

TABLE 5-2   OXYGEN DELIVERY SYSTEMS FOR SPONTANEOUSLY BREATHING PATIENTS

System	Oxygen Source	Flow Rate Required (L/min)	Approximate FiO$_2$	Advantages
Nasal prongs	100%	0.5 to 6 l/min	0.25–0.40 (each additional l/min raises FiO$_2$ by 4%)	Simple, comfortable; Allows patient to eat or drink
Simple mask	100%	5 to 8 l/min	0.35–0.50	Delivers a higher flow rate than nasal prongs
Venturi mask	100%	4 to 15 l/min	0.24–0.50	More precise control of FiO$_2$
Partial rebreather	100%	Varies	0.4–0.7	
Non-rebreathing	100%	Varies	0.6–0.9	Higher FiO$_2$
Anesthesia mask	100%	Varies	1.0	Highest available FiO$_2$
Blow-by oxygen	100%	Varies	Unknown and varies by proximity of the oxygen source	May be used for pediatric patients and the extremely claustrophobic patient

Nasal Prongs

Nasal prongs or nasal cannulae increase the FiO$_2$ about 3 percent to 4 percent for each l/min increase in oxygen flow, regardless of whether the patient is breathing nasally or orally (Figures 5-1 and 5-2). Flow rates in excess of 6 l/min are not well tolerated.

Complications of nasal prongs include drying of the nasal mucosa, bleeding from the nasal mucosa, and dermatitis of the face and lips. Pressure

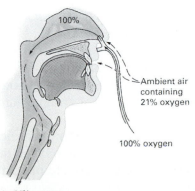

100%

Ambient air containing 21% oxygen

100% oxygen

24% to 44% oxygen concentration delivered

Figure 5-1 Nasal prongs.

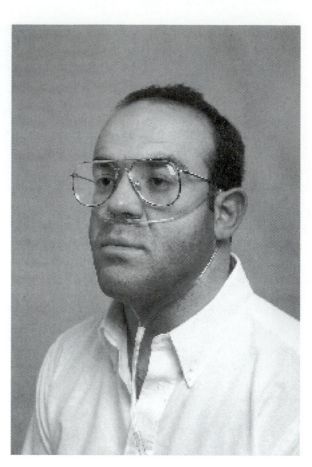

Figure 5-2 Nasal prongs in use.

ulcerations of the nose and ear creases may develop after long use. Rarely a patient will smoke with nasal prongs in place and the tubing will catch fire.

Generally nasal prongs are both comfortable and convenient. They can be left in place while the patient drinks or dines and are not easily dislodged.

Simple Oxygen Mask

The simple oxygen mask or simple face mask does not cause nasal drying or irritation, but is easily moved or dislodged. The FiO_2 delivered is variable and depends on the fit of the mask, the flow rate of the oxygen, and the patient's minute ventilation. A flow rate of at least 5 l/min is needed to flush CO_2 from the mask. Flow rates generally range from 6 l/min to 10 l/min and provide about 40 percent to 60 percent oxygen.

Side ports on the mask will allow room air to enter the mask and dilute the oxygen during inspiration (Figure 5-3). Delivery of more than 10 l/min will not increase the oxygen concentration delivered to the patient, because the ambient air is still sucked in from around the mask's edges and through the ports during inhalation.

Some patients (particularly children) will become claustrophobic and experience a smothering feeling when an oxygen mask is applied. A pediatric mask may be used over a tracheal stoma to provide oxygen to a patient with a permanent tracheostomy.

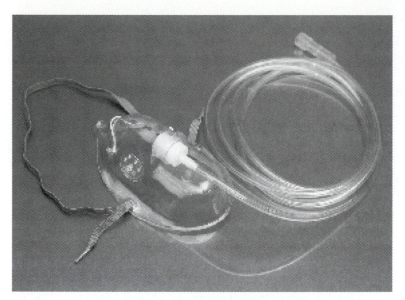

Figure 5-3 Simple oxygen mask.

Venturi Mask

The Venturi mask is a high-flow oxygen system (Figure 5-4). A rapidly moving jet of oxygen sweeps a known amount of air along with it (the Bernoulli principle) to provide a fixed FiO_2 to the patient. The FiO_2 is less dependent on the patient's minute ventilation or the oxygen flow rate than are other mask systems.

The diluter jets are color coded and are available to provide an FiO_2 of 0.24, 0.28, 0.31, 0.35, 0.40, and 0.50. When preparing to use the mask, the provider must insert the proper diluter jet into the mask. Some manufacturers have a dial on the mask that rotates the proper diluter jet into the oxygen stream.

The usual indication for a Venturi mask is in treatment of the chronic COPD patient who has longstanding CO_2 retention. As previously discussed these patients often depend on hypoxia for their drive to breathe and may benefit from careful regulation of their inspired oxygen concentration.

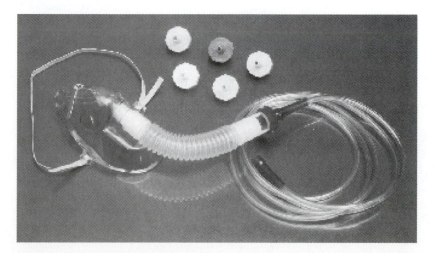

Figure 5-4 Venturi mask.

Like all oxygen masks, the Venturi mask can be dislodged and must be removed if the patient wants to drink or dine. They are less comfortable than nasal prongs and may cause claustrophobia.

Rebreather Oxygen Masks

Rebreather oxygen masks with a reservoir include both the partial rebreathing mask and the non-breathing mask (Figure 5-5). These systems add inhalation valves and a reservoir bag to a simple oxygen mask. A minimum oxygen flow of 5 l/min to 6 l/min is required, and 10 l/min t 15 l/min provides higher oxygen concentrations.

The partial rebreather mask has a disk valve that covers the face mask's side ports. The valves on the side ports will decrease the inspiration of room air. Some air will still be inspired from around the edges of the mask.

The non-rebreather mask has the same one-way side ports as the partial rebreather mask (Figure 5-6). The mask has an added reservoir bag to hold oxygen. The reservoir bag is filled with oxygen and exhaled gases during exhalation and emptied during inhalation. The reservoir augments the flow of oxygen so that during inhalation less room air is added to the inspired oxygen. When the patient breathes in, the oxygen is taken from the low-resistance reservoir first and then from around the mask's edges.

The reservoir masks must fit tightly in order to be effective. They are not comfortable and are intended for short-term use only. If a patient requires one of these masks for more than a few hours, a serious consideration should be given to intubation.

Nebulizer Chamber

The nebulizer chamber is not strictly an oxygen delivery device, but must be mentioned because it is so frequently used in patients who have respiratory distress. The nebulizer holds 3–5 ml of fluid and may be attached to a large diameter tubing, bite piece, or to a face mask. It allows delivery of medications in aerosol form (nebulized). The nebulizer may be driven by either oxygen or air. In prehospital care, oxygen is almost universally used.

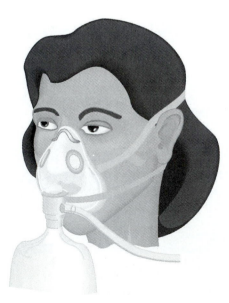

Figure 5-5 Rebreather mask.

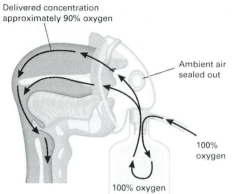

Delivered concentration approximately 90% oxygen

Ambient air sealed out

100% oxygen

100% oxygen

Figure 5-6 Nonrebreather mask.

Anesthesia Mask

The anesthesia machine may be used to ventilate the patient. This will require wide bore tubing and a 100 percent oxygen source. It can provide 100 percent oxygen (FiO_2 of 1.00) if a perfect seal is achieved on the face. This is obviously not a suitable device for the field and most emergency departments.

HeliOx Mixtures

Helium-oxygen mixtures (HeliOx™) are useful in the spontaneously breathing patient with a partial upper airway obstruction (epiglottitis, carcinoma of the larynx, laryngeal hematoma, severe asthma, or postextubation stridor).

SOURCES OF SUPPLEMENTAL OXYGEN		
Source	Percentage	FiO_2
Mouth-Mask ventilation	16–18% oxygen	0.16–0.18
Ambient Air—the real thing	20.84% oxygen	0.21
Nasal prongs	24–28% oxygen	0.24
Nasal cannula (goes in nose)	30% oxygen	0.30
Venturi Mask	35–45% oxygen	0.35–0.45
Non-rebreathing mask	85% oxygen	0.85
Bag-valve mask		
Without oxygen supplement	21% oxygen	0.21 (ambient air)
With supplemental oxygen	40% oxygen	0.40
With reservoir	95% oxygen	0.95
Anesthesia gas machine	100% oxygen	1.00
Aircrew pressurized mask	100% oxygen	1.00
May be able to deliver higher pressure than ambient		

Helium has a markedly lower density than nitrogen (0.14) and hence has less airflow resistance and turbulence in the airway. This means that much less work is required to breathe a helium-oxygen mixture than a nitrogen-oxygen mixture. Special flow meters are needed to correct for the low density of helium.

Typically, an 80 percent helium and 20 percent oxygen (80/20 helium-oxygen) mixture is administered by a non-rebreathing face mask until the obstruction has been resolved or the patient has an appropriate airway (surgical or tracheal intubation). There is no known toxicity, but like nitrogen, helium does not support life. Oxygen must be present.

The lower density of heliox will change the patient's voice. It is likened to a "Donald Duck" sound.

It is unlikely that Heliox mixtures will be used routinely in prehospital care. Prehospital providers may be exposed to Heliox mixtures during transport of critically ill patients with partial airway obstruction, such as epiglottis.

Ventilation Devices

There are three types of devices commonly used to ventilate a patient in prehospital care and in emergency departments. The bag-valve-mask (BVM) is the most widely used. The manually triggered, oxygen-powered ventilator is another device in popular use. More recently pneumatically powered, automatic ventilators can be found in the prehospital setting. Each of these will be described in detail.

Bag-Valve-Mask

This device is familiar to every emergency practitioner. It is required equipment in every ambulance and emergency department. While it is the most popular device for providing artificial ventilation, it has significant disadvantages.

- It requires substantial training in order to use correctly.
- It requires a very tight seal in order to ventilate the patient.
- It is easily dislodged during ambulance movements or CPR.
- It causes substantial gastric distention.
- It can force blood, fluids, debris, and vomitus into the airway.

The bag should be self-filling and should have no sponge rubber on the inner lining (old style Ambu bags) (Figure 5-7). The sponge rubber is difficult to sterilize

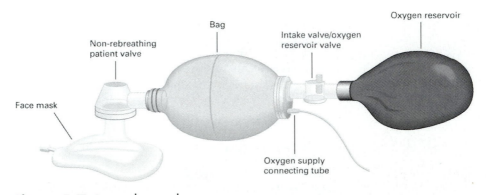

Figure 5-7 Bag valve mask.

and can be expelled into the patient's lung. The bag should be transparent. A clear transparent plastic permits the operator to see if there is vomitus or material within the bag. Most bag-valve-mask systems in the United States are disposable.

The bag must have a one-way valve that does not jam with vomitus or mucus and does not pop off. If the valve becomes plugged with mucus or vomit, it may not function at all or may function poorly. This failure may cause over pressure to the lungs or inadequate concentrations of oxygen to be delivered to the patient (Figure 5-8).

A pop-off valve limits pressure delivered to the lungs. When the pop-off valve functions correctly, the patient's lung will be protected from exposure to high pressure. Unfortunately, if the patient requires a high pressure to deliver oxygen to the lung, then the patient does not receive the full volume of gas within the bag. This situation may be encountered in COPD or asthma patients.

The valve should have a standard 15 mm adapter to fit either an endotracheal tube or a mask. The valve must also have a provision for delivery of supplemental oxygen.

The bag must also have a reservoir to allow high concentrations of delivered oxygen. The amount of delivered oxygen is dependent on the patient's ventilatory rate, the volume delivered to the patient with each breath, the rate of oxygen flow into the bag and into the reservoir, and the filling time for the reservoir. If all of these were equal, the type of reservoir would not matter. Unfortunately, all reservoirs are not equal, and the type of reservoir does matter. A reservoir of corrugated tubing is the least effective, while a 2.5 liter bag reservoir appears to be most effective.[2]

All BVM devices should be attached to a supplemental oxygen device at about 15 liters per minute. When attached to supplemental oxygen at 12–15 liters per minute, the bag-valve-mask will deliver 40 percent oxygen with a tight seal. When a reservoir is attached to the bag-valve-mask, the oxygen concentration is increased to 90 percent.

The mask should have a soft sealing device and should be transparent so the operator can see vomitus if the patient regurgitates during ventilation.

Various size masks and bags are available. Even when only adult patients are anticipated, it is wise to have adequate stock of both neonatal and pediatric masks and bag-valve units. Always select the mask that provides the tightest seal and conforms best to the patient's nose and mouth. The "Seal

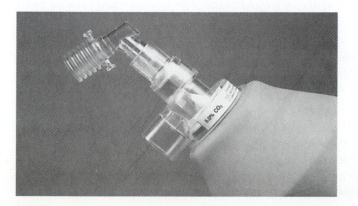

Figure 5-8 Bag with attached colormeter CO_2 detector.

Easy" mask from Respironics is particularly useful as it conforms with great ease to any difficult facial anatomy. The softness decreases leakage. A pediatric mask can be used to ventilate a tracheostomy patient.

Indications and Contraindications

The bag-valve-mask provides an immediate means to ventilate the patient. It also permits the operator to assess the compliance of the lungs. When a mechanical device is used, this clinical determination is lost.

Indications

- Absent or inadequate spontaneous respirations
- Preoxygenation when intubation is planned
- Short-term oxygenation when ventilation is temporarily compromised

Contraindications

- Inexperience of the operator (a rescuer who has little experience with the BVM will have better ventilation with mouth-to-mask ventilation)
- Suspicion of active or passive regurgitation
- Need to avoid head or neck manipulation (relative)
- Tracheo-esophageal fistula
- Tracheal fracture or laceration
- Facial fractures or trauma
- Disruption of facial dermal surfaces
- Oral bleeding or vomiting
- Full stomach (relative)

Equipment

- Fitted face mask
- Respiratory or resuscitator (Ambu-style) bag
- Oxygen supply (15 Liters per minute)
- Suction

Technique

An area of prehospital airway management that is typically neglected in training is appropriate use of a bag-valve-mask. During the airway management of an emergent patient is not the appropriate place to learn this technique. Although BMV technique offers no protection against aspiration, it can be used to oxygenate most patients.

Bag-valve-mask systems are awkward to use. The rescuer must provide both the head-tilt and chin-lift maneuver and maintain a perfect mask seal with one hand. The other hand is used to squeeze the self-inflating bag (Figure 5-9). This is difficult and taxing, even for a well-trained anesthetist or anesthesiologist.

The technique is often taught with CPR mannequins or intubation mannequins. These models are cumbersome and don't adequately simulate the soft tissues and slack jaw of a comatose patient. Only a few instructors will use water or soapsuds to show the student problems with seal and the effects of fluids and secretions on management with the bag-valve-mask unit.

The ideal model for teaching the use of a bag-valve-mask is the paralyzed patient in the operating room. This experience is often ignored, but will provide the student of any level with invaluable experience.

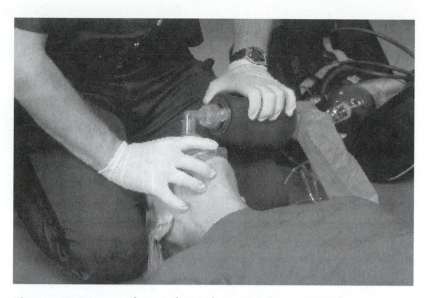

Figure 5-9 Bag-valve mask ventilation single person technique.

To properly use a bag-valve-mask

- Place an oral or nasal airway.
- The traditional method is to hold the mask in the left hand with the thumb and index finger gripping the mask while the third, fourth, and fifth fingers provide jaw extension and oppose the pressure from the thumb and index finger to create a tight seal with the mask.
  - Body of the mask fits into the left palm
- Place the narrow end of the mask on the bridge of the nose.
- Seat the chin section of the mask on the alveolar ridge.
- Seal the mask by pulling the jaw into the mask with the curled fingers of the left hand and tilting the mask slightly to the right. Maintain the airway by lifting the chin with the remaining fingers. Avoid placing pressure on the soft tissues under the chin. The left hand may be used for ventilation and the right to hold the mask, if the operator is more comfortable.
- Squeeze the bag firmly with the right hand. There is a learned skill in squeezing the bag effectively. Rapidly and forcefully squeezing the bag will promote gastric distention more than ventilation of the patient's lungs. Time delivered breaths with the patient's inhalations. Full compression of the bag is required for adequate ventilation.
- In tachypnea, alternate assisted breaths with the patient's inhalations.

If there is difficulty attaining a seal, secure the mask to the patient with both hands and have an assistant deliver the breaths with the bag. The two-person technique has been shown to be superior to the single-rescuer technique in multiple studies (Figure 5-10).

In bearded patients, surgical lubricant on the beard may enhance the seal. In edentulous patients, an oral airway is often needed.

Complications
The most important problem with a bag-valve-mask unit is that a lower tidal volume is delivered than with either mouth-to-mouth or the pocket

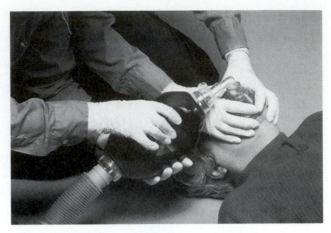

Figure 5-10 Two-rescuer technique for BVM.

mask.[3][4] The most common complication is failure to secure an adequate seal which causes inadequate delivery of oxygen.[5][6] As already noted, it is quite difficult even for an experienced practitioner to provide a perfect seal with one hand. This can be readily remedied by use of a two-hand seal and an assistant squeezing the bag.

Gastric distention is a very common problem found with use of a bag-valve-mask. Vomiting or difficulty ventilating the patient may result in extreme cases.

Assessing for Difficulties in Ventilation

Conditions that are associated with difficulties in ventilation with a bag-valve mask include

- A thick beard, preventing effective mask seal
- Facial trauma, including open cheek lacerations, fractures of the mandible, and large open facial wounds
- Facial burns
- The edentulous patient who has collapse of the facial muscles resulting in air leaks around the mask
- A distended abdomen or large chest wall, which can make chest excursion ineffective
- Severe bronchospasm with limited chest excursion
- Airway obstruction
- Obesity/bull neck
- Neck instability

Mouth-to-Mask Ventilation

Mouth-to-mask ventilation appears to offer some advantages over the bag-valve-mask system because both hands are free to hold the jaw forward and to maintain an airtight mask-to-face seal. Ventilation is then provided by the rescuer's own lungs. Delivered air volumes are as large as those seen with endotracheal intubation. The inspired FiO_2 is about 17 percent to 18 percent when exhaled air is used to ventilate the patient.

The pocket mask is a clear plastic device, often with a carrying case (Figure 5-11). Although pocket masks are sold for this express purpose, any anesthesia or resuscitation mask is appropriate. Pocket masks with supplemental

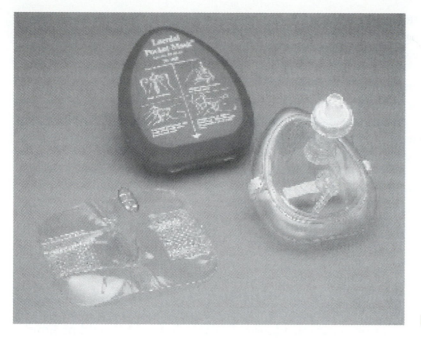

Figure 5-11 Pocket mask.

oxygen ports are available. Pocket masks may be either disposable or reusable. The reusable masks almost uniformly have a 15/22 mm adaptor that allows use of a bag-valve device.

Mouth-to-mask ventilation provides larger tidal volumes than bag-valve-mask systems.[7] The rescuer not only has both hands free to provide a good mask seal, he/she provides a larger volume than does a single hand squeezing a bag. It does deliver significantly lower oxygen and higher carbon dioxide concentrations.

Mouth-to-mask ventilation with a Respironics SealEasy mask system has been shown to easily reach target ventilation volumes.[8] The Laerdal Pocket Mask is another simple means of providing mouth-to-mask ventilation.[9] It is a soft, transparent vinyl mask with a portal for delivery of oxygen and a one-way valve for added security from contamination. A Guedel airway may be helpful with either of these masks.

With some masks, the oxygen concentration to the patient can be increased to greater than 70 percent. Unfortunately, only about 50 percent of the available masks have a portal for enhancement of oxygen concentration. If the mask does not have an oxygen port, then the rescuer can supplement his or her oxygen concentration with nasal prongs to enhance the oxygen concentration delivered to the patient.

The mask seal with two hands using a mouth-to-mask technique is usually superior to that provided by one hand and the bag-valve-mask technique. The same cautions about cervical trauma, facial trauma, beards, and "difficult anatomy" apply to the pocket masks as to the masks used with a BVM.

If mouth-to-mask ventilation is technically superior, why isn't it taught and used more freely? Mouth-to-mask ventilation is not used by most providers because they are afraid of disease transmission during mouth-to-mask ventilation. This could be avoided by routine use of a Pall Ultipore Breathing system filter or similar device to prevent exposure of the rescuer.[10] Use of extension tubing can increase the distance between the patient's mouth and the rescuer's mouth. (The connecting tubing will add to the dead space of air exchange. The emergency provider should be wary of any such device with a long extension tubing.)

Manually Controlled Ventilator

The manually controlled, pneumatically powered ventilator (also called the demand valve device manually triggered ventilator (MTV), or flow-restricted, oxygen-powered ventilation device) is operated by depressing a manual pressure-release button (Figure 5-12). When the button or valve is opened, oxygen flows to the mask. The device will deliver nearly 100 percent oxygen at up to 40 l/min. These devices are sturdy, compact, and easy to handle.

Many demand valve devices are equipped with an inspiratory release valve. The negative pressure generated by the patient on inspiration will trigger the valve. This allows use in a spontaneously breathing patient. The demand valve will supply more oxygen as inspiratory pressure increases. When inhalation stops, the demand valve shuts off the oxygen flow.

These devices have been documented to deliver pressures that can cause gastric insufflation or pneumothorax. This concern led to the 1986 American Heart Association recommendation that the flow rate should be limited to 40 l/min and a pop-off valve should be activated if pressures exceed 50 mL H_2O. Pressure is restricted to about 30 cm of water in most devices. The modified MTV now does not create the excessive pressures documented with the older MTV. This results in a decreased risk of gastric distention.

The devices deliver oxygen to the mask or endotracheal tube. It is the operator's responsibility to ensure that the mask is appropriately sealed and that the patient actually receives the oxygen flow. It affords no end of amusement to watch an ill-trained operator diligently squeezing the oxygen release button but failing to have a tight seal on the mask. One always hopes that the patient is spontaneously breathing in these cases.

The MTV does not give the operator any sense of the compliance of the lungs. If the patient develops a pneumothorax, the operator often does not

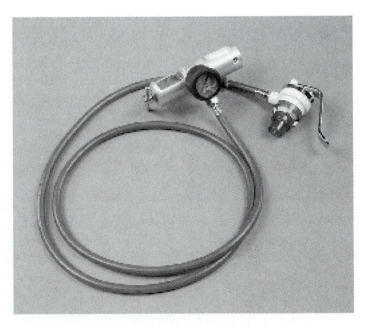

Figure 5-12 Oxygen powered manually triggered ventilator.

note the increased difficulty in ventilation when using this device. Since the device delivers oxygen at high pressure, pneumothorax and subcutaneous emphysema are somewhat more common when this device is used. Pneumothorax is particularly common when the demand valve is used in intubated patients.

Despite the previously mentioned modifications to the device, gastric distention remains a real problem. This may lead to difficulty ventilating the patient and to increased risk of vomitus.

Finally, this device uses a lot of oxygen. Small portable oxygen cylinders can be rapidly depleted by use of a demand valve.

The author does not much recommend the use of a demand valve. There are simply too many drawbacks to a high-flow system that does not give feedback to the operator about the patient's compliance and condition.

Automatic Transport Ventilator

There are several small ventilators designed for transport and prehospital care. These lightweight devices can maintain ventilation with minimal operator intervention. They are mechanically simple, are powered by the oxygen they deliver, and allow the operator to focus on other tasks (Figure 5-13). They can be quite useful or quite detrimental to the patient's well-being, depending on the operator's skill and diligence.

An automatic transport ventilator is clearly most effective when the patient is intubated. In the unintubated patient, the operator must still ensure that the mask is in place and appropriately sealed. In some rare situations where intubation has failed, is difficult, or impossible, the operator may seal the mask with both hands and allow a transport ventilator to provide ventilation. Positioning of a face mask with elastic straps or similar devices during transport is fraught with hazard and should be condemned.

Although other ventilatory devices such as the COPA, LMA, and Combitube may theoretically be used with a ventilator, the possibility of

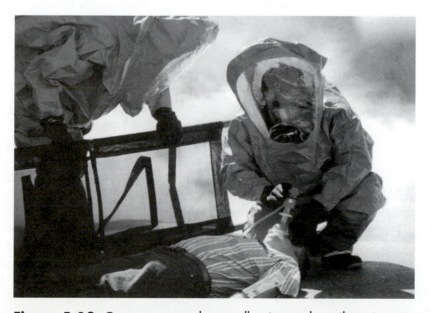

Figure 5-13 Oxygen powered manually triggered ventilator in use.
Source: Oxylator, courtesy of Lifesaving Systems, Inc.

movement within the confines of an ambulance or during transfer in an emergency department makes them problematical at best.

The compact ventilator usually has two or three controls: the ventilatory rate, the tidal volume, and possibly inspired oxygen concentration. Some models have intermittent mandatory ventilation capacity, so that they can be used in the spontaneously breathing patient to intermittently assist their ventilation.

When automatic transport ventilators are compared with bag-valve ventilation during transport situations, the automatic transport ventilator provides a more consistent ventilation. The ventilator simply doesn't suffer from fatigue and distraction.

Although ventilators in an intensive care unit have alarms, the transport ventilator does not usually have an alarm. This means that the operator must be diligent in ensuring that tubes are not displaced or disconnected. The oxygen supply must be carefully checked to ensure that the ventilator stays operational.

Many of these devices have a pressure-relief valve (pop-off valve). This, as with a bag-valve device, is a double-edged sword. It will prevent barotrauma by opening when the airway pressure exceeds a set level. It will do so by venting some of the tidal volume. This means that the patient who has an increased compliance from pulmonary edema, pulmonary contusion, bronchospasm, pneumothorax, or adult respiratory distress syndrome will not be appropriately ventilated.

An adult transport ventilator is not usually suitable for children and vice versa. When transporting children, ensure that the ventilator can be properly adjusted for the child being transported or use a bag-valve device.

CPAP and Similar Modalities

Continuous positive airway pressure (CPAP) maintains a positive airway pressure during the entire respiratory cycle. CPAP prevents early airway closure during expiration and increases the functional residual capacity, thus improving oxygenation and decreasing the work of breathing.[11][12]

CPAP may be applied with a face mask, a nasal mask, or an endotracheal tube. When used with a face or nasal mask, the patient must be alert, cooperative, and have an intact gag reflex. Typically, this tight-fitting mask is strapped on the patient and positive pressure is applied with a CPAP machine equipped with one-way valves and a reservoir bag.[13]

CPAP was originally used for patients with diffuse lung disease and a low CO_2. It has been used in emergency medicine for patients with cardiogenic pulmonary edema, COPD, pneumonia, and inhalation lung injury.[14] In patients with cardiogenic pulmonary edema, CPAP improves the patient's oxygenation, reduces the work of breathing, and may reduce the blood pressure.[15][16] In some patients, CPAP may decrease the need for urgent intubation.

Complications of CPAP include facial discomfort, gastric distention, nausea and vomiting, reduced cardiac output, increased intracranial trauma, and barotrauma. The patient must be able to remove the mask if he or she vomits.

END NOTES

[1] Aubier, M., Murciano, D., Milic-Emili, J., et al. "Effects of the administration of oxygen on ventilation and blood gases in patients with chronic obstructive pulmonary disease during acute respiratory failure," in *Am Rev Respir Dis* 1980;122:747

[2] Campbell, T. P., Steward, R. D., Kaplan, R. M., et al. "Oxygen enrichment of bag-valve-mask units during positive-pressure ventilation," *Ann Emerg Med* 1988;17:232.

[3] Hess, D., and Baran, C. "Ventilation volumes using mouth-to-mouth, mouth-to-mask, and bag-valve techniques," in *Am J Med* 1985;3:292–296.

[4] Elling, R., and Politis, J. "An evaluation of emergency medical technicians' ability to use manual ventilation devices," in *Ann Emerg Med Services* 1982; 7:44–46.

[5] "Standards and Guidelines for Cardiopulmonary Resuscitation and Emergency Cardiac Care," in *JAMA* 1986;225:2905–2960.

[6] Hackman, B. B., Kellermann, A. L., Everitt, P., and Carpenter, L. "Three-rescuer CPR: The method of choice for firefighter CPR?," in *Ann Emerg Med* 1995;26:25–30.

[7] Harrison, R. R., Maull, K. I., Keenan, R. L., and Boyan, C. P. "Mouth-to-mask ventilation: A superior method of rescue breathing," *Ann Emerg Med* 1982;11:74–76.

[8] Giffen, P. R., and Hope, C. E. "Preliminary evaluation of a prototype tube-valve-mask ventilator for emergency artificial ventilation," in *Ann Emerg Med* 1991;20:262–266.

[9] Harrison R. R., Maull, K. I., Keenan, R. L., and Boyan, C. "Mouth-to-mask ventilation: A superior method of rescue breathing," in *Ann Emerg Med* 1982;11:74–76.

[10] Thomas, A. N., O'Sullivan, K., Hyatt, J., and Barker, S. J. "A comparison of bag mask and mouth mask ventilation in anaesthetized patients," in *Resuscitation* 1993;26:13–21.

[11] Stock, M. C., Downs, J. B., and Corkran, M. L. "Pulmonary function before and after prolonged continuous positive airway pressure by mask," in *Crit Care Med* 1984;12:973.

[12] Duncan, A. W., Oh, T. E., and Hillman, D. R. "PEEP and CPAP," in *Anesth Intensive Care* 1986;14:236.

[13] Hoff, B. H., Flemming, D. C., and Sasse, F. "Use of positive airway pressure without endotracheal intubation," in *Crit Care Med* 1979;7:559.

[14] Meduri, G. U., Conoscenti, C. C., Menashe, P., et al. "Non-invasive face mask ventilation in patients with acute respiratory failure," in *Chest* 1989; 95:865.

[15] Katz, J. A., and Marks, J. D. "Inspiratory work with and without continuous positive airway pressure in patients with acute respiratory failure," in *Anesthesiology* 1985;63:598.

[16] Rasanen, J., Vaisanen, I. T., Heikkila, J., et al. "Acute myocardial infarction complicated by left ventricular dysfunction and respiratory failure. The effects of continuous positive airway pressure," *Chest* 1985;87:158.

Chapter **Six**

Tracheal Intubation

Endotracheal intubation is the insertion of a tube in the trachea. Tracheal intubation is the definitive method of airway management. Endotracheal intubation allows the greatest control of the airway. It is a skill that requires extensive training and is subject to degradation if not practiced appropriately.

Indications

Historically, intubation has been taught to field providers for use in the patient who has a cardiac arrest and has neither pulse nor respiration. There is no question that these patients need rapid airway maintenance. This indication is noncontroversial and is described in ACLS, ATLS, and PALS textbooks of resuscitation.

Patients who also can clearly benefit from emergency endotracheal intubation include those in respiratory arrest who still have a pulse, patients with severe respiratory depression from whatever cause, selected patients in pulmonary edema, and those with inhalation injuries.

Patients for whom the benefit of urgent endotracheal intubation is less clear and the risk is greater are those with anticipated cardiovascular or respiratory collapse from sepsis or severe trauma, patients with a head injury who have a patent airway and are breathing but are in a state of agitated delirium, patients with drug overdoses who become combative when stimulated, and patients with respiratory failure who are still breathing but "running out of steam."

Although the technique of airway intubation is straightforward to teach, the greater challenge for emergency physicians is to help EMS personnel develop the clinical judgment needed to select appropriate patients for intubation.

Indications

- Hypoxia
- Hypercarbia
- Altered mental status (head injury, drug overdose)

- Altered respiratory effort
- Inability to protect airway
- Anticipated cardiovascular or respiratory collapse (sepsis, severe trauma, etc.)
- Anticipated respiratory obstruction (epiglottitis, respiratory burns, major oral or facial injuries)

Contraindications

Contraindications

- Tracheal fracture or disruption
- The patient does not wish to be intubated

Assessing for the Difficult Intubation

> *If you are properly prepared for the difficult airway,*
> *it becomes increasingly difficult to find a difficult airway.*

The frequency of difficult intubations is not clear. This is partly due to who defines "difficult." Reports in the anesthesia literature suggest that anywhere from 6 percent to 15 percent of intubations are rated difficult by the anesthesiologist. In emergency medicine, there is no question that the less controlled environment of the field or the emergency department will lead to more frequent difficult intubations.

Prolonged efforts to intubate can result in hypoxia and cardiac decompensation. Pharyngeal stimulation during the attempt at intubation can cause profound bradycardia or asystole. Prolonged attempts at intubation can provoke laryngospasm and bronchospasm.

It is helpful to have some prior warning that a difficult intubation may occur. Unfortunately, there is little help from predictive factors in the literature. Indeed, in over 1,200 prospectively studied patients, 84 were predicted to have a problem with the airway—and only 22 of these actually did (25 percent).[1]

Several factors can predispose to a difficult intubation. These include poor technique, anatomic variations, coincident diseases, trauma, and patient preparation.

Poor Technique

Suboptimal technique can turn an intubation into a disaster. In the haste to secure the airway, standard pre-intubation procedures are often neglected. A well-prepared patient will better tolerate a prolonged attempt or multiple intubation attempts. Standard noninvasive monitoring offers immediate feedback about how the patient is responding to the procedure.

Ensure that the patient has IV access and is getting pre-oxygenated with 100 percent oxygen. This will provide an oxygen reserve to bridge the apneic period during intubation.

Ensure that you have the best position that you can get during the intubation. Obviously a field intubation in cramped quarters is going to be more difficult than intubation in a well-lighted ambulance or emergency department. If you are easily ventilating the patient with simple techniques, consider waiting until lighting and conditions are better.

Ensure that the patient is in "sniffing" position if possible.

The most common mistake made during intubation is levering or "cranking back" on the laryngoscope handle in order to lever the tip of the blade and provide better visibility. This maneuver may demonstrate the glottis better, but it decreases the size of the oral opening and may destroy the teeth. If the laryngoscope blade is lifted forward and upward, the glottic opening will be visualized better and the oral opening will be wider. This allows more room to manipulate the endotracheal tube into position.

Anatomic Variations

There are several anatomic features that are associated with increased difficulty in intubation. If these risk factors are found, then rapid sequence intubation should be avoided if possible. In general, the longer the neck and the more prominent the mandible, the easier the intubation will be.

Unfortunately, there is no single anatomic indicator that is uniformly reliable in predicting when intubation is going to be difficult. The emergency provider often does not have a choice whether or not to intubate the patient. When appropriate, an alternative technique may be incorporated that allows the patient the ability to protect his own airway and maintain spontaneous respirations.

The original method of airway evaluation was developed by Mallampati.[2] In this system, the visibility of the tonsillar pillars and the uvula is assessed when the patient is seated with the tongue fully protruding and the mouth wide open (see Figure 6-1). Dr. Mallampati noted that when the tonsillar pillars and the uvula were concealed, the difficulty of the intubation was also increased. In those patients where the tonsillar pillars and the uvula were readily seen, the patient was easily intubated. A prospective study by Dr. Mallampati and his colleagues resulted in three classes of visualization of the tonsillar pillars and the uvula.[3] This has been revised by Samson and Young with

TABLE 6-1 AN ACRONYM FOR AIRWAY ASSESSMENT

M	Mandible	Length of the mandible and any subluxation of the mandible should be assessed. Is the mandibular space wide enough?
O	Opening	Ease, symmetry, and range of the opening should be assessed. Can the patient open the mouth widely?
U	Uvula	Visibility of the uvula should be assessed (Mallampati classification). What structures can be seen in the open mouth?
T	Teeth	Note if the patient has adequate dentition and presence of any loose teeth or dental appliances. What structures will be damaged or loosened by laryngoscopy?
H	Head	Assess flexion, extension, and rotation of the head upon the neck. Can the patient assume the sniffing position?
S	Silhouette	Obesity, buffalo hump, kyphosis, large breasts should be identified. The massively obese patient should always be considered a difficult intubation.

Source: Adapted from Davies, J. M., Eagle, C. J. "Mouths," in *Can J Anaesth,* 1991;38:687.

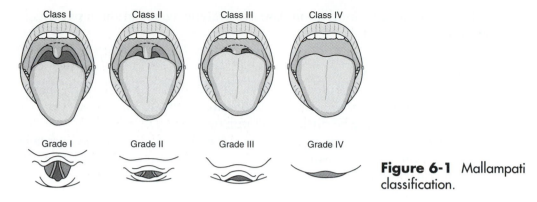

Figure 6-1 Mallampati classification.

a useful pictorial classification of the laryngoscopic views that correlate with Mallampati's pharyngeal structures.[4]

These and most of the subsequent classification schemes are designed for use in non-emergent patients. In many emergencies, having the patient sit up and protrude the tongue is simply not feasible. Assume that if you can't see any of the posterior pharyngeal wall that the intubation is going to be difficult!

Dentition

Protruding incisors, extensive caries, loose teeth that can be dislodged, and chipped teeth should all be noted. Edentulous patients with dentures may be easier to intubate and much more difficult to ventilate with a mask. In some cases, leaving the dentures in during ventilation and removing them just prior to intubation may be appropriate.

Small Oral Opening

If possible, the patient should be asked to open his or her mouth completely to ensure that there is adequate room to insert both a laryngoscope and an endotracheal tube into the oral cavity. A good general guideline is to make sure that there area at least three finger-breadths between the upper and lower central incisors when the mouth is fully opened. Patients with arthritis may not be able to open the jaw sufficiently. Patients with large teeth may have a small intraoral opening. A small opening compromises the space available for laryngoscopy and may make the intubation much more difficult.

When the patient has a smaller opening, use the narrower Miller blade, if possible. An assistant may tug on the corner of the mouth to enlarge the opening laterally. Use of a suction tip as a lip retractor may be helpful.

Short Mandible

A short mandible, as in retrognathia or micrognathia, will change the angle that the laryngoscope meets the epiglottis. There may be a short distance between the tip of the mandible and the Adam's apple. When this distance is less than three finger-breadths in an adult, the visualization of the glottis may be quite difficult. These patients may have a very difficult intubation.

Pediatric syndromes such as the Pierre Robin syndrome (macroglossia and micrognathia), fetal alcohol syndrome, or the Treacher Collins syndrome (hypoplasia of the facial, malar, and mandibular bony structures) also predispose to difficult intubation. Use of paralytic agents in these patients is hazardous in the field.

Anterior Larynx

The distance from the chin to the hyoid bone should be about three finger-breadths. Anything less than this distance may indicate an anterior larynx and, consequently, may be difficult to intubate.

Likewise, the space between the hyoid bone and the thyroid cartilage should be about two finger-breadths wide. Lesser distances are also suggestive of an anterior larynx. In these patients, positioning is critical.

Use Sellick's maneuver to posteriorly displace the glottis and allow easier visualization. The BURP maneuver can also enhance visualization of the cords. Backwards, Upwards, Rightwards Pressure (to the patient's right) will displace the glottis into the intubator's line of sight.

Immobile Neck

As noted earlier, the optimal position for intubation is slight flexion of the neck at the shoulder and extension of the head on the neck. Any condition that limits this mobility, such as contractures of the head and neck, arthritis of the neck, etc., will impair the ability to achieve alignment of the oral, pharangeal, and tracheal lines.

The most common cause of the immobile neck is cervical immobilization for suspicion of trauma. Management of this problem is covered in a separate section.

Patients with rheumatoid arthritis may have instability of the atlantoaxis joint. If it is possible, the examiner should try to find the limits of neck movement prior to attempting intubation. Note if this movement causes neurologic symptoms.

Distortion of Anatomy

Trauma may distort normal landmarks or displace the normal structures with swelling, subcutaneous air, or bleeding. Particularly noteworthy is trauma to the larynx and anterior trachea caused by direct impact (clothesline injuries).

Surgery of the head and neck may also distort normal anatomic landmarks. This is quite common after radical neck dissections for cancer. A patient with a tracheostomy may or may not be able to be intubated orally. If a tracheostomy scar is present, the operator should try to find out why the tracheostomy was performed. A prior tracheostomy may require a smaller than usual tube for intubation. These alterations of normal anatomy may make intubation difficult or impossible.

In adults, severe rheumatoid arthritis, burn contractures, or acromegaly can make intubation difficult. The anatomy may be shifted and the neck may be immobile.

Morbid Obesity

In addition to the factors already mentioned, morbid obesity is an independent predictor of a difficult intubation. A short, thick, or fat "bull" neck will certainly make intubation more difficult.

Orotracheal Intubation

Technique

Equipment

Equipment Needed

- Laryngoscopy blade and handle
- Bag-valve-mask
- Oxygen delivery system
- Endotracheal tubes and stylet
- Suction apparatus
- Tube placement verification device
- Magill forceps
- Monitoring equipment
- Oral and nasal airways

The Laryngoscope The basic components of a laryngoscope include the handle, the blade, and the light source (Figures 6-2 and 6-3).

Blades Multiple types of blades are available to suit the preferences of operators. The most common of these blades are the Macintosh curved blade and the Miller straight blade. Each is available in a variety of sizes for infants, children, and adults. The largest laryngoscope blades are size 4 (straight blade 190 mm long, curved blade 158 mm long). Shorter blades are smaller numbers and are available for smaller adults, children, infants, and newborns. The average-sized adult will be intubated with a size 3 curved or straight blade. The larger sizes of blades are useful in the morbidly obese patient. A Miller 0 blade is often used in infants, and a Miller 2 is used for all patients over a year old.

Other common blades include the straight Wis-Forreger or Wisconsin blades. Disposable curved and straight blades are made by a variety of manufacturers. The practitioner usually finds one or the other type more comfortable and the choice of blade is usually up to the operator. Every practitioner should be familiar with both types of blades, since the desired type may not be available or working at the time that is needed. It is probably better to err

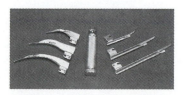

Figure 6-2 Laryngoscope and blades.

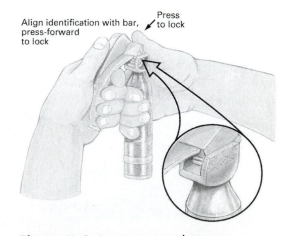

Align identification with bar, press-forward to lock

Press to lock

Figure 6-3 Laryngoscope being put together.

on the side of selecting a blade that is slightly too large rather than a blade that is too small.

When using the curved blade, the tip is placed in the vallecula, anterior to the epiglottis. The key to proper insertion of the curved blade is to visualize the epiglottis, not the larynx and vocal cords. Once the epiglottis has been identified, slide the blade into the pharynx so that it rests in the vallecula anteriorly and superiorly to the epiglottis. If the left arm is now lifted, the epiglottis is moved upwards and anteriorly and the vocal cords are easily exposed.

The curved blade usually offers a wider separation of the oral and soft palate tissues and gives the laryngoscopist more room to manipulate the tube or use the Magill forceps to remove foreign bodies or position a tube (Figure 6-4). A major drawback of this blade is that the laryngoscopist may not see the vocal cords as well, providing some "gentle amusement" when only the "bubbles" can be seen and hence intubated.

When using the straight blade, the tip is placed beneath the epiglottis so that the blade lifts the epiglottis and exposes the vocal cords (Figure 6-5). The long axis of the blade provides a direct line of sight into the cords. It offers the laryngoscopist the opportunity to consistently see the tube pass through the cords. It is very important not to obscure this visual line of sight with the tube. Insert the tube laterally and advance obliquely toward the glottis.

The obvious disadvantage is that the opening through which the laryngoscopist views the cords is smaller than with a curved blade. This provides the experience of being able to visualize the cords well and not be able to maneuver the tube through the cords. In pediatric patients, the straight blade may be placed in the vallecula and the epiglottis raised indirectly.

Blades with fiberoptic light delivery are significantly brighter than bulbs that become encrusted and scratched over time. The fiberoptic systems also are available in disposable models.

If the light fails, consider the loose bulb first, a burned out or failed bulb second, and the batteries third. Tighten the bulb. If that does not work, then replace the blade with a similar size blade. If the laryngoscope is still nonfunctional, then replace the handle with the spare or replace the batteries.

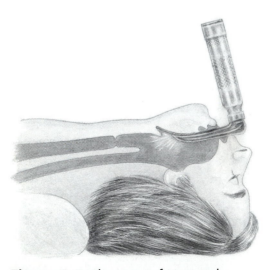

Figure 6-4 Placement of Macintosh blade.

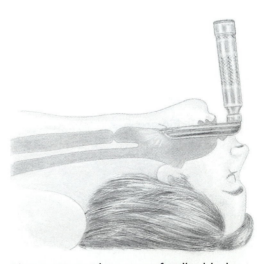

Figure 6-5 Placement of Miller blade.

Occasionally, both bulb and batteries can fail, but with two handles and two blades, this "quad" failure is quite remote.

Handles There are two main categories of laryngoscope handles: The L type and the U type. The U-type handle was introduced by Chevalier Jackson, but has been virtually abandoned in favor of the L-shaped laryngoscope. The U-type laryngoscope is found only in operating rooms and is used only rarely in that environment. The L-type laryngoscope is lighter, less bulky, and is the only type found in emergency medicine practice.

Most L-type handles have the blade at right angles to the handle, but there have been several modifications in the angle of attachment for ease of use in special clinical situations. The most famous of these is the Polio blade used to intubate patients who are in an iron lung.

The blade can be permanently attached to the handle or have a detachable hook-on mount. The detachable mount allow different blades to be used with the same handles. The mount contains a switch that turns on the light source when the blade is lifted into a working position.

The battery capacity of L-type handles are also manufactured in a variety of styles with single AA batteries all the way to D cell batteries. One of the most useful is the AA cell handle. Although this is often found on the pediatric crash cart, the author keeps one in a belt pack, giving a readily available "known good" spare and readily available spare batteries. The D size may have more electrical capacity but is just too big for most hands to hold comfortably.

The Endotracheal Tube The cuffed endotracheal tube was invented by Trendelenburg in 1871.[5] In 1910, Elsburg first used the endotracheal tube to ventilate a patient for open thoracic surgery.[6] Modern endotracheal tubes must meet the standards of the F-29 Committee on Anesthetic and Respiratory Equipment, American Society of Testing and Materials (ASTM) (Figure 6-6).

The ideal endotracheal tube would be pliable and nonkinkable, inert and nonreactive to tissue, very thin to minimize the external diameter while maximizing the internal diameter. It would have a cuff that could prevent any secretions or stomach contents from being aspirated. The cuff would be

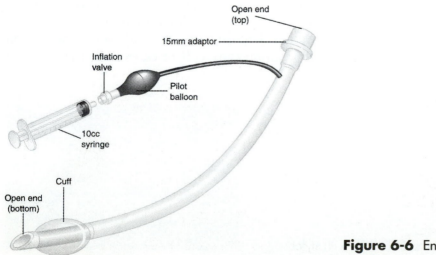

Figure 6-6 Endotracheal tube.

harmless to the tracheal mucosal, despite a long duration of intubation. Such a cuff would also be tough so that it could be manipulated by Magill forceps or thrust through the nose without tearing and leaking. An ideal tube would have a distal CO_2 sensor to ensure that it was placed in the trachea.

We don't have this tube yet. Most tubes in EMS service are made out of polyvinyl chloride and are disposable. This substance is nonirritating and soft. Many special endotracheal tubes exist, including Endotrol trigger tubes for difficult intubations, foil-wrapped tubes for laser surgery, spiral imbedded tubes that are not kinkable, and special tubes for jet ventilation.

Key aspects of the tube include the internal diameter, the length, and the type of cuff. The tube size refers to the internal diameter of the tube. The tubes vary in length with larger ID tubes being longer. Outside tube diameters vary as the thickness of the wall of the tube is proportional to the ID of the tube.

A rule of thumb is to use a 7 mm or 7.5 mm tube in an adult female, an 8 mm tube in an adult male for nasal intubation, and about 0.5 mm to 1 mm larger for oral intubation. Some elderly men with larger tracheas may require a 9.5 mm or 10 mm oral tube, although the need for this size tube is rare. Calculation of the tube size of a pediatric tube is covered in the section on pediatric intubation.

Each tube will be packaged with an adaptor matched for the bag-valve device. This conical adaptor will have a standard 15/22 mm connector on one end and a sized connector for the tube on the other. The adaptor will be stamped with the size of the tube it is designed for (for example, 8.5 mm). A tube adaptor that is more than 0.5 mm smaller than the ID of the tube should not be used.

All modern endotracheal tubes have a second outlet, or "Murphy eye," at the distal end of the tube, beyond the cuff. This outlet is designed to allow continued ventilation should the end of the tube become blocked or be shoved against an occlusive structure. When a stylet is used with the tube, ensure that the tip of the stylet does not protrude through the Murphy eye and cause airway trauma (Figure 6-7).

The distal end of the tube is beveled to ease passage through the vocal cords. The direction of the bevel is of some importance when passing a tube through the nose, although this is controversial.

The cuff can be either high-volume, low-pressure (5 cc to 10 cc) or the older low-volume, high-pressure cuff. The low-volume, high-pressure cuff gives better protection from aspiration. Unfortunately, the additional protection comes with a high price. The high-pressure cuff often exceeds the capillary

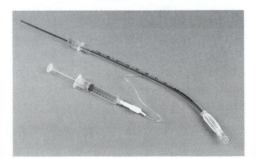

Figure 6-7 Tube with stylet.

pressure in the tracheal mucosal. This causes ulceration after less than 24 hours of use. Tracheal ulceration can be followed by formation of tracheal granulomas, tracheal stenosis, and pseudo membranes. On the other hand, the soft, pliable, low-pressure cuff can allow aspiration if the patient vomits. Overinflation of the cuff can also cause tracheal damage. The soft cuff, however, can be used for extended periods. The low-pressure cuffs can also allow tube pistoning in the trachea, which can lead to potential mainstem bronchial intubation.

The cuff is inflated through a one-way valve that is designed to accept a syringe. A pilot balloon between the one-way valve and the inflating tube for the cuff shows whether the cuff is inflated. The cuff must always be checked for integrity before insertion in a patient.

If either kind of cuff is inflated in the larynx, the pressure can cause damage to the recurrent laryngeal nerve. This damage is frequently bilateral, with resultant vocal cord spasm.

Foam-filled cuffs (Kamem & Wilkinson) maintain a lower tracheal wall pressure. In order to insert the tube, the air is evacuated from the cuff, compressing the foam. After insertion, they are left open to ambient pressure to allow the foam to expand. These tubes are good for long-term intubation, but are rarely used in emergency medicine. They may be more difficult to insert into the poorly visualized vocal cords.

Technique
- ALWAYS WEAR GLOVES AND EYE PROTECTION!
- Oxygenate the patient. Attach the bag-valve-mask to an oxygen supply at about 15 l/min. The oxygen supply should be checked before every shift and after every intubation. If the operator is using portable oxygen, ensure that the bottle is full. An e tank with less than 500 psi will quickly empty at 8 l/min to 10 l/min.
- Check suction apparatus. Suction apparatus should be readily available for every intubation. The suction apparatus should be checked at the start of every shift and cleaned and re-set after every intubation. Batteries should be checked for portable suction when the rest of the suction apparatus is cleaned. Yankauer or tonsil tips should be available as well as tracheal suction catheters. The presence of working suction at the start of the intubation can mean the difference between harmless vomiting and fatal aspiration.
- Check ETT tube cuff for leaks. Before intubation is attempted, the appropriate size tube should be selected, the cuff tested, the tube lubricated, and if desired, a stylet inserted. A 10 cc syringe used for testing should be attached to the tube.
- Check blade and handle for functioning.
  - This should be done prior to every shift and again before every intubation.
- Put head in sniffing position.
- Pre-oxygenate with mask ventilation.
- Have an assistant apply cricoid pressure (Sellick's maneuver or BURP maneuver).[7]
- Remove oral airway.
- Hold laryngoscope handle in left hand.

- Open mouth as wide as possible.
  - Use scissorlike motion with thumb and second fingers of right hand (thumb on mandibular teeth, middle finger on maxillary teeth).
- Place laryngoscope blade in right side of mouth.
- Sweep tongue to the left with the blade while advancing the blade.
- Position the blade correctly.
  - Under the epiglottis—straight blade
  - In the vallecula—curved blade
- Lift the laryngoscope handle upward and away from the operator to expose the vocal cords.
- Pass the tube through the vocal cords.
- Inflate the cuff of the endotracheal tube.
- Position the tube so that the tube is about 23 cm to 24 cm at the teeth in adults. Although Magill forceps are not often needed for the oral intubation, they may be helpful with intubation of the far anterior larynx.
- Verify tube placement with at least three clinical and one instrument method. The routine use of a tube placement verification device will prevent most esophageal intubations from causing devastation to the patient. These devices should be used even in the field. The author prefers the Nellcor EasyCap II device. It is simple, reliable, relatively inexpensive, and small enough to fit into a belt pack or jump bag.
- Release the cricoid pressure.
- Secure the tube.
- Place an oral airway or bite block in the awake patient to avoid biting obstruction of the tube.

As a rough guide to time the intubation technique, the operator should take a single deep breath when he or she starts the procedure. If the patient cannot be intubated before the operator has to take a breath, then the intubation attempt should stop and the patient should be ventilated. This maneuver is not designed to add stress to the intubation, but to simply remind the operator that the patient needs to breathe. Failure to intubate during this 30–45 second period means that the patient needs to breathe as badly as the operator!

The use of preoxygenation before the intubation is also important. This preoxygenation will ensure that the nitrogen is washed out of the lungs and will extend the allowable apneic time until the oxygen in the lungs is used up. Attach the bag-valve-mask to an oxygen supply at about 15 l/min. Have an assistant apply the mask to the patient and ventilate the apneic patient or assist the patient who is spontaneously ventilating. Active ventilation may distend the stomach and cause vomiting.

In patients with a short, thick neck, the Macintosh blade may give somewhat better visualization of the glottic opening. These patients often have a more posterior tongue and epiglottis.

In children and infants, the straight blade may be more useful. The child has a large head, small epiglottis, and short distance from pharynx to epiglottis. The curved blade may not displace the epiglottis as well as the straight blade. This is more of a theoretical advantage than practical, as some individuals prefer the curved blade even when intubating a neonate.

Lift the laryngoscope handle upward and away from the operator to expose the vocal cords. The vector angle is about 45–55 degrees from the patient's trachea. Do not use the blade as a pry bar, as this will certainly damage the teeth and will be far less effective in exposing the cords (Figure 6-8).

The forearm may be "braced" against the patient's forehead and the handle lifted with wrist extension. This is a useful adjunct in practitioners who have decreased shoulder and upper arm strength.

Placing the blade in the middle of the tongue and failure to move the tongue to the left are the two most common problems that prevent a good view of the cords. Placing the laryngoscope blade in the middle of the tongue allows the tongue to fold over the sides and obscures the view of the cords. If the tongue is not pushed to the left, then it may be possible to see the cords, but not possible to place the tube through the cords.

In endotracheal intubation of the adult when visualization of the glottis is difficult, two simple maneuvers may be of use:

First: Place a folded towel under the occiput to flex the neck, aiding in alignment of the axes of the neck and mouth. This brings the patient's head into the sniffing position.

Second: Sellick's maneuver—compression of the larynx and trachea may not only facilitate visualization of the glottis, but prevent aspiration of vomitus. Sellick's maneuver should be released only when the tube is confirmed to be in the trachea.

Verify tube placement with visualization of passage of the tube through the cords, endtidal CO_2 device, auscultation of the chest wall, chest expansion, chest x-ray and pulse-oximeter, or all of these techniques, depending on the locale of the intubation. (See section on Adjuncts-verification of tube placement.)

Tape the tube securely. In a trauma situation or cardiac arrest, be sure that someone has complete responsibility for tube security and positioning before you let go of the tube and move to another task.

Inflate the cuff with the minimum volume that will completely occlude the lumen of the trachea. This will minimize mucosal trauma.

Tape the tube with the 21–23 cm marker at the maxillary tooth line. Smaller patients should have the shorter depth. Calculations for the tube depth in a child are demonstrated in the pediatric section. An oral tube should never be taped to the mandible, since the mandible is mobile and can change the depth of the tube.

Be wary of devices that go completely around the neck, particularly in the patient with head or neck trauma. They require movement of the neck in

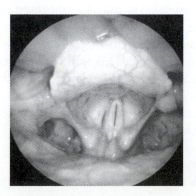

Figure 6-8 Visualization of larynx.

order for appropriate placement and may restrict venous overflow from the head leading to increased intracranial pressure.

Place an oral airway or bite block in the awake patient to avoid biting obstruction of the tube.

After placing an endotracheal tube, check for loose or missing teeth. A fractured or dislodged tooth is the most common complication of intubation. Any newly missing teeth must prompt a chest x-ray to ensure that the patient has not aspirated the tooth. This is particularly true in children who are shedding deciduous teeth and in the elderly with poor dentition.

Awake Oral Intubation

If the patient also has a condition that will make either intubation or mask ventilation a difficult proposition, the operator should consider awake oral intubation. In this case, a moderate dose of sedative is given to the patient, the airway is anesthetized with liberal amounts of topical anesthesia, and the patient is intubated with a laryngoscope, while completely awake.

Awake means that the patient is able to follow the operator's directions and understand what is happening. This also means that the operator must take uncommon pains to educate the patient about each step and what will be required. This patient will be able to give the operator complete feedback on the procedure, so uncommon skill will be required of the operator. The patient must be completely cooperative for this procedure to function.

This is not the same as using sedation to obtund the patient enough to permit intubation. It is exceedingly dangerous to obtund the patient with respiratory distress. The patient now may be unable to protect his or her own airway and at risk for aspiration. Since all sedative agents can cause both respiratory depression and hypotension, the operator may have an apneic hypotensive patient after the sedative has been given.

The classic situation requiring an awake intubation is the "clothesline" neck injury or the patient with penetrating neck injury. Although the anatomy may be normal, it may also be distorted to the point that initial attempts at intubation will be unsuccessful. Bag-valve-mask ventilation may cause subcutaneous emphysema and result in worsening the situation. Intubation is indicated because airway compromise is quite likely. If the intubation is unsuccessful, then the situation may be worsened with bag-valve-mask ventilation. This patient may be best served with an awake intubation, or at least an awake visualization of the cords.

Anesthesia may be provided by nebulizing lidocaine in a hand-held nebulizer. Good airway anesthesia may be obtained in about 5–10 minutes with a nebulizer solution of 4 percent lidocaine.

Alternatively, a lidocaine spray device can be used to spray the lidocaine directly on the cords and pharynx. This will require patience.

The laryngoscopy can then be performed. After the patient's cords have been visualized, then the tube may be passed. If desired, the patient can now be completely sedated and paralyzed and the tube passed. Visualization of the cords will demonstrate that intubation is possible.

Blind Oral Endotracheal Intubation

Blind oral endotracheal intubation refers to the situation where the vocal cords can't be seen. The intubation proceeds with the airway landmarks guiding the tube into position. Essential landmarks that must be visualized include the esophagus, arytenoids, and the epiglottis.

Other techniques that have been helpful in this situation follow.

Magill Forceps

Although the Magill forceps were designed to help with nasal intubation, it can be very useful in the difficult oral intubation. The distal tip of the endotracheal tube is directed anteriorly towards the glottis. An assistant can help with either holding the laryngoscope or advancing the tube while the intubator concentrates on advancing the tip into the larynx.

Stylet

A stylet is a useful adjunct for oral intubation. It will help keep a soft tube in the appropriate shape to facilitate manipulation and insertion through the cords. The stylet gives rigidity to the tube and allows greater control of the tip of the endotracheal tube. It is particularly helpful in the patient with a far anterior larynx or in the patient with a short fat "bull" neck where head positioning is difficult.

The stylet should have a blunt tip and be coated with soft plastic. Lubricating the stylet may allow it to be withdrawn from the tube without withdrawing the tube from the cords. Inability to remove the stylet is a particularly frustrating indication for immediate extubation and reintubation.

Ensure that the stylet is recessed at least 2 cm from the tip of the tube. If the stylet protrudes from the tube, it can cause serious damage to the soft pharyngeal tissues or the cords.

Directional Control Tip Endotracheal Tube

The Endotrol endotracheal tube allows the intubator to alter the distal curve of the endotracheal tube during the intubation. These tubes are slightly softer and more flexible than the standard endotracheal tube. When using the Endotrol tube, don't use a stylet.

Complications

Failure to intubate

- Hypoxia
- Hypercarbia
- Cardiovascular instability
- Cardiac arrest

Intubation of the Esophagus

The most common serious complication associated with endotracheal intubation is unrecognized esophageal intubation. As multiple EMS providers, emergency physicians, and even anesthesiologists have discovered, it is not possible to sustain life with gastric ventilation. The intestinal mucosal simply won't transport oxygen to the blood in any reasonable quantity. It is far better to assume that the intubation was not a success and ventilate by mask during the resuscitation than to wait for deoxygenation, bradycardia, and subsequent cardiopulmonary arrest. There is no place for an ego when managing the airway.

> *By the very bowels of Christ, I beseech you.*
> *Know that ye might be wrong!*
> Oliver Cromwell, Lord Protector of England.

Complications Associated with Difficult Airways

*   Hypoxia
*   Cervical spine injury
*   Hypercarbia
*   Cardiac arrhythmias
*   Increased intracranial pressure
*   Aspiration of vomitus and gastric contents
*   Dislodged and broken teeth, both permanent and deciduous
*   Soft tissue lacerations and avulsions
*   Local swelling from trauma

Bronchial Intubation

Asymmetric breath sounds usually mean that the tube has been inserted into the bronchus and only one lung is being ventilated. When breath sounds are heard on only one side, the cuff should be deflated and the tube withdrawn until breath sounds are equal. Delayed repositioning of the tube can cause hypoxia and possibly unilateral pulmonary edema. If breath sounds continue to be unequal after the tube has been repositioned, then the patient may have a hemothorax, pneumothorax, or a main stem bronchus obstruction.

Laryngospasm

Laryngospasm, when both vocal cords are approximated, allows no passage of air. It reuslts when the patient has inadequate relaxation and sedation and may represent an attempt by the body to prevent aspiration. If the operator attempts to force a tube through the laryngospasm, it can cause hemorrhage, destruction of one or more vocal cords, arytenoid dislocation, and late granuloma formation. A late complication of this trauma is possible tracheal or laryngeal setnosis.

Laryngospasm can be best prevented by judicious use of RSI techniques for intubation. With an adequate dose of paralytic agent, it is impossible to have laryngospasm. It can be treated by gentle bag-mask ventilation and by use of succinylcholine. Two percent or 4 percent lidocaine can be sprayed directly on the cords or sprayed through a cricothyroid puncture.

Dental Damage and Lacerations to Tongue, Lips, and Gums

As noted, this is the most common complication of laryngoscopy. Protruding incisors, loose teeth that may be dislodged, and all chipped or broken teeth should be noted prior to the intubation attempt. If teeth are dislodged, retrieve them immediately. If the teeth cannot be located easily, a chest x-ray is mandatory. A swallowed tooth is not a problem, but a tooth in the lung rapidly leads to a recurrent pneumonia.

Major Airway Trauma—This Is an Avoidable Complication

A more uncommon, but devastating complication is perforation of the pharynx with a subsequent mediastinitis or perforation of the trachea with formation of massive subcutaneous emphysema. These two complications can be prevented with gentle and precise technique.

Blind Nasotracheal Intubation

The technique of blind nasotracheal intubation was developed by Rowbotham and Magill during WWI (Figures 6-9, 6-10, 6-11).[8] Until the advent of RSI, blind nasotracheal intubation was considered to be a standard technique of intubation that should be routinely used in all patients with potential neck injuries.[9] It is no longer considered the method of choice for emergency intubation in the trauma patient, but since it requires little extra equipment and may be used as an awake intubation technique, it still belongs in all emergency provider's armamentarium.

Advantages

The advantages of blind nasal intubation follow.

Reduction of Movement

Nasal intubation is described as allowing the operator to avoid extension of the neck. If the patient is awake, neurological status may be documented after the intubation. (This putative advantage may be found more in the literature than in real practice. Certainly, the assumption that a blind nasal intubation can be performed without neck or head movement is rarely valid.)[10]

Ease of Intubation

Awake nasal intubation may be easier in the patient with a short stocky neck, morbid obesity, or who is unable to open the mouth. For acute epiglottitis, nasotracheal intubation is preferred by many clinicians. This technique in the patient with epiglottis should be done in the operating room with both anesthesia and ENT standing by.

Long-Term Intubation

Nasal intubation is better tolerated than oral intubation and there is less movement of the endotracheal tube. (Again, this may be a putative advantage, since sinusitis occurs frequently with long-term nasal intubation.)

Reduction of Aspiration Risk

Nasal intubation aggravates the gag reflex less than oral manipulations and may decrease the risk of vomitus and subsequent aspiration. The patient cannot bite the tube or manipulate it with his/her tongue.

Blind nasal intubation is possible in the sitting position. This may be appropriate for the massively obese patient or the patient with congestive heart failure.

Disadvantages of Nasotracheal Intubation

Nasotracheal intubation is technically more difficult than oral intubation and frequently takes longer. It is not an appropriate technique for patients with nasal or midface trauma. Nasotracheal intubation often precipitates epistaxis. It is possible to nasally intubate the patient who is apneic, but it is much more difficult.

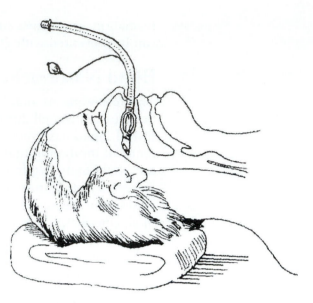

Figure 6-9 Nasal intubation technique—insertion of tube straight back into nares.

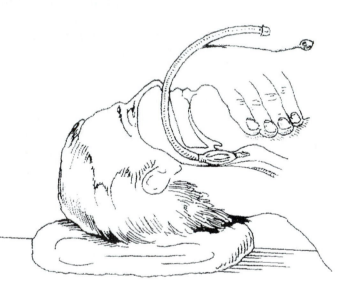

Figure 6-10 Nasal intubation technique—insertion of tube into oral pharynx.

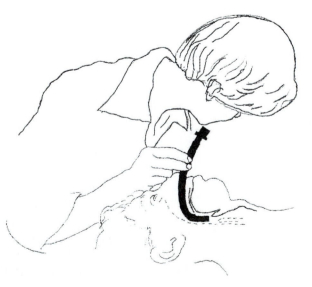

Figure 6-11 Nasal intubation technique—listening for breath sounds.

Method

Equipment

Equipment

- Laryngoscopy blade and handle
- Bag-valve-mask
- Oxygen delivery system
- Endotracheal tubes
  - Use of a "trigger" tube may make the intubation easier. The tube is more pliable, and it is easier to control the position of the distal end of the tube.
- Suction apparatus
- Tube placement verification device
- Magill forceps
- Monitoring equipment
- Translaryngeal anesthesia equipment
- Lidocaine jelly or Cetacaine
- Vasoconstrictor such as 0.25 percent phenylephrine, oxymetazoline (Afrin™) or 4 percent cocaine. This will make the procedure easier and will markedly decrease the incidence of epistaxis.

Blind Method

The nose can be anesthetized with any of several agents: lidocaine jelly, cocaine solution, Cetacaine. If a vasoconstrictor is used with the anesthetic, not only is the procedure easier, it is accompanied by far less bleeding. Topical anesthetics can be supplemented with phenylephrine, cocaine, or oxymetazoline to decrease the edema and ease tube passage.

Alternatively, in patients with intact protective airway reflexes, consider using translaryngeal anesthesia. A small amount of lidocaine instilled through the cricoid membrane with a 25-gauge needle will decrease cough and possibility of laryngospasm.

Warming the tube in hot water prior to the procedure will make it more pliable and easier to pass. As already noted, a trigger tube is more pliable and has the advantage of control of the distal end of the tube. The tube should be liberally lubricated prior to insertion.

Failure to lubricate the tube adequately or choosing a tube that is too large can lead to either epistaxis or to a torn cuff on the tube (or both). Ensure that the endotracheal tube adaptor is firmly seated in the tube before a tube is used for nasal intubation. Loss of the tube in the nostril can make subsequent intubation quite difficult and give the ENT surgeon an opportunity to voice a few new invectives in the operating suite. Most of these invectives will be to the detriment of the intubator that "lost" the tube in the nose.

It is probably easiest for a right-handed person to intubate from the patient's left side. This allows the right hand to be used for the intubation, with the left hand applying cricoid pressure. By leaning slightly forward and listening to the breath sounds, the operator may more easily guide the tube into proper position.

The tube is slid straight back into the nostril, parallel to the floor of the nasal cavity. The floor of the naris is almost horizontal. The most common error in inexperienced operators is to attempt to follow the nasal passages upwards, directly into the frontal sinuses. A slight resistance may be felt until the tube turns the corner into the posterior pharynx.

The operator slowly advances the tube and listens to the breath sounds from the tube. As long as the trachea and the tube are aligned, these breath sounds are present. If the breath sounds disappear, then either the tube has slid into the pyriform fossa or the operator has intubated the esophagus. Pull the tube back until breath sounds reappear and re-advance the tube.

As the tube is advanced past the anterior turbinates, the operator should direct the tube toward the floor of the nose. This advance should be slow and cautious.

Watch for signs of fogging as the tube approaches the vocal cords. The patient's voice may change as the tube engages the vocal cords, if the patient is still able to speak. When the tube is passed through the cords, the patient will lose the ability to phonate. The patient will often have a cough as the tube passes through the cords and enters the trachea. At this point, inflate the tube and verify the position. If the tube slides down easily, it may have passed in the esophagus. If the patient does not have cervical spine trauma, extending the patient's head may allow the tube to be more easily advanced in the proper position.

If the tube is inserted into a pyriform sinus or the vallecula, breath sounds may be heard but may change character. A tube placed in the right nostril advances diagonally into the left piriform sinus. Pull the tube back and re-advance it. As the tube is re-advanced, twist it from one side to the other. If neck mobility is not a problem, flexing or extending the head may also change the angle of the endotracheal tube and allow passage into the trachea. Remember that a tube passed into the right nostril will cross over to the left and plan maneuvers accordingly. If the patient's neck can't be moved, an assistant may try pushing the larynx toward the side opposite the nostril.

Direct Method

If the tube can't be passed blindly and the patient doesn't have any neck trauma, the tube can be positioned with direct laryngoscopy. If the patient stops breathing during the procedure, the tube must be passed under direct vision. An assistant should push the tube forward while the operator visualizes the cords and directs the tip with a Magill forceps (Figure 6-12). Never grasp the tube by the cuff, as the forceps can easily rip the thin cuff.

If the patient can't be moved, the operator can try to manually reposition the tube.[11] The index and long fingers are slid over the tongue posteriorly until the epiglottis is felt. The endotracheal tube is trapped between the fingers and pulled to the posterior border of the epiglottis. The endotracheal tube can then be advanced in the midline and guided into the larynx.

After the tube has been placed through the cords

- Inflate the tube with only enough pressure to ensure a seal.
- Verify position as for an oral endotracheal tube.
- Secure the tube to the nose.

Precautions and Complications

The method should be used with caution in patients who are hoarse, have dysphonia, or are known to have tumors of the neck or vocal cords. Performance of blind nasotracheal intubation is much easier in a spontaneously

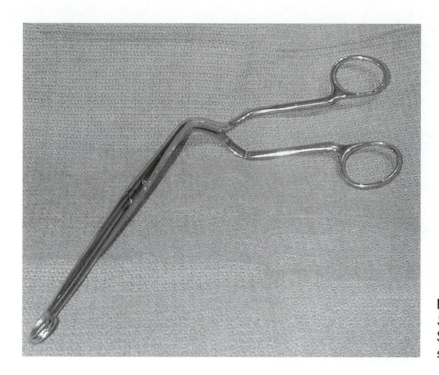

Figure 6-12 Magill forceps.
Source: Photo by Charles Stewart and Associates; www. storysmith.net.

breathing and unconscious or relatively cooperative patient—it is not possible to intubate the combative patient with this technique. Most emergency providers consider apnea to be a contraindication to this technique, but there are multiple reports of successful BNI in patients with deliberate apnea.[12][13]

This technique limits the size of the tube to the size of the nares and may mean that the operator has to use a slightly smaller tube. In most patients, this is a theoretical disadvantage.

Esophageal Intubation

Since this is a "blind" technique, placement of the tube in the esophagus is relatively common with BNI. In most cases treatment of this complication involves simply noting the cessation of breath sounds, withdrawing the tube slightly, and reinserting it. The operator must confirm that the tube is appropriately placed with three clinical and one instrument method. Unrecognized esophageal intubation has been noted in patients who have very poor respiratory efforts or who become apneic during the procedure.

Epistaxis

Severe epistaxis has been frequently noted as a consequence of blind nasotracheal intubation.[14] The presence of polyps, trauma, or aberrant anatomy contributes to this complication. Inexperienced operators will frequently use a tube too large for the opening or will advance the tube into the turbinates.

Use of phenylephrine or oxymetazoline (Afrin™) nasal spray can decrease the incidence of epistaxis by constriction of the nasal mucosal vessels.

Submucosal Dissection and Other Trauma

Submucosal dissection by the tube can cause or aggravate epistaxis. The patient may complain of severe pain as the nasal lining is torn and the tube advanced submucosally. A bulge in the area behind the tonsillar pillars may be noted on oral examination. A retropharyngeal hematoma may form and be the site for abscess formation. Both antibiotic and surgical therapy may be required for management of this complication.

Inadvertent polypectomy may be caused by an unskilled and forceful insertion of the nasotracheal tube.[15] Turbinate destruction is a rare complication of nasotracheal intubation.[16]

The adenoids are found along the posterior wall of the nasopharynx. They are prominent until puberty. In the child, the adenoids may block nasal intubation, bleed, or even shear off and block the lumen of the endotracheal tube.

Movement of the Patient

As noted earlier, the assumption that blind nasal intubation can be performed without movement of the cervical spine is unwarranted. Flexion or rotation of the neck is often needed to insert the tube. Flexion may be minimized by use of a "trigger" type endotracheal tube, but still may be required.

Success Rate of the Procedure

Perhaps the most damning complication of this procedure is the low success rate and the prolonged time to intubate. In most literature, the success rate of nasal intubation ranges between 66 percent and 95 percent.[17] This is unacceptably low. The success rate can be markedly bettered by manipulation of the tube with Magill forceps during direct vision. Unfortunately, this may require an unacceptable time to intubate and may damage the cuff of the tube, requiring replacement of the tube.

Infections

A final consideration for nasotracheal intubation is the prevention of infectious sequelae. Most emergency practitioners do not ever see or discuss with the intensivist or patient the sinusitis that is associated with even relatively short duration of nasal intubation. Severely traumatized, critically ill patients are at highest risk. Sinusitis in these patients can progress to meningitis or cerebral venous thrombosis if the complication is not rapidly diagnosed and treated.

Diagnosis of postintubation sinusitis is suggested by fever, purulent draining, headache, and tenderness to sinus percussion. Plain film radiographs or computed tomography may show fluid collections. Treatment is removal of the nasal tube followed by appropriate antibiotic coverage with cephalosporins, ampicillin and chloramphenicol, or aminoglycosides.

Contraindications

Nasal intubation is contraindicated in patients with neck hematomas, in patients with severe facial trauma, basilar skull fractures, and those patients with severe coagulopathy. The patient who has an increased intracranial pressure may be worsened by nasal intubation.

Nasal intubation most often takes significantly longer than oral intubation. It should be performed with great reservation on any patient who needs rapid intubation. Despite overly optimistic claims to the contrary, nasal intubation requires several minutes to complete successfully. It is a poor choice for the patient in respiratory failure such as the COPD or asthmatic patient in extremis and the patient who can't be well oxygenated during the protracted intubation attempt.

Foreign Bodies in the Upper Airway

The method should be used with caution in patients who are hoarse, have dysphonia, or are known to have tumors of the neck or vocal cords. It is contraindicated in patients with anatomically disturbed airways or neck anatomy. It should not be used in patients who have increased intracranial pressure.

Combative Patients

As previously mentioned it is not possible to intubate the combative patient with this technique, and this also makes it much less useful. BNI in a combative patient carries significant risks of vomiting, aspiration, nasal hemorrhage, and periglottic trauma. The trauma that surrounds this effort in the combative patient may make subsequent attempts at intubation difficult or impossible. Since anxious anoxic children often fit into this category, BNI is essentially contraindicated in these children.

Contraindications to BNI

- Apnea (relative)
- Bleeding disorders (relative)
- Basilar skull fractures
- Combative patient
- CSF rhinorrhea
- Epiglottitis
- Foreign bodies in the upper airway
- Severe facial fractures

If the patient becomes combative during the procedure, then the attempt should be abandoned. Thorough explanation of the procedure prior to the start may avert this situation.

Apnea

Most emergency providers consider apnea to be a contraindication to this technique, but there are multiple reports of successful BNI in patients with deliberate apnea.[18][19]

Head Trauma

Use of NG tubes, and occasionally nasotracheal tubes, have been associated with perforation of the cribriform plate and inadvertent cranial intubation in isolated cases. Although this is probably quite rare, with any nasal intubation in a patient who has had head trauma, it is a possibility. **If the patient has a known basilar skull fracture, BNI is absolutely contraindicated.** BNI should be used with great caution, if at all, in patients with facial fractures. If BNI is performed in the presence of a nasal or a facial fracture, there is a risk of causing more damage and substantially more epistaxis.

Aids to Nasal Intubation

Success rates in nasotracheal intubation have ranged from as high as 92 percent to as low as 65 percent.[20] [21] Complications likewise range from nearly 70 percent of patients to as low as 3 percent of patients—with most rates ranging from 8 percent to 33 percent.[22] [23] [24] A better record of successful intubation is usually found in a more controlled environment than the emergency department.

Many aids to nasotracheal intubation have been proposed, including rigid stylets and tongue extrusion techniques. The author has had better success with directional endotracheal tubes such as the "trigger" tube, when they are available.

Perhaps the best aid to nasotracheal intubation is proper preparation of the nose with a vasoconstricting agent, such as cocaine or epinephrine. Even the use of Afrin will significantly shrink the mucous membranes and decrease the chances of epistaxis and increase the probability of successful passage.

Use of the flexible lighted stylet or the flexible fiberoptic laryngoscope may aid in intubation of the apneic patient (see following). With the exception of the flexible fiberoptic laryngoscope, none of these aids has markedly improved the intubation rates of skilled operators.

Stylet Guided Intubation

Lighted Stylet

Intubation with a lighted stylet depends upon transillumination of the soft tissue of the neck with a light placed in the larynx (Figure 6-13).[25] It requires neither flexion nor extension of the neck in order to insert an endotracheal tube. It is useful when the patient's cords can't be seen, or the neck can't be moved.

Method

Orotracheal intubation is performed with a standard endotracheal tube that has been shortened to 25 cm. This tube is placed over a lubricated surgical flexlight (Concept Corporation, Clearwater, Florida—Tubestat).[26] The light extends to the end of the shortened endotracheal tube.

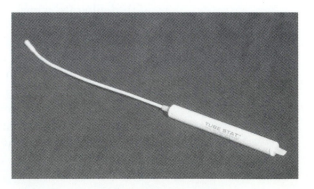

Figure 6-13 Intubating lighted stylet. *Source:* Photo by Charles Stewart and Associates; www.storysmith.net.

The equipment for intubation is prepared, and the patient is properly oxygenated. The patient's tongue should be grasped with a gauze pad and pulled forward. The curved stylet-tube combination is slid along the back of the tongue and past the epiglottis.

A bright glow in the midline at the level of the Adam's apple indicates that the tube is in the correct position. Esophageal placement will show little light in most subjects. A bright glow in the submental area indicates that the tip of the tube has been positioned in the vallecula. If the tip of the tube is lateral, in the pyriform fossa, then the lighted stylet will cause a lateral glow in the neck. Some newer lighted stylets will have the light blink to help with visualization.

After the tube is in the correct place, it is slid off of the stylet and secured in the usual fashion. Appropriate placement of the endotracheal tube is confirmed with the customary techniques.

This technique was successful in patients in whom routine intubation techniques had failed. It has also been used as an adjunct to blind nasotracheal intubation.[27] This technique may allow the operator to blindly insert a nasal tube in the apneic patient.

Complications and Precautions
Inability to Visualize the Light If the ambient lighting is extreme—as in direct sunlight—this method becomes difficult. In the original paper describing the technique, two of the three unsuccessful attempts were in sunlight. In an emergency department, simply extinguishing the overhead lights for a few seconds may solve this problem. In the field, a blanket can be thrown over the heads of the intubator and the patient.

Blood and vomitus may further obscure the light at the end of the tube. Charcoal will completely obstruct the light source.

Esophageal Intubation In very thin patients, visualization of a midline glow may be found in esophageal intubation. Since this is a blind technique, the operator must ensure that the tube placement is correct.

Loss of the Light Bulb In one case in the original paper, the light bulb at the end of the flexible stylet was dislodged. This required bronchoscopy for retrieval. Newer lights from the manufacturer have a shrink-fit plastic that improves strength and reduces this risk.

Fiberoptic Intubation
Since fiberoptic-lighted and remotely visualizing devices became available, we have been able to look in almost any orifice or body cavity (Figure 6-14). The larynx is no exception, and instruments are readily available for looking into the throat and upper airway. These devices range from fiberoptic laryngoscopes to fiberoptic bronchoscopes in both adult and pediatric sizes. They may be classified as fiberoptic bronchoscopes, laryngoscopes, or nasopharyngoscopes. A fiberoptic ET tube guide is now available, which is a simplified fiberoptic laryngoscope.

A scope that is used for intubation should be long enough to easily reach well into the trachea. The nasopharyngoscope will usually only reach to the cords and is not well suited for intubation. The laryngoscope has a smaller diameter and will both pass through the nose and accommodate a smaller

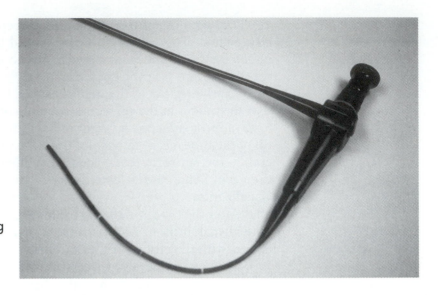

Figure 6-14 Fiberoptic intubating laryngoscope. *Source:* Photo by Charles Stewart and Associates; www.storysmith.net.

endotracheal tube. The laryngoscope is usually stiffer and less likely to kink when used for intubation.

If the scope has a suction port, it can also be used to insufflate high-flow oxygen to clear secretions from the visual field and promote oxygenation during the procedure.

The primary advantage of the flexible fiberoptic technique is in negotiation of difficult anatomy. The fiberoptic laryngoscope allows the operator to orally or nasally intubate the patient without flexion of the neck and without the disadvantages of the blind techniques. A secondary advantage is in the ready diagnosis of the patient with an inhalation injury.

Although the technique is not simple, it can be mastered with practice. It is not as quick as some of the other techniques mentioned. Passage of the tube takes about 1–5 minutes depending on the experience and skill of the intubator.

A fiberoptic laryngoscope can be readily obscured by fairly small amounts of vomitus, blood, or secretions. Since the fiberoptic laryngoscope is often considered to be the "last resort," by the time that a fiberoptic laryngoscope is employed, the patient already has bleeding, trauma, and subsequent swelling. Finally, the fiberoptic scope is an expensive and relatively delicate instrument.

The fiberoptic scope or stylet may be quite appropriate in the patient where the glottis can be visualized but where lack of mandibular mobility or edema make direct insertion of an appropriately large tube difficult or impossible. The thin fiberoptic stylet with a preplaced endotracheal tube is inserted though the cords with direct visualization or by using the fiberoptic view piece. Once the fiberoptic stylet is in place, the lubricated standard endotracheal tube can be slid over the fiberoptics into the trachea.

Indications: When Fiberoptics May Be Most Useful

- Cervical spine trauma—limits movement of the neck
- Laryngotracheal trauma—allows assessment of the severity of the injury and limits further injury

- Cervical hematoma—allows visualization despite distortion of the airway
- Thermal injury—allows assessment of the thermal injury to the trachea and bronchi

Contraindications

- Apnea/Agonal respirations—unless the operator is highly skilled, this procedure takes too much time for the patient's condition.
- Heavy bleeding, secretions, or vomitus—this will obscure vision. Charcoal vomitus, in particular, will destroy the ability of the operator to see.
- Severe agitation—If the patient can't be controlled, then they must be paralyzed and sedated.
- Complete upper airway obstruction—Proceed directly to a surgical airway.

Fiberoptic Laryngoscopy Will Be Made Difficult by

- Lack of knowledge and experience
- Nasal obstruction
- Basilar skull fracture
- Secretions
- Blood
- Vomitus
- Charcoal

Method
The basics of the techniques are

1. Handle the instrument carefully. Don't twist or bend it sharply. To do so will break the fibers.
2. Prepare the laryngoscope with a tube over it. The 5.5 mm laryngoscope will easily hold a 7.5 mm tube over it without difficulty. 4.0 mm laryngoscopes (Olympus) have recently been developed with both suction and oxygen delivery ports. With smaller adults and children, use of a pediatric bronchoscope may allow placement of a smaller diameter tube. If using the instrument for an oral intubation, use a bite block to prevent damage to the fibers.

Nasal Technique Prepare the patient as if they were going to get a nasotracheal intubation. Suction the patient nasally and pharyngeally. The neck may be left in neutral position. Since the fiberoptic laryngoscope may add some bulk or increase the trauma, ensure that both vasoconstricting agents and lubrication are provided.

After proper lubrication and use of a topical vasoconstrictor, pass the tube and laryngoscope along the floor of the nares posteriorly to the posterior pharynx. Ensure that the turbinates are not damaged.

As the posterior pharynx is reached, the tube must be curved towards the epiglottis. During passage of the tube/scope combination, the epiglottis may be visualized. After the curve has been negotiated, the cords can often be visualized. (See Figure 6-2.)

Oral Technique Again, use a bite block to prevent possible damage to the scope. When advancing the scope, keep the airway lumen, the glottic opening, and the tracheal lumen centered in the visual field. When the scope is advanced, any peripheral structures will be lost to visualization. Nasal and oral suctioning is mandatory prior to placement of the scope.

Remember that the anatomic structures will appear further away than they really are due to the telescoping effect of the optics.

The endotracheal tube can be advanced using the scope as a stylet. If the endotracheal tube sticks at the glottis, rotate the tube 90 degrees and try again.

If the patient is being intubated as part of management of a suspected inhalation injury, the laryngoscope can be passed throughout the cords and the carina can be seen, in many patients. If there is blood in the airway, passing the tube first into the hypopharynx may protect the scope somewhat from loss of the visualization. If no bleeding or secretions are present, passing the scope first will allow more certain placement of the tube.

Pass the entire assembly through the cords and slide the tube into the trachea. Withdraw the scope and ensure that the tube is not dislodged during the proceedings. Ventilate the patient and anchor the tube as usual.

Complications

By far the most major complication of use of a fiberoptic laryngoscope is delay in oxygenation caused by an inexperienced operator. Skill with the fiberoptic laryngoscope should be gained during elective or semielective intubation rather than during an emergency. Attempting to view landmarks from a new perspective with a new instrument, while dodging bits of debris, secretions, and blood, is not calculated to be either quick or elegant.

Fiberoptic laryngoscopes require free air space in order to visualize the structures. Vomitus, secretions, and blood will readily obscure either the viewing field or the light source. This competing fluid should be removed by nasal and oral suctioning prior to use of the fiberoptic laryngoscope. Likewise, marked pharyngeal edema will obscure both passage and vision. Patients in these situations are not good candidates for use of the fiberoptic laryngoscope or its analogues.

The suction port of the laryngoscope or bronchoscope, if available, can be used to clear limited amounts of mucus, secretions, or blood. Alternatively, the suction port can be attached to an oxygen supply; use the oxygen flow to sweep the area clear.

Since the anatomy can be identified positively, proper insertion of the endotracheal tube can be verified and inadvertent esophageal intubation is rare.

> *Fiberoptic intubation requires skill, an airway free of blood and edema, and experience . . . of these, the most important is probably experience. In the middle of a dire emergency is probably not the time to try to get that experience.*

NG Tube/Suction Catheter as a Stylet

A helpful technique that is infrequently used is the use of a NG or suction tube as a guide through the cords.[28] This is most helpful where the nasotracheal tube has been passed up to the cords but can't be passed through them. A NG tube or suction tube can then be slipped through the ET tube and passed through the cords. Using the smaller tube as a guide, the ET tube is then re-advanced in the proper position.

Retrograde Intubation

A variant of the stylet guided technique is retrograde guided intubation as described by Waters in 1963 for use in patients with drastically altered anatomy (Figure 6-15).[29] It is particularly useful in the patient with facial trauma and a suspected neck injury, in whom a blind nasotracheal intubation is unfeasible. In this technique, a transtracheal needle or a needle passed through the cricothyroid membrane is used to thread a long wire stylet cephalad through the cords. The guide wire is retrieved in the oropharynx and a tube threaded over it. The tube is then passed into the trachea past the vocal cords. Conceivably, the guide wire could be passed through a nostril and the entire process used to pass a nasotracheal tube. Successful pediatric use in a 14-month-old infant has been described.[30]

The technique may be valuable where vomitus or bloody drainage obstructs the view or obscures the light in standard intubation. The author has used it for a patient with activated charcoal emesis that completely obscured the light of a standard laryngoscope—despite adequate suction. Retrograde guide wire intubation does take time to perform but is far more useful than

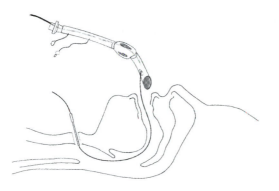
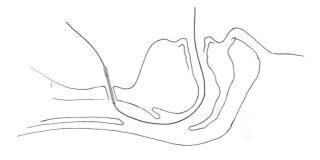
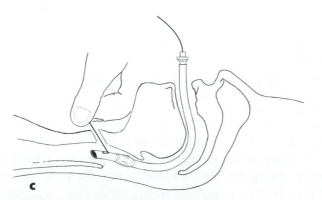

Figure 6-15 Retrograde intubation.

repeated unsuccessful attempts at standard or blind nasal intubation in the difficult patient.

Optimally, the guide wire needs to be long enough to pass well outside the mouth. Both Intracath central venous pressure catheters and Seldinger guide wires have been used for this technique. Most guide wires in vascular kits are barely long enough to attempt this technique.

Contraindications

The guide wire can't be used when the patient has a complete upper airway obstruction. It is not likely to be successful in the setting of severe trauma to the larynx or laryngotracheal separation.

Complications appear to be related to the needle stick required and are usually minor. Obviously, the guide wire and needle shouldn't be passed through a soft tissue infection or abscess over the cricothyroid area. Likewise, a coagulopathy may cause a hematoma at the site of the needle stick.

Technique

Identify the cricothyroid membrane. (While the cricothyroid membrane is the usual place to insert the retrograde stylet, anywhere along the trachea is useable if the guide wire is long enough.)

Insert a 16–18 gauge needle into the cricoid membrane. Direct the needle at about 30–40 degrees angled towards the head.

Pass the guide wire from the larynx to the oral cavity. Although a through the needle catheter can be used, a soft tipped guide wire is more appropriate.

When the end can be easily seen in the oral cavity, pull out enough to thread onto the ETT tube.

Secure the proximal guide wire at the skin with a hemostat.

Thread the distal side hole (Murphy's eye) of an endotracheal tube and out the proximal end.

Pass the tube along the guide wire into the larynx while the guide wire is held taut.

Ensure that both ends of the guide wire are secured while trying to pass the tube so that the guide wire will not be pulled free from the neck.[31]

The guide wire can be either cut or pulled through the cricothyroid membrane and removed through the proximal end of the ET tube. Use mild to moderate pressure on the ET tube so that it will go forward through the larynx and into the trachea when the guide is released.

If the ET tube falls back into the hypopharynx when the guide is released, then the operator must start over.

Digital or Manual Intubation

Manual intubation, or more correctly digital intubation, has been used for centuries (Figure 6-16).[32] It fell into disfavor when Chevalier Jackson introduced laryngoscopy and direct vision of the vocal cords.[33] It may have a limited place in the patient who needs endotracheal intubation in the field or where equipment has broken during the procedure.[34 35]

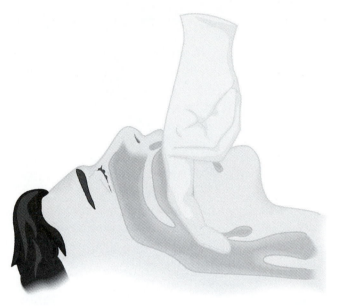

Figure 6-16 Digital intubation feeling the landmarks.

Indications

- Cramped quarters or extremely awkward position
- Upright patient
- Copious oral secretions or vomitus
- Inability to visualize the vocal cords
- Suspected cervical spine trauma
- Equipment failure or lack of laryngoscope

Technique

The intubator faces the patient from the foot end of the bed and standing to the shoulder of the patient. The index and long fingers are inserted into the patient's mouth and walked past the base of the tongue until the epiglottis is palpated. When the epiglottis can be felt by the tip of the long or middle finger, the endotracheal tube is passed into the mouth from the side by the dominant hand and then passed between the fingers over the epiglottis and into the trachea. The tip of the tube can be coaxed anteriorly with the tip of the index finger towards the tracheal opening and between the cords. If the patient is breathing, air movement may further guide placement.

Complications

The most feared complication of this procedure is to the operator—being bitten by the patient. This can be prevented by use of a bite block or oral airway inserted laterally along the molars.

As in all blind intubation techniques, esophageal intubation is a real possibility. This is an innocuous complication if it is promptly recognized by the standard techniques for checking tube placement (Figure 6-17).

Digital intubation predisposes to LEFT mainstem bronchial intubation.[36]

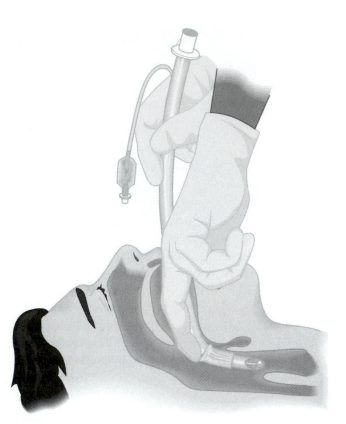

Figure 6-17 Digital intubation passing the tube.

Adjuncts to Intubation

Securing the Tube

A wide variety of elaborate tracheal tube holders ranging from inexpensive to relatively dear are available (Figure 6-18). There is no good study that shows a clear benefit over standard adhesive tape. Umbilical tape may be used in patients with burns.

The author uses a 2 foot long, 1 inch wide strip of adhesive tape with backing to prevent the sticky surface from sticking to the hair. This strip is passed completely around the head just at the level of the ear lobe. The front ends of the tape are split and then wrapped around the tube in opposite directions. An additional chevron of tape is applied to keep the tube in the corner of the mouth.

Be careful to ensure that the mouth remains unobstructed and that pressure on the lip is avoided. There should be some motion of the lip and the tape should permit inspection of the mouth.

A nasotracheal tube should be anchored lightly at the upper lip so that the tube curves inferiorly. This avoids pressure on the alae of the nose and along the nostrils.

Changing Tracheal Tubes

Occasionally, the intubation is successful but the cuff has been damaged during the intubation. In this situation, the endotracheal tube can be removed and reinserted. If the intubation was simple, this is an appropriate procedure. If there was any difficulty with the intubation, an alternative technique is to change the endotracheal tube over a 60 cm flexible stylet. This procedure is quite similar to retrograde stylet intubation.

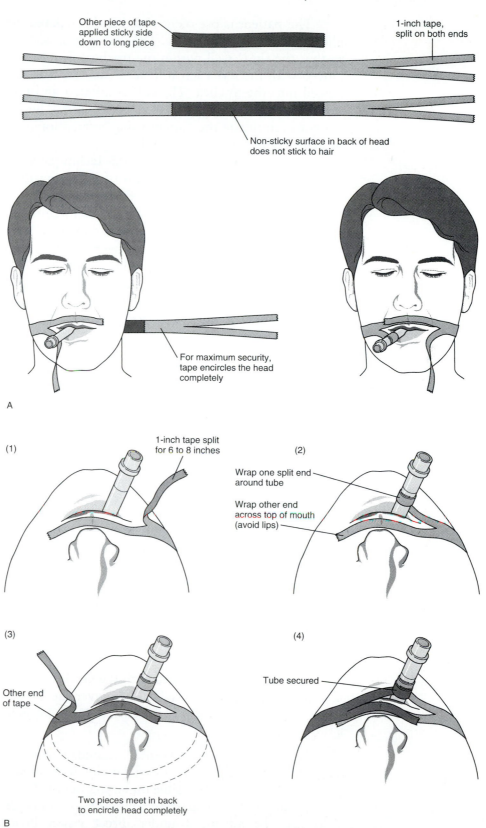

Other piece of tape applied sticky side down to long piece

1-inch tape, split on both ends

Non-sticky surface in back of head does not stick to hair

For maximum security, tape encircles the head completely

A

(1)   1-inch tape split for 6 to 8 inches

(2)   Wrap one split end around tube

Wrap other end across top of mouth (avoid lips)

(3)   Other end of tape

(4)   Tube secured

Two pieces meet in back to encircle head completely

B

Figure 6-18 Securing a tube. *Source:* Roberts J. R. and Hedges J. K., eds. *Clinical Procedures in Emergency Medicine,* 3rd ed. Philadelphia: W. B. Saunders Company, 1997.

The patient is pre-oxygenated and resedated. Sellick's maneuver is applied to the cricoid cartilage. The device is passed through the existing tube so that the tip is well within the trachea. The first endotracheal tube is removed with the stylet left in place. The new tube is slid over the stylet and passed into the trachea. The cuff is inflated and the position of the tube is verified. The new tube can then be secured. The operator must always be ready to reintubate the patient using conventional techniques if there is any difficulty reinserting the new tube.

The most common failure of this technique is to partially or completely withdraw the stylet in the process of removing the first tube. The time to change the tube should not exceed 30 seconds.

The tube should never be forced. If force is required to push the new tube into the trachea, the cords may be damaged. If force is required, then the patient should be reintubated in conventional fashion.

An 18 French Salem sump tube may be used in the adult for a tube exchanger. The proximal end of this tube is wider than the distal end, so the proximal 6–8 cm must be cut off. The plastic tube should be lubricated with water soluble lubricant before use. Even with lubrication of the Salem sump, a hemostat may be needed to force the NG tube through the new endotracheal tube.

Gum Bougie Stylet (Eschmann tracheal tube introducer)

The Eschmann tracheal tube introducer [also called the gum elastic bougie (GEB)] is a flexible, resin-coated, braided polyester device that has been in a clinical use in operating rooms for about 30 years.[37] (See Figure 6-19.) Although it has been frequently noted in the anesthesia literature, this device has not seen frequent use in either emergency departments or in the field in the United States.

The GEB is 60 cm long, with graduations at each 10-cm interval. The first 25 cm of the bougie is angled to approximately 40 degrees. The angle allows the operator to both keep the tip of the GEB in the midline and keep the operator's hand out of the field of view. The gum elastic bougie is small enough to be used with an endotracheal tube of 6.0 mm or more in internal diameter.

Use of the GEB is a three-step process:

1. Intubation of the trachea with the GEB
2. Passage of the endotracheal tube over the GEB into the trachea
3. Removal of the GEB and securing the endotracheal tube

Intubation times between 21 seconds and 45 seconds, with a 100 percent success rate, were reported for this technique in 26 patients in whom only the epiglottis was visible on laryngoscopy.[38]

In patients with part of the glottis or only the epiglottis visible, the GEB can be advanced under direct vision beneath the epiglottis and "walked" off the vocal folds through the rima of the glottis. Successful placement of the GEB into the trachea can be ascertained on the basis of three signs:

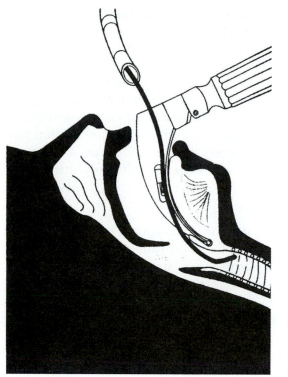

Figure 6-19 Technique of Eschman gum bougie. *Source:* Nocera A. A flexible solution for emergency intubation difficulties. *Ann. Emerg. Med.* 1996;27: 665–667.

1. The "clicks" of the bougie over the tracheal rings
2. The holdup of the bougie at approximately 45 cm as it catches in a small bronchus
3. The rotation of the bougie as it enters a bronchus

The clicks as the operator advances the GEB over the tracheal rings are felt in about 90 percent of cases.[39] Holdup of the GEB at about 45 cm will always occur in an endotracheal placement of the bougie.

If the patient needs ventilation during or after the bougie has been inserted, the bougie can be left in place. The flexibility of the bougie allows it to be bent over the side of the patient's mouth. The small size of the bougie does not interfere with the seal of the mask, allowing ventilation by bag-mask during the procedure.

After the operator has inserted the GEB, the assistant lubricates the bougie and then slides an endotracheal tube over it. The assistant holds the end of the GEB as the operator advances the endotracheal tube over the bougie. The passage of the tube over the GEB may be eased by leaving the laryngoscope in place and by rotation of the bevel of the endotracheal tube posteriorly.[40 41]

When the endotracheal tube is believed to be in position, the operator stabilizes it in place and the assistant withdraws the GEB through the endotracheal tube. After the endotracheal tube is inserted, position is verified using the techniques described in Chapter 7. The endotracheal tube is then secured using the usual techniques.

Complications of the device include

1. Esophageal intubation
2. Sore throat
3. Hoarseness

A single case of hemopneumothorax has been reported in the European literature following GEB assisted intubation.

The GEB retails for $68 in the United States from SIMS, Incorporated. Use of the GEB is abundantly described in the anesthesia literature, although it is not currently carried or used in most emergency departments and field airway kits in the United States. It may be appropriate to investigate the GEB as a rescue device in the emergency department and prehospital settings. The GEB takes little storage room in either intubation tray or field intubation kit. Because the device requires no set-up time, it can be rapidly deployed as a rescue emergency device in cases of difficult intubation.

Analgesia and Sedation

Laryngoscopy in a conscious patient has been described as if someone is using a crowbar to open the mouth and then shoving it down your throat.[a] The upper airway has substantial nerve supply with branches of the fifth, seventh, ninth, and tenth cranial nerves. Cough and gag reflexes are activated in most patients with light touch. Even when the patient is critical and sedatives are given, if they are not given in appropriate doses, the patient can recall vivid details of an uncomfortable procedure.

Orotracheal intubation is markedly easier to perform when the musculature of the oropharynx is completely relaxed. This is most certainly true when the emergency provider is under pressure and the circumstances are less than ideal. With the advent of rapid sequence intubation techniques and protocols, there is little excuse for inadequate sedation and analgesia of the patient who is going to be intubated.

Sedatives cannot be safely given in high enough dose or quickly enough to intubate the patient without risking hypotension and respiratory depression. To cite "safety" of the technique of simply giving a modest amount of sedative rather than using an appropriate dose of both sedative and muscle relaxant is to ignore the growing body of literature supporting safety, efficacy, and speed of rapid sequence intubation. The combination of a sedative and a paralytic agent is superior to the use of a sedative alone. This is the basis of the technique of rapid sequence intubation.

Indications for Intubation

Resuscitation
Cardiac arrest

Respiratory Failure
Chest trauma, flail chest, pneumothorax, pulmonary embolus, airway obstruction (croup, epiglottitis, deep space infection of the neck, bilateral recurrent laryngeal nerve palsy, foreign body in the neck)

Asthma, congestive heart failure, COPD

---

[a]One of my patients described this sensation in detail for me during the wee hours of the night. It seems that he had been recently intubated for a severe episode of pulmonary edema. The intubator had used "brutane" for anesthesia, and the patient was fully conscious during the entire attempt. The physician was well meaning, but incompletely trained. The patient was not nearly as obtunded as the physician had presumed with only 3 mg of Diazepam IV.

Protection of the airway
Unconscious patient

Stroke, head trauma, diabetes, drug overdose, other causes of coma

Full stomach
Bleeding in the airway
Paralysis for any other reason

Control of carbon dioxide
Head injuries
Increased intracranial pressure
Respiratory failure

Steps to Improve Intubation Success

1. **Ensure that the patient is in the proper position.** Place the patient in the sniffing position, if possible. This sometimes requires more than simple elevation of the head. For the obese patient, elevation of both head and shoulders may be needed.
2. **Improve the view with laryngeal movement.** Use the right hand to move the larynx so that the glottis is best seen. This is usually backwards, upwards, and to the right (BURP maneuver), but may be up, down, or to the left. Once the proper position has been determined, the assistant can reproduce this position while the operator intubates the patient.
3. **Change blades.** Changing blades may help. The Miller blade is superior with a long, floppy epiglottis, but the Macintosh blade is better for the patient with tongue swelling or a floppy tongue. If the patient has a receding chin or anterior position of the larynx, then a Miller blade is more appropriate.
4. **Carefully consider before RSI.** Remember that long-acting agents will mean that you have to ventilate the patient for a long time if you can't intubate the patient. If succinylcholine has been given and ventilation can be maintained, the patient will be able to breathe spontaneously in 4–5 minutes. Also remember that you may not be able to intubate the paralyzed patient with facial or neck trauma, and a surgical airway may be needed. Patient safety should not be compromised for the ego trip of the difficult intubation.

End Notes

[1] Barwise, J. A. "Evaluation of the emergency airway."http://anesthesiology.mc.Vanderbilt.edu/resweb/eamg/Eamg2.htm, retrieved 04/10/2000.

[2] Mallampati, S. R. "Clinical sign to predict difficult tracheal intubation (hypothesis)," in *Can Anaesth Soc J* 1983;30:316.

[3] Mallampati, S. R., Gatt, S. P., Gugino, L. D., et al. "A clinical sign to predict difficult tracheal intubation: a prospective study," in *Can Anesth Soc J.* 1985;32:429.

[4] Samson, G. L. T., and Young, J. R. B. "Difficult tracheal intubation: A retrospective study," in *Anaesthesia* 1987;42:487.

5 Meade, R. W. *A history of thoracic surgery.* Springield, MA: Charles C Thomas, 1961, p. 15.

6 Ravitch, M. M. "Progress in resection of the chest wall for tumor with reminiscences of Dr. Blalock," in *Johns Hopkins Med J* 1982;151:43.

7 Sellick, B. A. "Cricoid pressure to control regurgitation of stomach contents during induction of anaesthesia," in *Lancet* 1961;2:404–406.

8 Iserson, K. V. "Blind nasotracheal intubation," in *Ann Emerg Med* 1981;10:468–471.

9 Iserson, K. V., Sanders, A. B., and Kaback, K. "Difficult intubations: Aids and alternatives," in *Amer Family Phys* 1985;31:99–112.

10 Ligier, B., Buchman, T. G., Breslow, M. J., and Deutschman, C. S. "The role of anesthetic induction agents and neuromuscular blockade in the endotracheal intubation of trauma victims," in *Surg Gynecol Obstet* 1991; 173:477–481.

11 Korber, T. E., and Henneman, P. L. "Digital nasotracheal intubation," in *J Emerg Med* 1989;7:275–277.

12 Fassolt, A. "Blind nasal tracheal intubation in the muscle relaxed patient," in *Anaesthesist* 1986;35:505–508.

13 Maltby, J. R., Cassidy, M., and Nanji, G. M. "Blind nasotracheal intubation using succinylcholine," in *Anesthesiology* 1988;69:946–948.

14 Dingley, A. R. "Nasal intubation: Dangers and difficulties from the rhinological aspect," in *Br Med J* 1943;1:693.

15 Binning, R. "A hazard of blind nasal intubation (letter)," in *Anaesthesia* 1974;29:366–367.

16 Wilkinson, J. A., Mathis, R. D., and Dire, D. J. "Turbinate destruction—a rare complication of nasotracheal intubation," in *J Emerg Med* 1986; 4:209–212.

17 O'Brien, D. J., Danzl, D. F., Hooker, E. A., Daniel, L. M., et al. "Prehospital blind nasotracheal intubation by paramedics," in *Ann Emerg Med.* 1989;18:612–617.

18 Fassolt, A. "Blind nasal tracheal intubation in the muscle relaxed patient," in *Anaesthesist* 1986;35:505–508.

19 Maltby, J. R., Cassidy, M., and Nanji, G. M. "Blind nasotracheal intubation using succinylcholine," in *Anesthesiology* 1988;69:946–948.

20 Danzl, D., and Thomas, D. M. "Nasotracheal intubation in the emergency department," in *Crit Care Med* 1980;8:677–682.

21 Dronen, S. C., Merigian, K. S., Hedges, J. R., et al. "A comparison of blind nasotracheal and succinylcholine-assisted intubation in the poisoned patient," in *Ann Emerg Med* 1987;16:75–77.

22 Gillespie, N. A. "Blind nasotracheal intubation," in *Anesth Analg* 1950; 29:217–222.

23 Gold, M. I., and Buechel, D. R. "A method of blind nasal intubation for the conscious patient," in *Anesth Analg* 1960;39:257–263.

24 Harvey, D. C., and Amorosa, P. "Traumatic nasotracheal intubation," in *Anaesthesia* 1986;41–442.

25 Vollmer, T. P., Steward, R. D., Paris, P. M., et al. "Use of a lighted stylet for guided orotracheal intubation in the prehospital setting," in *Ann Emerg Med* 1985;14:324–328.

[26] Ellis, D. G., Stewart, R. D., Kaplan, R. M., et al. "Success rates of blind orotracheal intubation using a transillumination technique with a lighted stylet," in *Ann Emerg Med* 1986;15:138–142.

[27] Verdile, V. P., Chiang, J. L., Bedger, R., et al. "Nasotracheal intubation using a flexible lighted stylet," in *Ann Emerg Med* 1990;19:506–510.

[28] Dryden, G. E. "Use of a suction catheter to assist blind nasal intubation," in *Anesthesiology* 1976;45:260.

[29] Waters, D. J. "Guided blind endotracheal intubation," in *Anesthesia* 1963; 18:158–162.

[30] McNamera, R. M. "Retrograde intubation of the trachea," in *Ann Emerg Med* 1987;16:680–682.

[31] Akinyemi, O. O. "Complications of guided blind endotracheal intubation," in *Anesthesia* 1979;34:590–592.

[32] Stewart, R. D. "Tactile orotracheal intubation," in *Ann Emerg Med* 1984; 13:175–178.

[33] Collins, V. J. *Principles and practice of anesthesiology.* Philadelphia, PA: Lea & Febiger, 1952, p. 288.

[34] Hudon, F. "Intubation without laryngoscopy," in *Anesthesiology* 1945; 6:476–482.

[35] Hardwick, W. C., and Bluhm, D. "Digital intubation," in *J Emerg Med* 1984;1:317–320.

[36] White, S. J. "Left mainstem intubation with digital intubation technique. An unrecognized risk," in *Am J Emerg Med* 1994;12:466–468.

[37] Nocera, A. "A flexible solution for emergency intubation difficulties," in *Ann Emerg Med* 1996;27:665–667.

[38] Nolan, J. P., and Wilson, M. E. "Orotracheal intubation in parents with potential cervical spine injuries. An indication for the gum elastic bougie," in *Anaesthesia* 1993;48:630–633.

[39] Kidd, J. F., Dyson, A., and Lasso, P. "Successful difficult intubation: Use of the gum elastic bougie," in *Anaesthesia* 1988;43:437–438.

[40] Dogra, S., Falconer, R., and Lattro, P. "Successful difficult intubation: Tracheal tube placement over a gum elastic bougie," in *Anaesthesia* 1990; 45:714–776.

[41] Viswanathan, S., Campbell, C., Wood, D. G., et al. "The Eschmann tracheal tube introducer (gum elastic bougie)," in *Anesth Rev* 1992;19:29–34.

Chapter **Seven**

Verification of Endotracheal Tube Placement

Introduction

There is no sin in an esophageal intubation but there is much sin in not recognizing such a placement. Unrecognized esophageal intubation is catastrophic for the patient and a career-limiting maneuver for the paramedic or physician. Since the stomach is not designed for gas exchange, gastric ventilation does not support life very long.

Multiple methods of verification of correct tube placement have been taught. Each and every one of these methods has failed in clinical practice. The astute paramedic or physician will always use a combination of at least three of these clinical methods and will verify the tube placement by at least one of the instrument techniques. This is particularly important when the patient's ability to breathe has been removed with a paralytic agent.

The judicious clinician will also reverify tube placement when clinical conditions deteriorate. Remember that when the patient's neck is flexed, extended, or rotated, the tube will move within the trachea. It is possible to extubate the patient with sufficient movement of the patient's neck. This may occur after central line placement or radiographs of the chest or neck, or motion of the patient for other procedures or transport.

The patient's clinical condition may also deteriorate if equipment is detached or fails, if the patient suffers a catastrophic event such as increasing shock or pulmonary embolus, or if the patient develops a pneumothorax.

Verification of tube placement should be repeated at the slightest suspicion that the position of the tube has changed or the patient's clinical condition is deteriorating.

Clinical Verification of Tube Placement

Inspection

In the perfect intubation, the tube will be seen to pass through the cords and after the tube is placed, the tube will mist when the patient takes a breath or is ventilated.

Visualization of the Cords

Unfortunately, in the stress of an emergency intubation, with vomitus or blood, poor lighting, and with difficult anatomy or cervical immobilization, direct visualization of the tube's passage through the cords and trachea is all too often a fond aspiration.[1]

Misting of the Tube

Misting of the tube is inadequate as a verification technique, since even minimal fluid in the stomach can sufficiently humidify the expired gases to ensure misting.

Expansion of the Chest

Likewise, it is difficult to look for even expansion of the chest without any gastric distention in the immobilized patient with potential chest trauma. It is nice to see, but you can't be depended on as the only sign of a good intubation.

Patient Able to Speak

Again, if the patient is able to speak with an endotracheal tube in place, the tube is in the wrong place. Apposition of the cords and phonation is impossible with a chunk of plastic between them. Obviously this technique is useless in the patient in cardiac arrest, the unconscious patient, the patient who has been paralyzed, and the patient with severe hypotension.

Breath Sounds

In the perfect patient, the breath sounds will be heard equally when the tube is in appropriate position in the trachea. Air meeting water (fluid) causes bubbling, which implies the tube is in the esophagus or stomach. The breath sounds should be auscultated in the precordium, both axilla, and the epigastrium (Figures 7-1 and 7-2).

Unfortunately, auscultation is not completely reliable. In aircraft or moving ambulances, auscultation may be difficult or impossible. In the obese patient, few sounds may be heard in any body cavity. When the stomach has been dilated by mask ventilation, the gastric gurgle may be lost as a sign of esophageal intubation.

Stomach Sounds

In the small child, normal breath sounds may be heard when listening over the stomach. If breath sounds but no bubbling is heard over the stomach, do not pull the tube but complete the rest of the assessment; listen for two breaths on the right third intercostal space in the midaxillary line and compare to two breaths on the left side in the same place.

In the spontaneously breathing patient, auscultation of the chest may be fruitless in evaluation of the tube position. If the patient has had an esophageal intubation and is spontaneously breathing, then breath sounds

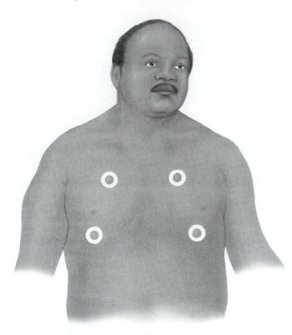

Figure 7-1 Places to listen for in auscultation of chest (anterior).

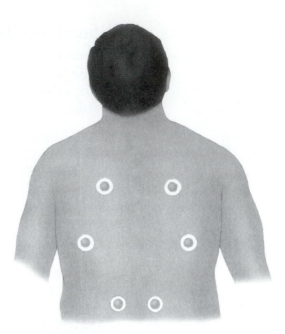

Figure 7-2 Places to listen for in auscultation of chest (posterior).

will be heard as the air bypasses the improperly placed tube. Airflow in the tube will be absent, however.

Instrumentation Methods of Verification

Pulse Oximetry

Pulse oximetry provides a noninvasive and continuous means of determination of the arterial oxygen saturation. Oxygen saturation monitors are produced by a number of companies and are widely available in handheld, tabletop, and even clip-on varieties. The more modern monitors have better sensitivity at low blood pressure and oxygen saturation levels.

The pulse oximeter measures the reflectance of two wavelengths of red light. At 660 nm, reduced hemoglobin absorbs about ten times as much light as oxyhemoglobin. At the infrared wavelength (940 nm), the absorption is about equal. Pulse oximeters measure the ratio of oxygenated hemoglobin to deoxygenated hemoglobin and calculate the percent of oxygenated hemoglobin. They may be misled during periods of low flow (vasoconstriction due to cold or shock), by movement, severe anemia, artificial nails, nail polish, or by altered hemoglobins such as carboxyhemoglobin or methemoglobin. In dark-skinned patients, signal readings from 3 percent to 5 percent high have occasionally been noted.

Despite these potential inaccuracies, pulse oximetry reading reflects a fairly reliable, noninvasive, and continuous monitoring of the oxygen saturation. It is most reliable when sequential readings over time give a trend analysis.

Continuous pulse oximetry monitoring should be mandatory for all critically ill patients, trauma patients, and patients with acute cardiopulmonary disorders such as asthma, bronchiolitis, COPD, CHF, or myocardial infarction, or with an altered sensorium from any cause. Continuous pulse oximetry may be the first indication of hypobolemia or shock as vasoconstriction develops.

Clinically, the clinician can see the oxygen saturation rise or fall as the patient's oxygenation status changes. For example, during a prolonged and difficult intubation attempt the oxygen saturation will fall well before other clinical signs of deterioration. Conversely, if the patient has been adequately preoxygenated, then an unhurried approach to the intubation may be used because the saturation monitor will demonstrate when the patient's functional residual capacity of oxygen has been depleted.

If the oxygen saturation is rising, or stays at an acceptable level in a paralyzed patient, then the endotracheal tube is certainly in the appropriate place. Unfortunately, most pulse oximeters are not accurate in the patient with profound shock or cardiac arrest.

Desaturation may be delayed because the patient has been well preoxygenated before rapid sequence intubation and thus mislead the intubator for several minutes. Indeed, desaturation may occur when the intubator has relaxed and is consequently less vigilant than just after the intubation. When the situation is now recognized, the patient may be in dire straits, and the initial pulse oximeter reading has led the clinician astray.

Use of pulse oximetry during intubation will decrease the incidence and duration of hypoxemia and may alert the clinician to an esophageal intubation before other clinical indications. This device should be available on every ambulance and in every emergency department.

Carbon Dioxide Detectors

End tidal carbon dioxide measurements or a disposable colorimetric device (CO_2 detector) can be used to confirm appropriate tube placement (Figure 7-3).[2] These devices work by measurement (colorimetric or direct measurement) of the carbon dioxide produced by the body and eliminated by the lungs. The

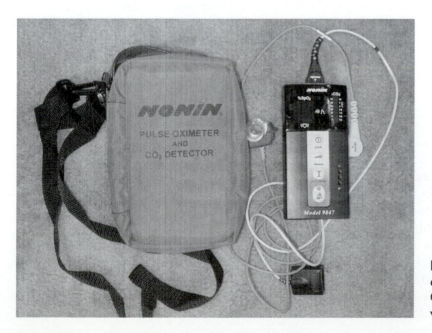

Figure 7-3 Nonin CO_2 detector and pulse oximeter. *Source:* Photo by Charles Stewart and Associates; www.storysmith.net.

theory is that if the ET tube is improperly placed in the esophagus, then there should be no carbon dioxide in the exhaled gas.

The use of a capnometer allows the detection of CO_2 in the exhaled air to be recorded and graphed continuously (Figure 7-4). This waveform provides information about tube placement and ventilation.

The end-tidal CO_2 detector works so well in the operating room that its use there is considered standard care by anesthesiologists.[3] In 1990, the American Society of Anesthesiologists extended this standard to any anesthetic practice involving airway management, irrespective of location.[4] Given the precedent of the American Society of Anesthesiologists, failure to use some form of end-tidal CO_2 detection during field intubation followed by an unrecognized esophageal intubation may invite litigation.

Unfortunately, a capnograph (at least currently available models) is neither durable nor portable and hence not usable for field medicine. There are few such devices available outside of the operating suite, even in well-equipped and busy emergency departments. A less expensive, more durable capnometer device combined in the same package with a pulse oximeter may be a singularly useful tool during field intubation.

Colorimetric End-Tidal Monitor

A colorimetric end-tidal monitor uses an indicator that changes color in response to $ETCO_2$ concentration (Figure 7-5).[5] This indicator may be built into the bag-valve system, or may be an additional device inserted between the endotracheal tube adaptor and the valve of the bag-valve system. If the indicator remains purple after the monitor is attached to the endotracheal tube, carbon dioxide concentration is low (<0.3%). If it turns bright yellow, the concentration is high (>2.0%). A beige color represents intermediate concentration (0.5–1.0%).

CO_2 detectors have been shown to fail in the patient who has suffered a cardiac arrest or is in profound shock, the severely hypothermic patient, and in the patient who has recently consumed a carbonated beverage. False

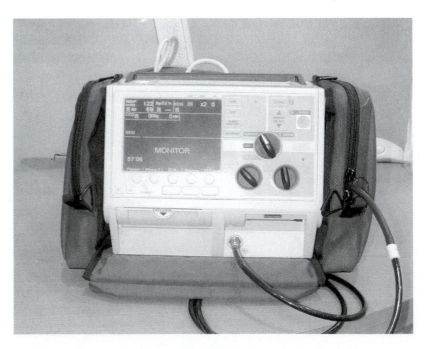

Figure 7-4 Zoll capnometer
Source: Photo by Charles Stewart and Associates; www.storysmith.net.

Nellcor-Puritan-Bennet EasyCap II Colorimetric CO2 Detector

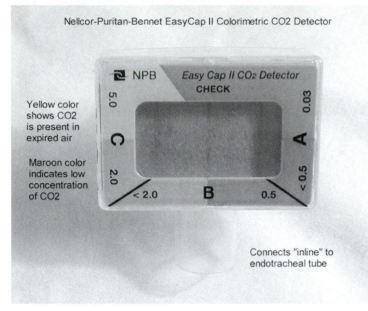

Yellow color shows CO2 is present in expired air

Maroon color indicates low concentration of CO2

NPB   Easy Cap II CO₂ Detector
CHECK

Connects "inline" to endotracheal tube

Figure 7-5 Nellcor EASYCAP CO_2 detector. *Source:* Photo by Charles Stewart and Associates; www.storysmith.net.

positives occur when the stomach contains a CO_2-containing beverage, so that CO_2-containing gas is moved back and forth with ventilation. False negatives occur when the patient does not produce CO_2 with ventilation. This situation may occur in cases of cardiac arrest, profound hypothermia, or severe hypovolemic shock. The false negative may expose the patient to repeated attempts at laryngoscopy and intubation.

In one prospective study, the sensitivity of this device in detecting proper endotracheal placement in the cardiac arrest patient was only 85 percent.[6] This means that as many as 15 percent of properly placed endotracheal tubes (in cardiac arrest patients) would be inappropriately removed when this device was exclusively depended on. These conditions occur far more frequently in emergency medicine practice than in the operating room.

A study that included 227 patients assessed the reliability of colorimetric monitoring in the prehospital setting.[7] In patients with spontaneous circulation, the device invariably remained purple in cases of esophageal intubation. A color change consistently indicated that the tube was well placed.

Colorimetric CO_2 detectors fail in the patient who has had a cardiac arrest receiving closed chest massage.[8][9] Under these conditions, a color change consistently indicated the presence of a properly placed tube. The results were less dependable if the device did not change color. In the absence of a color change, approximately one-third of the tube placements were esophageal while two-thirds were tracheal. Similar results were obtained in another study of patients with and without cardiac arrest who were intubated in a prehospital or ED environment.

A colorimetric carbon dioxide detector costs about $20. This is good insurance for the paramedic and should be routinely employed in every intubation.

The colorimetric CO_2 detectors have a fairly long shelf life (about 15 months). Once opened, the device will function for up to 5 hours. It is not considered reusable. In high humidity, the life span may decrease to as little as 15 minutes.

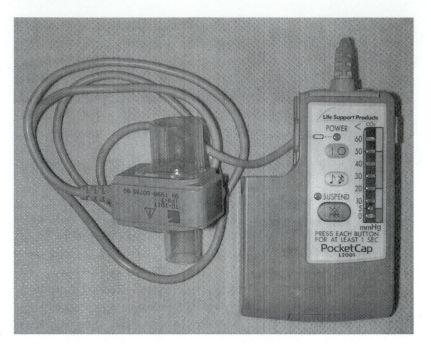

Figure 7-6 Digital capnometer. *Source:* Photo by Charles Stewart and Associates; www.storysmith.net.

Another similar CO_2 device is the MiniCAP III by MSA Catalyst Research, Owings Mills, Maryland. This device is a battery-operated capnometer that emits a flash and beep during each breath that contains CO_2. An alarm sounds for each breath that does not contain CO_2. It is both small, relatively inexpensive, and reusable. Reliability and sensitivity is about the same as the Easy Cap II. A singular advantage is that qualitative devices have alarms that sound if CO_2 detection ceases for more than a few seconds (Figure 7-6).

Esophageal Detector Devices

There are two different kinds of esophageal detector devices (EDD). Both involve the aspiration of a large volume of air rapidly through the endotracheal tube in order to determine whether an endotracheal tube is located within the esophagus or the trachea. The rigid structure of the trachea would mean that air would flow freely to the esophageal detector device. The soft tissues of the esophagus collapse and prevent rapid refill through the device.

Syringe aspiration esophageal detector devices have recently been used to confirm tube placement.[10,11] These devices use the rapid refill of a syringe or equivalent through the endotracheal tube as "proof" that the tube is in the airway, rather than the esophagus (Figure 7-7). Rapid flow of air when the syringe is aspirated would indicate a tracheal intubation, while resistance against aspiration would indicate an esophageal intubation.

Bulb aspiration devices use a round compressible plastic globe, similar to the bulb on an infant nasal syringe or a turkey baster for the same purpose (Figure 7-8). The bulb is compressed and deflated by hand. Keeping pressure on the bulb, the end is attached to the endotracheal tube and then the pressure is released rapidly. If the tube is in the esophagus, inflation is delayed. If the tube is in the trachea, inflation should be quite prompt.

In adults, there is a reasonable assurance that the tube is *not* in the esophagus, but the EDD may misidentify endobronchial or mainstem intu-

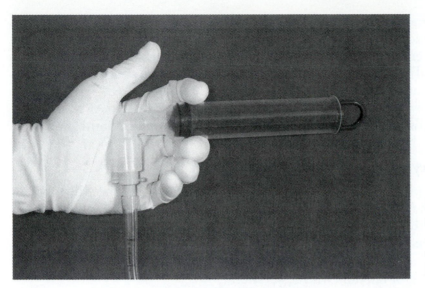

Figure 7-7 Syringe type esophageal detector device. *Source:* Positube esophageal detector device, courtesy of Jim Flory, Paraproducts.

bation as esophageal. C. D. Marley and his colleagues showed that the esophageal detection device correctly identified 100 percent of esophageal intubations (but only 35 of 40 ET intubations).[12] In a prospective study by W. A. Jenkins and his colleagues, this technique correctly identified 88 endotracheal tube placements and 2 esophageal misplacements.[13] There is no study that assures that these devices will be effective in the deliberate air leak associated with uncuffed tubes used in a pediatric airway.

Since an esophageal detector device costs only about $10 and has virtually unlimited shelf life, it is also very good insurance for the paramedic. Either an EDD or a carbon dioxide detector, or both, should be used in every field intubation with RSI. Catastrophe is easy to prevent by using one or both of these devices. There is quite simply no excuse for an unrecognized esophageal intubation.

Chest X Ray

The radiograph will be the gold standard by which the legal field judges our performance. Unfortunately, a radiograph takes several minutes to obtain and process and the patient needs appropriate and adequate ventilation

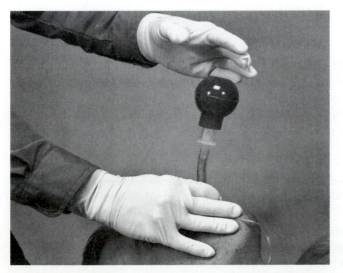

Figure 7-8 Bulb type esophageal detector device.

while the radiograph is processed. The device simply isn't appropriate for field emergency medicine.

In the emergency department, the chest x ray is most often taken portably and a lateral view is usually not obtained in an emergency situation. If a lateral is not obtained, an esophageal tube placement may be missed. The tube may simply overlay the trachea, but actually be in the esophagus. An AP film is quite useful for ensuring that the patient does not have a bronchial intubation.

Ten Ways to Verify an Intubation

1. Tube placement through the cords. The operator must see the tube between the cords. Obviously not applicable in most nasal intubations.
   - If the patient can speak, then the tube isn't in the correct place. Speaking is not possible with a chunk of plastic between the vocal cords.
2. Misting of the tube with respiration
3. Movement of the chest with respirations
4. Auscultation of the chest (You should hear breath sounds on *both* sides of the chest)
5. Auscultation of the stomach (You shouldn't hear gurgles here)
6. Capnometer or CO_2 colorimeter
7. Esophageal detector device
8. Clinical improvement
9. Rising or stable O_2 saturation (See above—this is truly just another way of saying "clinical improvement")
10. Chest X ray (This really requires a lateral view for completeness so an esophageal tube superimposed over the trachea won't be misread)

Remember, please . . . that there isn't any one of these methods that hasn't failed. The responsible clinician will verify tube placement with at least three clinical methods and one "instrument" method, and always, always, recheck the tube if the patient gets worse at any time.

Reasons for Acute Deterioration of the Intubated Patient

Think **DOPE**

- **D**isplacement of the tube (It isn't where it should be!)
- **O**bstruction of the tube (mucous plug, biting)
- **P**neumothorax, PE, pulselessness (cardiac arrest or shock)
- **E**quipment failure (No oxygen, failure of the ventilator, disconnected tubing)

END NOTES

[1] White S. J., Slovis C. M. Inadvertent esophageal intubation in the field: Reliance on a fool's "gold standard." *Academic Emerg Med* 97;4:89–91.

[2] Macleod B. A., Heller M. B., Gerard, J., et al. Verification of endotracheal tube placement with colorimetric end-tidal CO_2 detection. *Ann Emerg Med* 1991;20:267–270.

[3] Ginsburg W. H. When does a guideline become a standard? The new American Society of Anesthesiologists guidelines give us a clue. *Academic Emerg Med* 1993;21:1891–1896.

[4] American Society of Anesthesiologists. Standards for basic anesthetic monitoring. Approved by the House of Delegates on Oct. 21, 1986, and last amended on Oct. 21, 1998.

[5] Anton W. R., Gordon R. W., Jordan T. M., Posner K. L., Ceney F. W. A disposable endtidal CO_2 detector to verify endotracheal intubation. *Ann Emerg Med* 1991;20:271–275.

[6] Bhende M. S., Thompson A. E. Evaluation of an end-tidal carbon dioxide detector during pediatric cardiopulmonary resuscitation. *Pediatrics* 1995; 95:395–399.

[7] Ornato J. P., Shipley J. B., Racht E. M., et al. Multicenter study of a portable, handsize, colorimetric $ETCO_2$ detection device. *Ann Emerg Med* 1992;21:518–523.

[8] Garza M. End tidal CO_2 detector questions arise. *J Emerg Medical Services* 1991;16:22–23.

[9] MacLeod B. A., Heller M. B., Gerard J., Yealy D. M., Menegazzi J. J. Verification of endotracheal tube placement with colorimetric end-tidal CO_2 detection. *Ann Emerg Med* 1991;20:267–270.

[10] Zaleski L., Abellow D., Gold M. I. The esophageal detector device, does it work? *Anesthesiology* 1993;79:244–247.

[11] Marley C. D. Jr., Eitel D. R., Anderson T. E., Murn A. J., Patterson G. A. Evaluation of a prototype esophageal detection device. *Acad Emerg Med* 1995;2:503–507.

[12] Marley C. D. Jr., Eitel D. R., Anderson T. E., Murn A. J., Patterson G. A. Evaluation of a prototype esophageal detection device. *Acad Emerg Med* 1995;2:503–507. OP CIT.

[13] Jenkins W. A., Verdile V. P., Paris P. M. The syringe aspiration technique to verify endotracheal tube position. *Am J Emerg Med* 1994;12:413–416.

Chapter **Eight**

Surgical Airways

A surgical airway is better than a pretty neck in a corpse.
(Far easier to explain, too!)

Cricothyrotomy

Cricothyrotomy is an incision of the cricothyroid membrane and insertion of an airway directly into the trachea below the vocal cords. The surface anatomy of the cricothyroid membrane allows easy location of the landmarks. The area has few blood vessels and few critical structures, so cricothyrotomy is safer, technically easier, and has fewer complications than classic tracheostomy. It may be the procedure of choice for patients with laryngeal or pharyngeal obstruction. It is used in patients with facial and neck trauma as a field airway in some localities.[1][2][3][4]

Indications and Contraindications

Clinical conditions where cricothyrotomy may be indicated include trauma to the upper airway with associated bleeding, obstructive lesions of the upper airway, massive emesis, spasm of the jaw or vocal cords, laryngeal stenosis, and structural deformity of the upper airway. Some authorities feel that the "patients who are completely obstructed or in extremis are best managed by establishing an airway via the cricothyroid membrane."[5][6][7]

Indications

- Extensive orofacial trauma
- Known cervical trauma (relative and controversial)
- Upper airway obstruction due to edema, hemorrhage, or foreign body
- Unsuccessful endotracheal intubation

Contraindications

- Ability to secure an airway by less invasive techniques

  Cricothyrotomy should not be done when an oral or a nasal airway can be achieved easily and safely.

- Transection of trachea with retraction of distal end into the mediastinum

  This is the single indication for emergent low tracheostomy or midline sternotomy.

- Child under the age of 8.
- Significant damage to the cricoid cartilage or larynx (fractured larynx)
- Indication for tracheostomy below the site of damage

Massive Neck Edema

Massive neck swelling requires modification of the technique, since normal landmarks may be absent. This represents only a relative contraindication to the procedure in an acutely ill patient.

The hyoid bone can be used as a landmark in a patient with massive neck edema. The midpoint of the body of the hyoid is also the midpoint of the neck. An 18 gauge spinal needle can be used to find the hyoid bone. The needle is inserted into the neck below the chin, intersecting with a line connecting the earlobes and the angle of the jaw. If the hyoid bone is not found, then adjust the angle of the needle.

Some authors measure the distance between the point of the jaw and the angle of the jaw and divide this in half. They then use this distance to measure the distance from the point of the jaw to determine where the needle is inserted. Since this distance is only an approximation, measurements seem unnecessarily complicated during an acute procedure.

When the hyoid bone is found, the needle is left in position and a number 11 scalpel is used to cut down along the needle. A skin hook is used to retract the hyoid bone anteriorly and superiorly. A vertical skin incision is made below the skin hook. The incision is carried down to expose the cricoid cartilage, and the remainder of the procedure for a cricothyrotomy is followed.

Underlying Laryngeal Disease

In patients who have known or strongly suspected laryngeal pathology, such as chronic inflammation, cancer, or epiglottitis, cricothyrotomy will be more difficult, take longer, and carry a much higher risk of long-term complications. A large hematoma from a stab wound or gunshot wound may preclude performance of the procedure because of increased bleeding and distortion of the anatomy. The operator must proceed very carefully in these patients; temporizing to a controlled environment is appropriate, if possible.

Bleeding Diathesis.

A coagulopathy increases the hazard of any surgical procedure. If the patient is taking anticoagulants, the risk of bleeding increases, but there is no study that shows that anticoagulation would preclude this procedure. Coagulopathy, either iatrogenic or familial, is a relative contraindication. Most bleeding is fortunately from skin vessels and is readily controlled.

Children Under about 8 Years of Age

Cricothyrotomy is absolutely contraindicated in the child less than 5 years old. The anatomy of the cricoid membrane and the larynx is simply unable to support passage of a tube of sufficient caliber to support life without destruction of the membrane and possibly the cricothyroid cartilage. There is an increased incidence of subglottic stenosis in children following cricothyrotomy. It should be performed with extreme caution in children from 5 years old to 8 years old. Although the anatomy is more like the adult's, it may still present significant problems.

In this age group, emergency tracheostomy under controlled operating room conditions should be considered. Oral tracheal intubation with inline immobilization should be considered. Needle jet ventilation may temporize until a more definitive airway can be created.

Underlying laryngeal disease and cricothyrotomy in young children are associated with an increased rate of subglottic stenosis.

Anatomy

The cricothyroid membrane covers the space between the cricoid cartilage and the thyroid cartilage superiorly (Figure 8-1). The membrane is about 10 mm high and 22 mm wide. The vocal cords are located about a centimeter above the cricoid membrane.

Overlying the cricoid membrane is the skin and cervical fascia. There is little between the skin and the cricoid membrane, unless trauma has infused edema, subcutaneous air, or blood into the subcutaneous tissues.

There are several anatomic and physiologic features that make the cricothyroid membrane the appropriate choice for a surgical airway. The membrane is immediately subcutaneous in location. It has no overlying muscles or fascial layers. There are few important vessels in this area. The superior cricothyroid vessels run transversely across the upper third of the cricothyroid membrane. If the procedure is performed in the lower third of the cricothyroid membrane, these vessels will be avoided. The anterior jugular veins run vertically and are found laterally to the cricothyroid membrane. If a vertical incision is used, then these vessels will not be encountered.

Despite the fact that there are few important vessels, and even with flawless technique, a number of small skin and subcutaneous vessels will be found

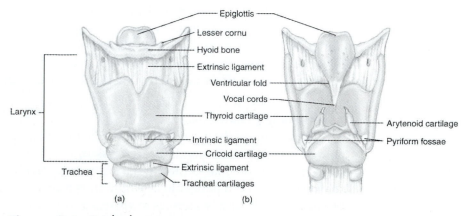

Figure 8-1 Crichothyrotomy anatomy.

during this procedure.[8] The emergency provider performing a cricothyrotomy must be prepared for bleeding as a complication. This bleeding is generally more annoying than dangerous and hemostasis can usually be achieved by pressure after the airway is inserted. (Somehow it seems that the books always leave out the "suck and blot, suck and blot" steps in this procedure.)

The thyrohyoid space is sometimes mistaken for the cricothyroid membrane. The hyoid bone and laryngeal prominence (Adam's apple) are located above the cricothyroid space. The hyoid bone should be identified and avoided when performing this procedure.

Procedure

There are two accepted techniques for cricothyrotomy: the classic technique and Brofeldt's rapid 4-step technique.[9] Although the classic technique is widely accepted, the rapid 4-step technique has gained widespread advocacy among emergency providers. The rapid 4-step technique is considered simpler because it involves fewer steps, requires fewer instruments, approximates the operator's positioning for orotracheal intubation, and stabilizes the larynx at the cricothyroid membrane rather than the thyroid cartilage (Figures 8-2-8-4).

Equipment: Standard Technique

- Scalpel (#11 blade and #15 blade) (minimum equipment)
- Tracheal dilator (Trousseau or Delaborde)
- Scissors (Mayo or Metzenbaum)
- Hemostats (at least 2)
- Tracheal hook
- Local anesthesia of choice
- Kelly clamp
- 5 mm–6 mm cricothyrotomy tube (5 mm–6 mm tracheal cannula can be substituted) (minimum equipment)
- Suction equipment including tracheal suction catheter
- Bag-valve-mask
- Oxygen delivery equipment
- Tracheal tape
- Sterile towels
- Gloves

This equipment should be assembled, sterilized, prepositioned, and located where it will be most likely used—the "trach or crick tray."

Positioning: Standard Technique

The patient should be supine with the neck in a neutral position. If possible, the patient's neck should be hyperextended by placing a towel roll under the shoulders. While these maneuvers improve the ability to locate the anatomy, they are often contraindicated in those cases where cricothyrotomy needs to be done most urgently.

The operator stands on the right side of the patient. If the patient is a trauma patient, then an assistant at the head of the bed should protect the position of the neck. The assistant holds each side of the patient's head and ensures that there is no movement of the neck during the procedure.

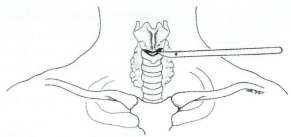

Figure 8-2 Location of incision.

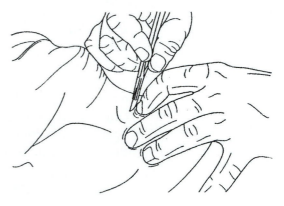

Figure 8-3 Making incision using forefinger as a guide.

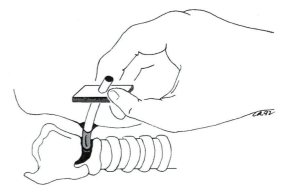

Figure 8-4 Insertion of a cricothyrotomy tube.

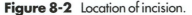

Technique: Standard Technique

1. *Clean, prepare, and drape the anterior neck if time permits.* The area should always be cleansed with an appropriate skin cleanser.
2. *Palpate the cricothyroid membrane below the thyroid cartilage in the midline.* Identify the landmarks. The cricothyroid membrane is directly below the skin between the thyroid and the cricoid cartilages. The edge of the thyroid cartilage should be identified, and the shield of the cricoid membrane lies immediately inferior.

3. *Stabilize the thyroid cartilage with the nondominant hand.* Steady the larynx with the index finger and the thumb of the nondominant hand. Infiltrate the area with lidocaine and inject a small amount into the larynx.

4. *Make a vertical incision about 2 cm in length.* A vertical skin incision is made over the thyroid cartilage and extends down to the middle of the cricoid fossa. A vertical incision promotes dissection in the midline and rapid identification of the structures. The index finger of the nondominant hand should be on the base of the cricoid cartilage.

5. *Expose and incise the cricoid membrane in the midline.* After the anatomy has been exposed, puncture the cricoid membrane with the scalpel and make a transverse incision over the puncture site. Extend this incision to about 1 cm on each side of the puncture wound. Ensure that the knife is not pointed towards the patient's head during the incision as the cords are just cephalad of the cricoid membrane.

6. *Insert the tracheal spreader into the trachea and gently widen the opening.* The superior part of the cricoid membrane can then be retracted with a tracheal hook towards the head. Insert the dilator into the wound.

If the tracheal spreader is not readily available, use the butt end of the knife as a spreader. Rotate the scalpel 90 degrees to widen the opening in the cricothyroid membrane. Alternatively, a Kelly clamp may be used to dilate the wound. If a small retractor is available, this may be used in place of the tracheal spreader.

7. *Insert the tracheostomy tube and remove the tracheal spreader or retractor.* Open the wound wide enough to admit the cricothyrotomy tube and slide it in. For most adults, a number 6 cuffed tracheostomy or cricothyrotomy tube is the largest appropriate tube to use.

Then,

8. *Inflate the cuff with 5 cc of air.*
9. *Attach the bag-valve-mask and ventilate the patient.*
10. *Verify position of the tube as for an orotracheal intubation.*
11. *Control superficial bleeding with hemostats or direct pressure as needed.*
12. *Secure the tube to the skin with 2-0 Prolene suture.*

Alternatively, secure the tube with tracheostomy ties or umbilical tape.

Equipment: Rapid 4-Step Method
*   Scalpel with #20 blade
*   Tracheal hook (wide curve, blunt tip is recommended)
*   No. 4-6 Shiley tracheostomy tube

A singular advantage of the rapid 4-step technique is that the required equipment can fit into an operator's pocket. This is important when a rescue airway is needed. Since the technique depends on palpable clues rather than visualization, there is no need for supplemental suction devices or for light sources.

Positioning: Rapid 4-Step Method

The operator stands on the left side of the patient. With the operator's left hand the cricoid membrane is palpated using the index finger. The thumb and middle finger stabilize the trachea.

If the patient is a trauma patient, then an assistant at the head of the bed should protect the position of the neck. The assistant holds each side of the patient's head and ensures that there is no movement of the neck during the procedure.

Technique: Rapid 4-Step Method[10][11]

1. *The cricothyroid membrane is identified by palpation.* In the obese patient, or in those where neck trauma has distorted the landmarks, an incision through the skin and soft tissue may be used to clearly identify the cricothyroid membrane (Figure 8-5).
2. *A horizontal stab incision is made through the skin and cricothyroid membrane with the scalpel.* Using the right hand and a low grip on the scalpel handle, a horizontal stab incision is made into the inferior portion of the cricothyroid membrane. The scalpel should be pushed through the membrane at about a 60 degree angle, creating an incision about 1 inch (2.5 cm) long.
3. *The larynx is stabilized with the tracheal hook at the inferior border of the ostomy on the cricoid cartilage, providing caudal traction.* The hook is placed along the caudal surface of the blade, pushed into the wound, and then turned 90 degrees inferiorly. Traction is maintained with the left hand while the scalpel is removed from the wound. The hand motion and grip are similar to those used for holding the laryngoscope during intubation.
4. *The Shiley tube is placed in the trachea.* A cuffed tracheostomy tube or endotracheal tube is inserted into the incision with the right hand, the appropriate position is confirmed, and the tracheal hook is withdrawn. An endotracheal tube can be cut shorter, provided it is not cut below the cuff inflation tube. The modified endotracheal tube can be replaced when an appropriate tracheostomy tube is available. A 4-5 Shiley tube is appropriate for an emergency cricothyrotomy (Figures 8-6-8-7).
5. *The bag-valve system is attached.* The patient should be ventilated and tube position verified with the usual techniques.
6. *The tube is secured and hemostasis achieved.*

Complications

In 1921, Chevalier Jackson condemned "high tracheotomy" because of its increased incidence of complications.[12] His description of subglottic stenosis caused by cricothyrotomy caused it to be abandoned for nearly 60 years. He made his judgment based on referrals to him with failed cricothyrotomies, with no regard to the training and skill of the operator who first performed them. His comments have generated a flurry of arguments regarding cricothyrotomy. Fortunately, Dr. Jackson was working in the era before antibiotics and the development of soft cuffs for both endotracheal tubes and cricothyroidostomy appliances. Equally fortunately, his comments were describing the use of an elective cricothyrotomy for long-term airway support.

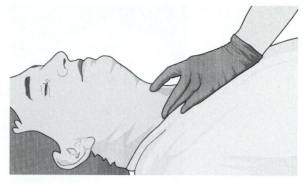

Step 1: Palpation

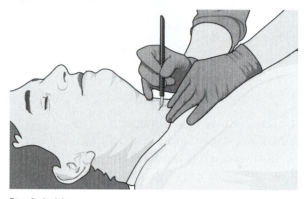

Step 2: Incision

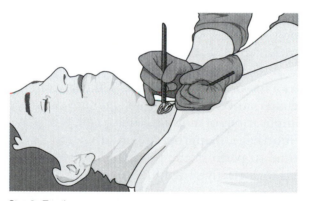

Step 3: Traction

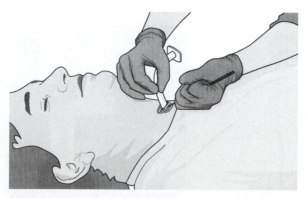

Step 4: Intubation

Figure 8-5 Rapid 4-step method technique. *Source:* Brofeldt, B.T., Panacek, E.A., Richards, J.R.: An easy cricothyrotomy approach: The rapid four-step technique. *Acad. Emerg. Med.* 1996;3:1060–1063.

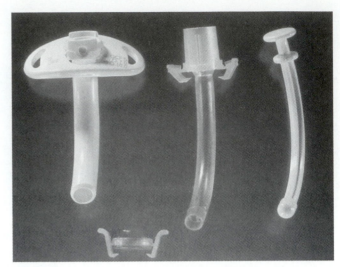

Figure 8-6 Cricothyrotomy cannula (uncuffed).

The classic study describing the safety of modern cricothyrotomy was conducted by Brantigan and Grow in 1975.[13] They performed 655 cricothyrotomies, both electively and in emergency situations, and found an extremely low incidence of complications, much lower than that reported with tracheostomy.

It is important for the emergency provider to realize that the debate has little application to the emergency procedure. The complication can be avoided by conversion of a cricothyrotomy to a tracheostomy within 72 hours, which takes the patient out of the purview of the emergency department and field emergency medicine.[14] Emergency cricothyrotomy is performed as a life-or-death procedure. A higher complication rate is acceptable since the alternative is a catastrophic failure to secure the airway.

Complications of most immediate concern to the emergency provider include hemorrhage, inappropriate or unsuccessful tube placement, and a prolonged time to perform the procedure. Emergency cricothyrotomy is more hazardous than elective cricothyrotomy with a 23 percent to 40 percent com-

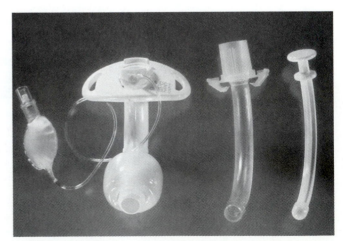

Figure 8-7 Cricothyrotomy cannula (cuffed).

plication rate for the former and only 6 percent to 10 percent incidence of complications during elective procedures.[15 16 17 18 19 20]

Inappropriate technique may cause laceration of arteries, veins, esophageal perforation, vocal cord injuries, laryngeal fractures, pneumothorax, pneumomediastinum, creation of false passages in the neck, and subcutaneous emphysema.[21 22] As with any tube in the airway, kinking, obstruction and plugging are possible complications.

Tracheal Injury

The standard technique teaches placement of the tracheal hook in the superior portion of the wound and stabilization of the thyroid cartilage. This maneuver potentially increases the risk of pretracheal intubation, increases the risk of vocal-cord injury, and increases the risk of bleeding from the superiorly located cricothyroid arteries. In the rapid 4-step technique, placement of the tracheal hook in the inferior aspect of the wound with cricoid stabilization is recommended because it may reduce the incidence of these injuries and because it mimics physician positioning for orotracheal intubation.

In the rapid 4-step technique the tracheal hook may damage the cricoid cartilage. The placement of the tracheal hook in the inferior aspect of the wound may increase the risk of injury to the cricoid cartilage as it is manipulated. The cricoid cartilage is much smaller but thicker than the thyroid cartilage. In the standard technique, the tracheal hook is placed on the larger but thinner thyroid cartilage. It is unclear which would be more susceptible to injury.

In the sole comparison study performed in cadavers, two cricoid cartilage fractures were noted.[23] This was thought to be artifactual due to cadaver preservation, but may represent a real risk if excessive traction is used to perform the procedure.

Esophageal Injury

Esophageal injury occurs when the scalpel penetrates the posterior trachea. This complication can be lethal.

In the standard technique, the operator should carefully expose the cricoid cartilage and the cricothyroid membrane. The depth of the incision may be controlled by holding the scalpel blade low (close to the blade) when cricothyroid membrane is incised.

The 4-step technique calls for a 1-step blind stab through the skin, fascia, and cricothyroid membrane, as opposed to the standard technique, in which the cricothyroid membrane is incised under direct visualization. This stab procedure is certainly time-saving compared with blunt dissection in the standard technique. However, control of depth of the incision is essential to preventing esophageal perforation. The operator must hold the scalpel low (very close to the blade) to prevent too deep of a puncture with the blade.

Massive Neck Swelling

This complication usually occurs from a cricothyrotomy tube misplaced in the pretracheal space and the subsequent introduction of subcutaneous air. It may occasionally occur with a leak around the cricoid opening or from a tracheal injury prior to the procedure.

Rarely, massive swelling occurs due to bleeding from vessels injured either in the original trauma or by the operator.

Asphyxia

Asphyxia, dysrhythmias, and cardiac arrest are related to both an inaccurately performed procedure and a procedure that takes too long. Cricothyrotomy should be performed successfully in less than 3 minutes.[24] Thirty to sixty seconds to perform the procedure is not an unusual time both in the emergency department and in the field.[25]

Bleeding

Incorrect skin incisions can contribute to both bleeding and incorrect tube placements. Transverse incisions have more complications in positioning than vertical incisions. If the desired anatomy is not found with a vertical incision, it can be simply extended in the appropriate direction.

Most bleeding about the site of the cricothyrotomy incision can be avoided if the operator uses a vertical incision rather than a transverse incision.[26] The operator must avoid making a blind stab in the area. Landmarks must be accurately located and visualized before the scalpel is applied. This should help prevent both hemorrhage and damage to the numerous structures such as the vocal cords, the thyroid, the tracheal rings, or the vessels and nerves around the cricoid cartilage. Never direct the knife towards the head. The vocal cords can be easily damaged and lie just cephalad to the cricoid membrane. The cricothyroid arteries are high in the cricoid membrane and a lower incision will also avoid these structures.

The rapid 4-step method focuses more on tactile clues than visual identification of the structures. Bleeding at the site of the procedure will not obscure the tactile positioning of the incision and the placement of the tube.

Control bleeding with direct pressure, cautery if available, or hemostats. Most bleeding is self-limited and from superficial vessels and will respond to direct pressure. Rarely, this complication can be lethal if major vessels are lacerated or the patient develops a massive neck hematoma.

Late Complications

Late complications include dysphonia, infection, subcutaneous and mediastinal emphysema, and subglottic stenosis. In modern medical practice, subglottic stenosis is a rare complication and most frequently found in patients who have an oral intubation for an extended period of time before the cricothyrotomy and in infants or small children.[27] [28] [29] [30] These devastating complications can be avoided by proper patient selection and appropriate care after the insertion of the tube.

Assessment of Difficulty of Cricothyrotomy

The most common anatomic abnormality that prevents cricothyrotomy is subcutaneous swelling or air obscuring the anatomy. This can be caused by direct trauma to the neck, trauma to the larynx, or even pneumothorax with dissection of air into the neck.

A short neck or excessive subcutaneous tissue will also increase the difficulty of cricothyrotomy. Morbidly obese patients may be quite difficult, even without trauma.

Cricothyrotomy Will Be Made More Difficult by

*   Lack of knowledge and experience
*   Short bull neck
*   Obesity

- Soft tissue neck injuries
- Subcutaneous air in neck
- Coagulopathy
- Confused and combative patient

Needle Cricothyrotomy and Transtracheal Jet Ventilation

The insertion of a needle into the cricothyroid membrane or the trachea proper for jet insufflation of high-pressure oxygen may be a viable alternative for the clinician who lacks surgical skill or training (Figure 8-8). It may also be used as an interim airway until more definitive measures can be accomplished at leisure. Percutaneous translaryngeal ventilation is far simpler and may be less hazardous than either cricothyrotomy or tracheostomy. Prophylactic transtracheal jet ventilation may be used while intubation is attempted in the anticipated difficult airway. This will allow the use of sedation or paralysis more safely.

Jet ventilation can occur through the cricoid membrane or the trachea itself. The term *transtracheal ventilation* by piercing the cricothyroid membrane is a misnomer. The cricothyroid membrane is part of the larynx, not the trachea. The term transtracheal jet ventilation should be properly reserved for a needle into the trachea. Since there is no advantage to use of the lower site, transtracheal ventilation should be saved for patients with trauma to the cricoid cartilage or the larynx.

Indications and Benefits

- Easier to perform than cricothyrotomy
- Often more rapid than cricothyrotomy
- Less risk of scar formation
- Extensive orofacial trauma
- Known cervical trauma (relative and controversial)
- Upper airway obstruction due to edema, hemorrhage, or foreign body
- Unsuccessful endotracheal intubation
- Age under about 8 years

Either form of transtracheal cannulation is quick, relatively atraumatic, and simple. Chest compressions may be continued during the insertion of the catheter. Retrograde air pressure can dislodge foreign bodies, clots, vomitus, or secretions. (This should be considered a benefit, not an indication for needle cricothyrotomy.)

After the airway has been established with a needle cannula, a formal cricothyrotomy can be performed with the needle as a guide.

The anatomic considerations for needle cricothyrotomy are the same as for a surgical cricothyrotomy. Transtracheal jet ventilation can be used while intubation is attempted in an anticipated difficult airway. This allows the use of sedation and even paralysis in otherwise contraindicated patients.

Contraindications

Unfortunately, if upper airway obstruction is complete, sufficient pressure may be developed in the lung to cause barotrauma, including mediastinal emphyseme and pneumothorax. Complete airway obstruction or transection of

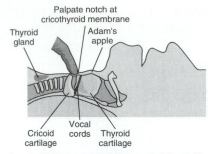

Step 1: Patient's neck is hyperextended, if possible, and cricothyroid membrane identified. Palpate.

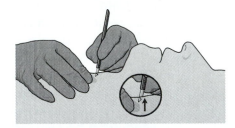

Step 2: Pinch 1 cm of skin and insert sharp tip of knife blade through skin. Cut in an outward motion.

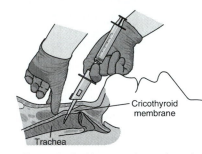

Step 3: The needle should puncture the membrane just beyond entry at approximately the same angle as the lower edge of the housing. Aspirate, easy moving syringe obturator denotes tracheal entrance.

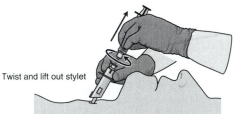

Step 4: The stylet and syringe are removed as a unit by twisting the luer adapter counter-clockwise and lifting out.

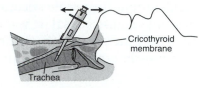

Step 5: The blunt needle is gently moved further into the trachea until the housing rests on the overlying skin. A freely rocking motion confirms proper depth of insertion.

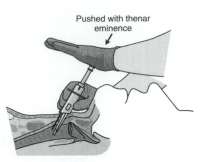

Step 6: In all cases, begin with the smallest airway (4.5 mm) and insert airway and obturator together PUSHING WITH THE THINNER EMINENCE resting against the cap of the obturator. Airway and obturator are PUSHED (not squeezed) downward into the needle, which is divided lengthwise and spreads apart to accommodate them.

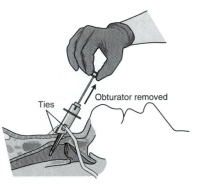

Step 7: Obturator is removed, leaving a clear passage for air to reach the lungs. If airway size requires change, this can be easily performed by leaving the housing and needle guide in place, while removal and insertion of airways are made. Ties are threaded through the brackets on the sides of housing.

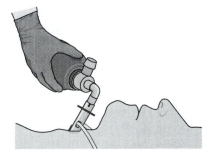

Step 8: System in operation: Bag valve or universal (15 mm) adapter may be fitted to the top of the housing. Expansion of lungs can also be started by mouth-to-mouth respiration, with fingers closing of the vents in the housing.

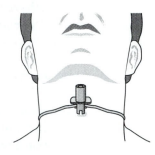

Figure 8-8 Needle cricothyrotomy insertion of needle.

the trachea is a contraindication for translaryngeal jet ventilation. An alternative method of securing the airway must be sought in this case.

A relative contraindication occurs for all invasive procedures that can be adequately managed by another less invasive technique. Other relative contraindications include bleeding disorders and infections about the site of the needle insertion. If the patient can be adequately managed with a bag-valve-mask combination, then translaryngeal jet insufflation is a poor choice.

Contraindications to Transtracheal Jet Ventilation

- Ability to secure an airway by less invasive techniques
- Significant cricoid cartilage injury
- Complete tracheal obstruction
- Tracheal transection with retraction of the distal trachea into the mediastinum

Procedure

The method consists of two basic steps:

Insertion of a cannula into the cricoid membrane
Ventilation with high-pressure oxygen.

The area should be briefly prepped with a skin cleanser.

Positioning for Cricoid Puncture

The technique works best if the patient's neck is fully exposed and with the laryngeal prominence further exposed by a towel roll placed under the patient's shoulders.

In trauma patients, these preparations may not be possible. If the patient is a trauma patient, then an assistant at the head of the bed should protect the position of the neck. The assistant holds each side of the patient's head and ensures that there is no movement of the neck during the procedure.

The operator should be facing the patient at the patient's right shoulder if he or she is right-handed. Using gloved fingers, palpate the cricothyroid membrane.

Equipment

Although this equipment can be fabricated in a few moments, it is best to have it ready *before* the patient shows up at the emergency department. One should not depend upon Yankee ingenuity at the time that a critical patient needs an airway.

- Oxygen delivery tubing (cut side hole about 2 cm away from the end or use a "Y" or "T" connector).[31]
- 14 gauge needle over catheter intravenous needle (either commercial insufflation device or standard IV needle is acceptable). If a larger size is available for adults, it will allow a more normal air exchange. A 4.0 mm percutaneous tracheal catheter device may be used and may provide appropriate oxygenation if only a bag-valve system is available.
- 50 psi oxygen source—this must be an unregulated wall outlet or similar device.[32] Oxygen-powered demand-valve devices are not adequate because they can only develop 60 cm water pressure.[33] A bag-valve system may be used but will require extraordinary work in order to deliver an appropriate volume of oxygen.

- Skin prep solution of choice
- 3.0 mm pediatric endotracheal tube with adaptor
- Sterile prep materials
- Sterile gloves
- Sterile 4 × 4 gauze pads

A Cook Critical Care "Melker Emergency Cricothyrotomy Catheter Set" has all needed equipment except oxygen supply and gloves. The Bivona Medical Technologies Nu-Trach (Figure 8-9) and Pedia-Trach devices also provide all needed equipment in a convenient package (Bivona Medical Technologies, Gary, Indiana) (Figure 8-10).

Technique

- Clean, prepare, and drape the anterior neck, if time permits.
- If appropriate, anesthetize the area with a lidocaine skin wheal over the cricoid membrane. Puncture the membrane and inject a little anesthesia into the trachea with the needle aimed towards the head.
- Palpate the cricothyroid membrane below the thyroid cartilage in the midline.
- Use a #14 gauge cannula through needle on a 3 cc to 5 cc syringe.
- Locate the cricoid membrane with one finger and direct the cannula towards the sternum.
- Stabilize the thyroid cartilage with the nondominant hand.
- Puncture the skin in the midline over the cricothyroid membrane.
- Direct the catheter inferiorly at 45 degrees to the skin plane.
- Aspirate while advancing the catheter. Stop when air is aspirated.
- Aspirate air to ensure that the needle is in the appropriate space. While carefully stabilizing the cannula-needle combination, remove the needle from within the cannula.
- Advance the catheter over the needle, down the distal trachea, and withdraw the needle.
- Use a finger of the other hand as a needle guard to help prevent inadvertent puncture of the posterior wall of the trachea. Hold the needle about 1.5 cm away from the needle point so that a sudden movement will not allow the needle to go any farther into the neck.

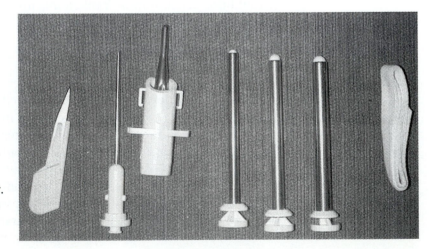

Figure 8-9 Nutrach kit.
Source: Photo by Charles Stewart and Associates; www.storysmith.net.

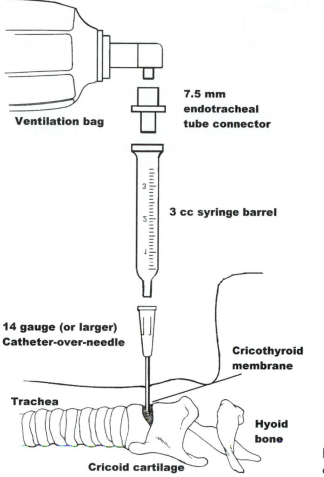

Ventilation bag

7.5 mm endotracheal tube connector

3 cc syringe barrel

14 gauge (or larger) Catheter-over-needle

Cricothyroid membrane

Trachea

Hyoid bone

Cricoid cartilage

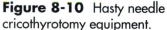

Figure 8-10 Hasty needle cricothyrotomy equipment.

- Attach a 3.0 pediatric endotracheal tube adaptor to the hub of the catheter. (Don't use the sometimes recommended 3 cc syringe barrel into which a connector from a 7 mm ETT is placed; it's just plain awkward.)
- Attach y connector to oxygen tubing and to pediatric endotracheal tube adaptor.
- Maintain oxygen flow at 15 l/min.
- Attach the oxygen and ventilate the patient with 1 second of pressure ventilation, followed by 4 seconds off.
- Allow sufficient time to permit exhalation through the small-bore cannula. This is particularly vital if the patient has a total obstruction above the cricothyrotomy.

When this procedure is done properly by a skilled operator, the airway can be open in 10 seconds. It requires less equipment and surgical set-up and makes a smaller scar with less bleeding.

To pierce the trachea below the larynx, the operator needs to stabilize the trachea with one hand. The other steps are quite similar. The only reason to penetrate the trachea in the lower position is to avoid an area of laryngeal trauma or infection. This is a distinctly unusual event.

Complications

Hypercarbia

Although many clinicians feel that insertion of a large-bore cannula into the cricoid membrane may provide enough ventilation for the traumatized patient, this is not correct. The patient must be ventilated with high-pressure oxygen through the cannula in order to avoid carbon dioxide retention. Inadequate ventilation occurs when the patient is ventilated with low-pressure oxygen or an inadequately sized catheter. Using proper technique and equipment, it has been shown that adequate ventilation can be maintained for as long as 75 minutes in adult patients.

Subcutaneous Emphysema

Perforation of the posterior trachea or insertion of the needle lateral to the trachea may occur. This may happen if the patient moves, the operator insufficiently guards the needle during insertion, or if the operator insufficiently identifies the landmarks and strays from the midline. An insertion posteriorly may occur and either perforate the esophagus or instill air into the subcutaneous tissues or the mediastinum. Accumulation of air can occur gradually over the course of 1 to 6 hours after transtracheal puncture.[34]

Vessel Perforation or Hemorrhage

Perforation of vessels may occur if the patient moves or the operator insufficiently identifies the landmarks and strays from the midline. Either the carotids or the internal jugular vessels may be damaged in this manner. Passage of a needle into the vascular thyroid instead of the cricoid membrane may be associated with significant bleeding and hematoma formation. The bleeding is usually superficial and self-limited. It may be controlled with direct pressure around the area.

Inability to Suction Secretions

Unfortunately, needles are usually too small to pass a suction catheter. This means that they may be readily obstructed by mucus and clots. High-pressure flow does keep the passage clear in most cases—but this may rarely cause an effective ball-valve obstruction.

Esophageal Perforation

Occurs when the needle penetrates the posterior trachea. This is a life-threatening emergency.

Tracheostomy

The term "tracheostomy" was coined by Lorenz Heister in 1718.[35] The tracheostomy is one of the oldest surgical procedures. A tracheostomy is portrayed on Egyptian tablets that date back to 3600 BC and the tracheostomy was mentioned in Hindu medical texts written in 2000 BC.

It is the author's opinion that the cricothyroid membrane puncture is the safest and simplest method for establishing a satisfactory surgical airway under most conditions. Even the most skilled surgeon would be unwise to attempt an emergency tracheostomy when a cricothyroid membrane puncture would admirably control the crisis. It is agreed by most cogent emergency providers that a classic tracheostomy should be performed rarely, if at all, in an emergency department.[36] The cricothyrotomy is used in patients with facial and neck trauma as a field airway in some localities.[37 38 39 40]

The tracheostomy was one of the first treatments for upper airway obstruction, but met with little success until the 1800s. Initially it was performed for choking caused by inhalation of foreign bodies, drowning, or trauma to the upper respiratory tract. The tracheostomy became popular in response to the diptheria epidemics. Abundant practice of the technique of tracheostomy for airway obstruction due to diptheria led to routine use of tracheostomies in children with this infection. In the early 1950s and 1960s, use of intubation and respiratory support began to supplant the tracheostomy. This revolutionized emergency and critical care of the airway from neonates to ninety-year-olds. Unless the patient has had an endotracheal tube for more than three weeks, endotracheal intubation has fewer complications and risks.

The poliomyelitis epidemic of the 1950s stimulated the use of tracheostomies for mechanical ventilation in patients paralyzed by polio. This led to similar use in the treatment of tetanus, cardiothoracic surgery patients, severe burns, and premature children. Today, the tracheostomy is rarely performed for emergent airway control, but is one of the most frequently performed surgical procedures in critically ill patients.[41]

Emergency tracheostomy is fraught with hazards and is not appropriate for the nonphysician or the physician who has not been trained in surgical techniques.[42] Anatomic considerations make the tracheostomy a relatively complicated and difficult field procedure. There are many complex structures in the neck, in close proximity to the trachea. These include the carotid arteries, the jugular veins, the recurrent laryngeal nerves, the thyroid gland, the tip of the lung, and the esophagus.

Indications for Tracheostomy

- May be appropriate for the child
- May be appropriate for the patient with transection of the trachea and retraction of the distal trachea into the chest
- May be appropriate for the patient with severe laryngeal trauma such as laryngeal fracture, cricoid fracture, and some burns
- Need for long-term artificial airway
- Need for continuous mechanical ventilation

Complications of the Tracheostomy

- Delay in securing an airway
- Bleeding
- Subcutaneous emphysema
- Malposition
  - Creation of a false passage
  - Accidental decannulation
- Pneumothorax
- Obstruction
- Chest and neck infections
- Esophageal laceration
- Late complications
  - Tracheal stenosis
  - Tracheal ulceration

- Scar formation
- Tracheoesophageal fistula
- Vocal cord paralysis

Indications

An emergent tracheostomy may be appropriate when the patient is an infant, but needle cricothyrotomy is generally recommended for this age group. The patient who has severe edema of the neck, particularly when there is a suspicion of laryngeal damage, may require a tracheostomy for airway management. The patient with a transected trachea and retraction of the trachea into the chest will require a tracheostomy.

Specific indications for a tracheostomy include obstruction of the upper airway below the cricoid membrane or involving the cricoid cartilage, such as facial trauma, and laryngeal trauma. Permanent obstruction (such as cancer of the larynx) above the level of the vocal cords is an indication for a non-emergent tracheostomy. Obstruction above the cricoid membrane, such as epiglottitis, is probably better managed by cricothyrotomy in the emergent situation.

Severe blunt trauma of the larynx may be the only noncontroversial indication for emergency tracheostomy. The injury can lead to laryngeal fracture or tracheal disruption with subsequent complete loss of the airway. In severe blunt trauma of the larynx, it may be impossible and potentially harmful to attempt to intubate the patient's trachea through the vocal cords because fragments from the thyroid and cricoid cartilage may be displaced and obstruct the airway.

Some authorities recommend awake fiber-optic intubation in this situation. With a readily available fiberoptic scope and a skilled intubator, this may be an alternative. This option is rarely available outside of a major trauma center.

A more common indication for a tracheostomy is long-term airway maintenance. Although this airway is not an emergency, care of the patient with a recent tracheostomy may be the responsibility of either the field provider or emergency physician.

Benefits of a tracheostomy in long-term mechanical ventilation include improved airway suctioning, increased patient comfort, fewer chronic laryngeal and tracheal complications, easier tube changes, and capability for oral feedings. There is a serious risk of tracheal damage if intubation is prolonged longer than about ten days to two weeks.[43] Ventilator patients may tolerate breathing through a tracheostomy better because there is less airway resistance. Bronchopulmonary care may require a nonemergency tracheostomy in some patients. A tracheostomy may be a treatment for some people with sleep apnea.

Complications

From the 1830s to the 1930s a tracheostomy was done only as a last resort for airway management. The survival rate for these operations was only 32 percent at that time.[44] Today, the morbidity and mortality associated with a tracheostomy performed in the operating room is quite low. The same is not true of emergent tracheostomies, which is the major reason why cricothyrotomy is preferred for emergency airway care.

Delay in Securing an Airway

A tracheostomy is a complex procedure requiring specialized equipment. There are few physicians who can perform this procedure in the operating room in the short time available to salvage a patient with an upper airway obstruction. Undue delay in securing the airway is a frequent complication of tracheostomies performed by those who are not familiar with the anatomy and the tools used for the procedure.

Hemorrhage

Serious bleeding is not an unusual complication of tracheostomy and should be a major concern during an emergency tracheostomy. The thyroid gland is perhaps the most vascular gland in the body and overlies the trachea. It has superior and inferior paired arteries that provide abundant opportunities for bleeding during the procedure. Other immediate bleeding may occur from trauma to the innominate artery, carotid arteries, subclavian arteries, anterior jugular veins, the jugular venous arch, and thyroid venous vessels. Delayed hemorrhage may occur when the cannula causes erosion in these vessels or in the brachiocephalic vein (particularly in children).

Subcutaneous Emphysema

Subcutaneous emphysema is commonly seen after a tracheostomy due to air leaks around the tube. It usually resolves without further treatment. The position of the tube, inflation of a cuff, and tightness of the tube within the stoma should all be checked if subcutaneous emphysema develops.

Malposition—Accidental Decannulation

This is a quite serious complication in the emergency department or the field. Hasty repositioning of the cannula may be difficult or create a false passage. The fistula tract has not formed into scar tissue and the fascial planes of the neck may be easily separated. In children, the small incision size makes for significant difficulty in reinsertion of a cannula. In patients with a "fresh" tracheostomy, recannulation should be performed under direct vision with operative lights and full equipment, or endotracheal intubation should be attempted.

Malposition—Creation of a False Passage

As previously mentioned, changing a tracheostomy tube or reinsertion of the tube may create a false passage if the procedure is done before the tract is well formed. If the posterior portion of the trachea is damaged, a tracheoesophageal fistula may be formed. The esophagus is more likely to be lacerated during a tracheostomy than during a cricothyrotomy.

Pneumothorax

A low tracheostomy may be associated with pneumothorax or pneumomediastinum. A tight tracheal tube-stoma fit will exacerbate the situation. Pneumothorax should be treated as in any other patient with observation or thoracostomy tube drainage depending on the clinical situation and transport considerations.

Obstruction

Obstruction of the tracheostomy cannula is an avoidable and potentially fatal complication. The most common cause of obstruction is the accumulation of dried and thickened mucus and crusts in the tube or the trachea. This complication can be prevented by adequate humidification and suction and ensuring that the patient is adequately hydrated. If suction fails to remove the obstruction, then remove the cannula and use forceps to remove the crusts. Explosive expiration may eject the crusts.

In very small children and obese patients, the chin may occlude the tracheostomy tube if the patient moves.

Chest Infections

Pulmonary infections are more common when the defenses of the upper airway are bypassed and the patient has an open wound in the neck.

Late Complications

Late complications can include occlusion of the tube as previously discussed, wound infections, tracheo-esophageal fistula from erosion of the cannula into the posterior trachea and then into the esophagus, and vocal cord paralysis. Even the incidence of these complications is increased when emergency tracheostomy is performed. Other late complications include residual stomas, disfiguring scars, and tracheal stenosis at the site of the scar.

Pediatric Considerations

Although the tracheostomy is much more appropriate for creating an emergency airway in the small infant than a cricothyrotomy, it is a technically difficult procedure and fraught with hazards.[45] Transtracheal jet ventilation is a technically easier procedure in the field and should be considered first. In the child, the air passages are smaller, the larynx is higher, and the thyroid cartilage is not as prominent. The recurrent laryngeal nerves are closer to the trachea. In extension, the mediastinal contents may enter the neck. The operator may find the dome of the pleura, the large vessels of the upper chest, and the thymus. A low tracheostomy may have truly fatal complications in the child.

Procedure

Detailed instructions for performing a tracheostomy are covered in ENT texts. The following general discussion of the technique is intended to acquaint the reader with the complexity of the task, rather than to specifically direct the performance of an emergency procedure fraught with hazard and accompanied with serious complications.

Position

The head should be hyper-extended. This moves the trachea closer to the skin incision. On the other hand it also may aggravate the patient's airway management problems. Hyperextension may not be possible in the patient with potential spinal trauma.

Technique

A horizontal incision is more cosmetic but a vertical incision allows for faster performance. The incision should be made midway between the cricoid cartilage and the suprasternal notch. The incision should be carried through the investing layer and the pretracheal muscles into the midline raphe. The pretracheal fascia is incised and separated.

The pretracheal muscles are laterally retracted and the thyroid isthmus is exposed. The thyroid isthmus is either retracted or cut. If the isthmus is wide, it should be clamped, cut, ligated, and retracted to the sides of the incision.

A tracheal window is then cut at the second or third tracheal rings. It is easier to insert the tube if a window of cartilage is removed.

The tube is then inserted into the trachea. A cuffed tube allows positive pressure ventilation in the adult. Uncuffed tubes are used in children for the same reasons that uncuffed tracheal tubes are used.

Verification of the tube's positioning is similar to verification of an endotracheal tube. Air movement in a tracheal tube by a spontaneously breathing patient is always a sign of appropriate placement.

The wound should be dry and have no bleeders. The tracheostomy wound should be minimally dressed. A dressing soaked with blood and mucus is a good source of infection.

Care of Tracheostomy

Although routine care of a tracheostomy is not an emergency procedure, the emergency provider may be called on to care for patients with other diseases who have a tracheostomy or may be asked for advice about a tracheostomy.

The most common complications associated with a tracheostomy that are seen by emergency providers are dislodged tracheal tubes, infections about the tracheostomy site, plugged tracheostomy tubes (granulomas or mucus plugging), and bleeding about the tracheostomy site.[46] Rare complications include late tracheal stenosis and tracheostomy.

Replacement of a Tracheostomy Tube

Replacement of a tracheostomy tube that has been in place for several weeks is often quite easy. The same cannot be said of the tube that requires replacement after only a few hours or minutes. That procedure may be as difficult as the original tracheostomy.

The most common complication of replacement of a tracheostomy tube is anterior dissection along the trachea. This occurs when the tube is forced between the soft tissues of the anterior neck and the trachea. Do not push the tube against resistance.

There are three choices of tracheostomy tubes available: cuffed, cannulated, and fenestrated.

In an emergency, cuffed tubes are generally used. Uncuffed tubes are more appropriate for smaller children for the same reasons that uncuffed endotracheal tubes are used. Uncuffed tubes may be easier to insert, but they provide less protection from aspiration and positive pressure ventilation is more difficult. When long-term tracheostomy is required, uncuffed tracheostomy tubes are usually used even when mechanical ventilation is required.

An inner cannula is used in many cases as it can be removed for cleaning and prevents tube blockage by secretions. Unfortunately, a cannula decreases the inner diameter of the tube and limits respirations. It is not appropriate for smaller children and infants.

A fenestrated tube has a hole in it that allows airflow through the vocal cords and upper airway to allow speaking. Fenestrated tubes are used in chronic care situations only. They do not provide as much protection from vomitus.

If a tracheostomy tube is not available, an ET tube can be used as a field expedient. If there isn't an ET tube around, a nasal airway will suffice until another method is available. In some cases, intubation with an endotracheal tube may be the appropriate management of the patient's airway.

- Use the same size tube as the tracheostomy tube that you are replacing
- Place the patient supine
  - A rolled up towel under the shoulders may expose the anatomy better
- Remove the old tube
  - Be sure to deflate the cuff if the tube has one
- Insert the obturator into the new tube
- Grasp the top of the tube with the thumb and forefinger and insert the tube into the stoma
  - Be sure to point the curve of the tube towards the chest
  - Do not force the tube
  - Lubrication with a water soluble lubricant may be helpful
- Remove the obturator
- Inflate the cuff (if any)
- Ventilate the patient
  - A pediatric mask and bag-valve system may be used to ventilate the patient through the tracheal stoma
- Check position as for an endotracheal tube with auscultation, observation of chest wall expansion, and end tidal CO_2
- Secure the tube

END NOTES

[1] Spaite, D. W., and Joseph, M. "Prehospital cricothyrotomy: An investigation of indications, technique, complications, and patient outcome." *Ann Emerg Med* 1990;19:279–285.

[2] Rosen, P., Dinerman, N., and Pons, P. "The technical imperative: Its definition and an application to prehospital care." *Topics Emerg Med* 1981; 2:79–86.

[3] Spaite, D. W., and Joseph, M. "Prehospital cricothyrotomy: An investigation of indications, technique, complications, and patient outcome." *Ann Emerg Med* 1990;19:279–285.

[4] Rosen, P., Dinerman, N., and Pons, P. "The technical imperative: Its definition and an application to prehospital care." *Topics Emerg Med* 1981; 2:79–86.

[5] Narrod, J. A., Moore, E. E., and Rosen, P. "Emergency cricothyrostomy—Technique and anatomical considerations," in *J Emerg Med* 1985; 443–446.

[6] Spaite, D. W., and Joseph, M. "Prehospital cricothyrotomy: An investigation of indications, technique, complications, and patient outcome," in *Ann Emerg Med* 1990;19:279–285.

[7] Rosen, P., Dinerman, N., and Pons, P. "The technical imperative: Its definition and an application to prehospital care," in *Topics Emerg Med* 1981; 2:79–86.

[8] Little, C. M., Parker, M. G., and Tanropolsky, R. "The incidence of vasculature at risk during cricothyroidostomy," in *Ann Emerg Med* 1986; 15:805–807.

[9] Brofeldt, B. T., Panacek, E. A., and Richards, J. R. "An easy cricothyrotomy approach: The rapid four-step technique," in *Acad Emerg Med* 1996; 3:1060–1063.

[10] Brofeldt, B. T., Panacek, E. A., and Richards, J. "An easier cricothyrotomy technique for emergency medicine: The rapid four-step approach [abstract]," in *Acad Emerg Med* 1994;1:A106.

[11] Brofeldt, B. T., Panacek, E. A., and Richards, J. R. "An easy cricothyrotomy approach: The rapid four-step technique," in *Acad Emerg Med* 1996; 3:1060–1063.

[12] Jackson, C. "High tracheotomy and other errors: The chief causes of chronic laryngeal stenosis," in *Surg Gynecol Obstet* 1921;32:392.

[13] Brantigam, C. O., and Grow, J. B. "Cricothyroidotomy: Elective use in respiratory problems requiring tracheotomy," *J Thoracic Cardiovasc Surg* 1976;71:72.

[14] Walls, R. M. "Cricothyrotomy," in *Emerg Clin NA* 1988;6:725–736.

[15] Erlandson, M. J., Clinton, J. E., Ruiz, E., et al. "Cricothyrotomy in the emergency department revisited," in *J Emerg Med* 1989;7:115–118.

[16] McGill, J., Clinton, J. E., and Ruiz, E. "Cricothyrotomy in the emergency department," in *Ann Emerg Med* 1982;11:361–364.

[17] Brantigean, C. O., and Grow, J. B. "Cricothyroidotomy revisited again," in *Ear Nose Throat J* 1980;59:289.

[18] van Hasselt, E. J., Bruining, H. A., and Hoeve, L. J. "Elective cricothyroidotomy." *Intensive Care Med* 1985;11:207–209.

[19] Esses, B. A., and Jafek, B. W. "Cricothyroidotomy: A decade of experience in Denver." *Ann Otol Rhinol Laryngol* 96:1987.

[20] Nugent, W. L., Rhee, K. J., and Wisner, D. H. "Can nurses perform cricothyrotomy with acceptable success and complication rates," in *Ann Emerg Med* 1991;20:367–370.

[21] Slobodkin, D., Topliff, S., and Raife, J. H. "Retrograde intubation of the pharynx: An unusual complication of emergency cricothyrotomy," in *Ann Emerg Med* 1992;21:220–222.

[22] Moncada, R., Demos, T. C., Dobrin, P. B., et al. "Complications of endotracheal intubation and tracheostomy," in *Res and Staff Phys* 1986; 32:42–49.

23 Johnson, D. R., Dunlap, A., McFeeley, P., et al. "Cricothyrotomy performed by prehospital personnel: A comparison of two techniques in a human cadaver model," in *Am J Emerg Med* 1993;11:207–209.

24 Roberts, J. R., and Hedges, J. R. *Clinical Procedures in Emergency Medicine.* Philadelphia, PA: Saunders 1991:40–59.

25 Johnson, D. R., Dunlap, A., McFeeley, P., et al. "Cricothyrotomy performed by prehospital personnel: A comparison of two techniques in a human cadaver model," in *Am J Emerg Med* 1993;11:207–209.

26 Mace, S. E. "Cricothyrotomy," in *J Emerg Med* 1988;6:309–319.

27 Boyd, A., Romita, M. C., Conlan, A. A., et al. "A clinical evaluation of cricothyroidotomy," in *Surg Obstet Gynecol* 1979;149:365–368.

28 Walls, R. M. "Cricothyrotomy," in *Emerg Clin NA* 1988;6:725–736.

29 Esses, B. A., and Jafek, B. W. "Cricothyroidotomy: A decade of experience in Denver," in *Ann Otol Rhinol Laryngol* 1987;96:519–524.

30 O'Connor, J. V., Reddy, K., Ergin, M. A., et al. "Cricothyroidotomy for prolonged ventilatory support after cardiac operations," in *Ann Thorac Surg* 1985;39:353–354.

31 Reich, D. L., and Schwartz, N. "An easily assembled device for transtracheal oxygenation," in *Anesthesiology* 1987;66:437–438.

32 Reed, J. P., Kemph, J. P., Hamelberg, W., et al. "Studies with transtracheal artificial respiration," in *Anesthesiology* 1954;15:28–41.

33 Yealy, D. M., Stewart, R. D., and Kaplan, R. M. "Myths and pitfalls in emergency translaryngeal ventilation: Correcting misimpressions," in *Ann Emerg Med* 1988;17:690–692.

34 Massey, J. Y. "Complications of transtracheal aspiration—a case report," in *J Arkansas Med Soc* 1971;67:254–256.

35 Frost, E. A. M. "Tracing the tracheostomy." *Ann Otol Rhinol Laryngol* 1976;85:618–624.

36 Stemmer, E. A., Oliver, C., Carey, J. P., and Connolly, J. E. "Fatal complications of tracheotomy." *Am J Surg* 1976;131:288–290.

37 Spaite, D. W., and Joseph, M. "Prehospital cricothyrotomy: An investigation of indications, technique, complications, and patient outcome." *Ann Emerg Med* 1990;19:279–285.

38 Rosen, P., Dinerman, N., and Pons, P. "The technical imperative: Its definition and an application to prehospital care." *Topics Emerg Med* 1981; 2:79–86.

39 Spaite, D. W., and Joseph M. "Prehospital cricothyrotomy: An investigation of indications, technique, complications and patient outcome." *Ann Emerg Med* 1990;19:279–285.

40 Rosen, P., Dinerman, N., and Pons, P. "The technical imperative: Its definition and an application to prehospital care." *Topics Emerg Med* 1981; 2:79–86.

41 Heffner, J. E., Miller K. S., and Sahn, S. A. "Tracheostomy in the intensive care unit: Part 1. Indications, technique, management." *Chest* 1986,90; 269–274.

42 Zetouni, A., and Kost, K. "Tracheostomy: A retrospective review of 281 cases." *J Otolaryngol* 1994;23:61–66.

[43] Whited, R. E. "A prospective study of laryngotracheal sequelae in long term intubation." *Laryngoscope* 1984;94:367–377.

[44] Tracheostomy. *http://medicine.creighton.edu/forpatients/trache/trache.html.* Accessed March 5, 2001.

[45] Soriano, S. G., Kim, C., and Jones, D. T. "Surgical airway, rigid bronchoscopy, and transtracheal jet ventilation in the pediatric patient." *Anes Clin NA.* 1998;16:827.

[46] Hackeling, T., Triana R., Ma O. J., and Shockley, W. "Emergency care of patients with tracheostomies: A 7-year review." *Am J. Emerg Med* 1998; 16:681.

Chapter **Nine**

Rapid Sequence Intubation

Philosophy

Intubation of the adult larynx and trachea is taught in every ACLS course and is required of every emergency provider. The minimal morbidity associated with short-term intubation justifies the procedure in most critically ill patients. Until recently, the procedure was either limited to moribund patients or the emergency provider was quite limited in the tools available to control movement and sedate the patient. (This state of affairs sadly applied to most emergency physicians as few as 10 years ago!) On the emergency provider's arrival, the patient could range from frankly moribund to simply "running out of steam," so 4 to 6 minutes could represent a very optimistic constraint before the patient finally ceased to breathe. When the patient was combative or awake, the clinician could choose to delay rather than risk a failed intubation. This delay was often to the patient's detriment. The reasons for this delay have completely changed with the technique known as RSI—Rapid Sequence Intubation. The proven effectiveness of this technique in the emergency department has swept most other techniques aside over the past 10 years.[1] The field application of RSI started first with air ambulance services, followed shortly by selected ground based ambulance services.

Rapid sequence intubation (RSI) is defined as the rapid (nearly simultaneous) administration of both a neuromuscular blocking agent and a potent sedative agent to facilitate intubation while decreasing the risks of aspiration, combativeness, and potential damage to the patient. It is the ultimate in emergency provider control, since when properly done, the patient literally can no longer breathe without the emergency provider.

RSI is the cornerstone of modern emergency airway management. There is ample evidence that both pediatric and adult patients emergently intubated with the principles of RSI have both lower complication rates and higher success rates than with all other techniques.

There are three major assumptions inherent in RSI. Every emergency provider MUST realize that the assumptions are an integral part of the technique.

1. The Patient Has a Full Stomach

Since emergency patients are rarely so considerate as to present with an empty stomach, a major precept of RSI is that the patient is about to vomit. Furthermore, the majority of these same patients present after receiving bag-valve-mask oxygen therapy and subsequent gastric distention. Since unconscious patients have decreased laryngeal closure reflexes and decreased lower esophageal sphincter tone, this further predisposes the patient to regurgitation and aspiration.[2] The mortality of regurgitation and subsequent aspiration is between 30 percent and 70 percent.[3 4] For those who don't die, the hospital stay is about three weeks, most of which is in the ICU. The technique of RSI is designed to prevent this major problem. While apnea can be managed by a period of bag-valve-mask ventilation and failure to intubate can be managed by a surgical airway, the risk of aspiration cannot be ignored.

2. The Operator Can Secure an Airway

Some form of airway can be secured even if the initial attempt(s) at intubation are not successful. The operator must be competent with bag-valve-mask ventilation. If the operator can't guarantee an airway, it will be fatal to the patient and a career limiting move for the operator.

FAILURE IS NOT AN OPTION!

Intrinsic to this assumption is the secondary postulate that the operator knows all of the available equipment, has it immediately available, and can both size it and employ it rapidly. This means that the operator is intimately familiar with several alternative airway devices and has *immediate* access to them. The operator must also be trained, willing, and appropriately credentialed to perform a cricothyrotomy in the event of a failed airway.

3. The Operator Can Resuscitate the Patient

Again, failure is not an option. If you don't have the equipment and knowledge for a full resuscitation of the patient, you shouldn't be taking away critical survival drives.

Rapid sequence induction is a very similar technique used by our anesthesiology colleagues to rapidly deliver general anesthesia in similarly unprepared patients at risk for aspiration of stomach contents. The anesthesia emphasis is on continued sedation and induction of general anesthesia once intubation is accomplished. Emergency medicine focuses on the procedure of intubation and maintenance of an airway and removes much of the sedation immediately following intubation. There is a significant difference in the use of paralytics and sedation to facilitate intubation and using them as the first steps in anesthesia (Figure 9-1).

There is no advantage to using RSI in the deeply comatose patient or the patient who has cardiac arrest. In every other patient, RSI is faster and safer than any alternative technique.[5 6 7 8] RSI should be considered in every nonarrested patient requiring emergency intubation.

In the patient with potentially increased intracranial pressure (ICP), RSI blunts further ICP increases due to laryngoscopy, coughing, or struggling during the intubation.

Contraindications to Rapid Sequence Intubation
- Spontaneous breathing with adequate ventilation
- Operator concern that both intubation and mask ventilation may not be successful
- Major laryngotracheal trauma
- Upper airway obstruction (such as epiglottitis)
- Distorted facial or airway anatomy
- Operator unfamiliarity with the medications used

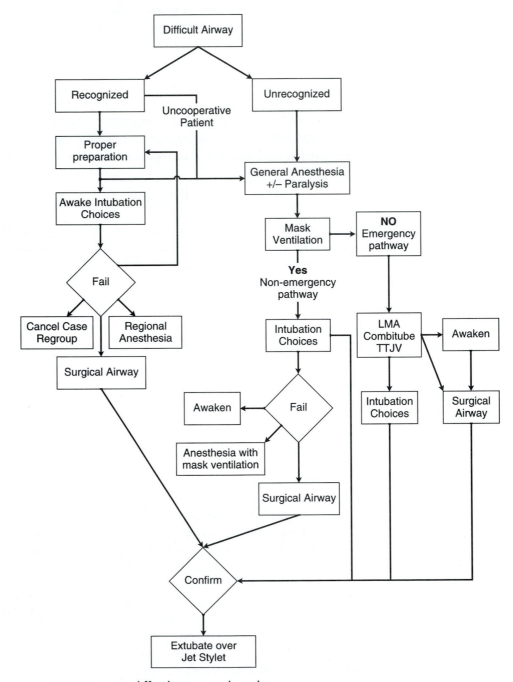

Figure 9-1 ASA difficult airway algorithm.

In these cases, the physician or paramedic should NOT paralyze the patient. If necessary, a surgical airway would be appropriate.

Procedure: Ten-Step RIS Technique

1. Assess the Risks

Ensure that at least the AMPLE history is available, if possible (Allergies, Medications, Past medical history, Last meal, Existing circumstances). The intubating physician or clinician should personally examine the neck, face, head, nose, throat, and chest, even when a full surgical team approach is used for resuscitation (Figure 9-2).

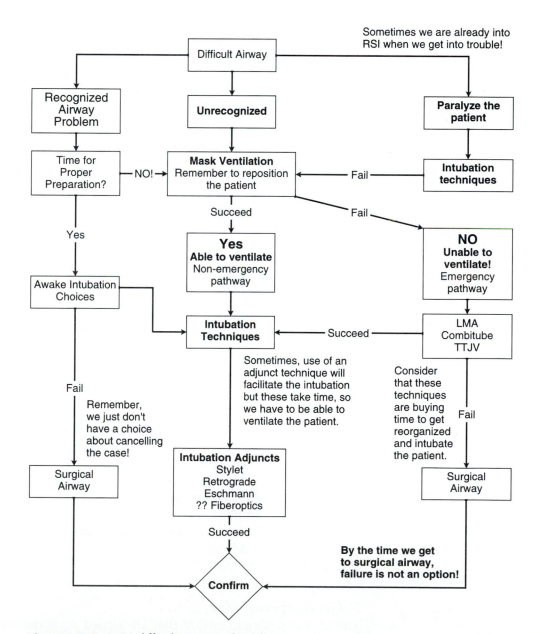

Figure 9-2 EMS difficult airway algorithm.

Conditions that can lead to problems with intubation include cervical immobilization, limited mouth opening, big tongue, high arched palate, buck teeth, receding chin, reduced submandibular space with little possibility to displace the tongue, thick neck, and, of course, the disrupted airway from blunt trauma to the face and neck. (See discussion in Special Problems section.) Distortion of anatomy or a requirement for a specific position to maintain upper airway patency may cause significant problems with rapid sequence intubation, particularly in patients who are dependent on upper-airway muscle tone or specific positioning to maintain the patency of the airway.

Ten-Step Technique for RSI

1. Assess the risks
2. Get equipment ready
3. Monitor the patient
4. Preoxygenate the patient
5. Medicate the patient
6. Sedation/Paralysis
7. Sellick's maneuver/BURP maneuver
8. Intubate the patient
9. Verify placement
10. Secure the tube

RSI Time Sequence—Depolarizing Route

T-5 min	Preparation
T-3 min	Oxygenation
T-2 min	Premedication
T-30 sec	Sedation
T-30 sec	Succinylcholine
T-15 sec	Cricoid pressure
T = 0	Intubation
T + 30 sec	Tube placement confirmation
T + 1 min	Additional sedation
T + 1 min	Additional paralysis

RSI Time Sequence—Nondepolarizing Route

T-5 min	Preparation
T-3 min	Oxygenation
T-2 min	Premedication
T-90 sec	Nondepolarizing agent
T-30 sec	Cricoid pressure
T-30 sec	Sedation pressure
T = 0	Intubation
T + 30 sec	Tube placement confirmation
T + 1 min	Additional sedation
T + 1 min	Additional paralysis

2. Get equipment ready

The operator should ensure that all needed equipment is opened, laid out, and fully functional before any medications are given to the patient.

Minimum immediately available equipment includes

- Appropriately sized bag-valve-mask with reservoir
- Suction (fully hooked up and working)
- Oxygen (hooked up to a bag-valve-mask)
- Laryngoscope with appropriately sized blades and functioning lights
- Appropriately sized endotracheal tubes (Have immediately available at least one size above and below the predicted size)
- Stylet for the endotracheal tube
- Stethoscope
- All pharmaceutical agents to be used in the procedure
- Alternative airway equipment at the operator's side

Equipment for an alternative airway should always be readily available in the immediate vicinity of the intubator. For an adult, this would mean that a cricothyrotomy kit is kept in the intubation kit. In the pediatric population, this should include both cricothyrotomy equipment for older children and jet ventilation equipment. Depending on the experience of the operator, an appropriately sized laryngeal mask airway could also be used.

This procedure should not be done solo. The operator must have an appropriate number of assistants to aid with the drugs, position the patient, and apply Sellick's maneuver. In patients with a possible spinal injury, the operator must have a dedicated assistant who can maintain in-line stabilization of the cervical spine throughout the entire procedure.

3. Monitor the patient

Cardiorespiratory monitoring is essential for all patients who are ill enough to need intubation. Heart monitoring, pulse oximetry, and blood pressure monitoring should be readily available for every responder who contemplates RSI (Figures 9-3–9-4). These monitors should be used as a routine measure in every patient where intubation is even considered as a possible procedure.

Cardiac monitoring may alert the operator to bradycardia, tachycardia, or dysrhythmia in apneic patients. Pulse oximetry is the best monitoring device available to show the operator if the patient develops hypoxia during an

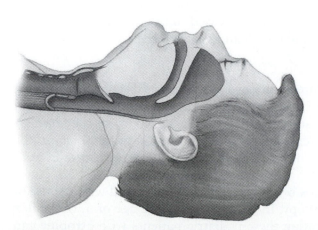

Figure 9-3 Sellicks maneuver.

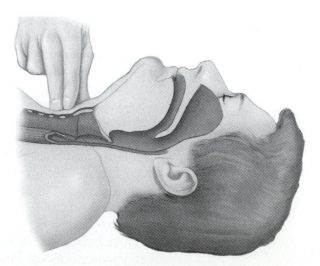

Figure 9-4 Sellicks maneuver with pressure.

intubation attempt. Unsuspected hypotension may be revealed with automated blood pressure monitoring.

4. Pre-oxygenate the patient

Once the patient is paralyzed, respirations slowly decrease until the patient is apneic. During this time, the patient can rapidly desaturate.

Preoxygenation replaces the patient's functional residual capacity of the lung with oxygen and washes out the nitrogen. This gives a limited time of security if the patient is apneic during the RSI sequence. If the patient is placed on 100 percent oxygen as soon as intubation is considered, then the patient has already been preoxygenated prior to the intubation.

In adults, preoxygenation will permit as much as 8 minutes of apnea before hypoxia develops. The child may not be able to tolerate apnea as long as an adult due to the smaller functional residual capacity and the higher basal oxygen consumption of the child. Medically compromised and obese patients also have a shortened window before desaturation occurs, often less than 3 minutes.

Even when rapid intubation is essential, simply asking the patient to take four or five deep breaths on a nonrebreather mask will remove much of the nitrogen and replace it with oxygen. In the unconscious patient, applying four fully assisted BVM with 100 percent oxygen will serve the same purpose. At least this much should be done in all patients to be intubated.

Rise of the $PaCO_2$ in apnea is not usually a significant concern unless the patient has a head injury or is severely compromised prior to the intubation. $PaCO_2$ will rise at about 3 mm Hg/min when the patient is apneic.

Ordinarily, a bag and mask should not be used to artificially ventilate the patient. Ventilations may be assisted in synchrony with natural respirations. When the patient is adequately preoxygenated, there is no need to forcibly ventilate the patient just prior to intubation. This habit markedly increases the risk of gastric insufflation and subsequent regurgitation. If bagging is necessary because of a failed intubation, then cricoid pressure should be continued at all times.

5. Medicate the patient

The first medications given should reduce the physiologic responses of the patient to the subsequent intubation. These responses include bradycardia, tachycardia, hypertension, hypoxia, increased intracranial pressure, increased intraocular pressure, and cough and gag reflexes.

Bradycardia

Infants and young children can develop profound bradycardia during intubation from medication effects, vagal stimulation, and hypoxia. Vagal stimulation may occur from stimulation of the oropharynx by the laryngoscope blade. Succinylcholine can also produce profound bradycardia in the infant. Hypoxia, of course, can rapidly cause profound bradycardia in both the infant and child.

Atropine blocks the reflex bradycardia that is associated with the use of succinylcholine and laryngoscopy. In children under the age of 5, this reflex is more pronounced. Pre-treating these pediatric patients with atropine can minimize vagal effects.[9][10] The appropriate dose is 0.02 mg/kg to a maximum of 1 mg. Even in the very small child, a minimum dose of at least 0.1 mg should be used. For effect at the time of intubation, atropine should be administered at least 2 minutes prior to intubation.

Pressor Response

The pressor response was first described in 1951. It is a transient increase in the blood pressure and pulse rate occurring as a response to stimulation of the oropharynx, larynx, and/or trachea. The pressor response can occur with any manipulation or instrumentation of the upper airway.

The pressor response usually peaks about 45 seconds after instrumentation and lasts about 5 minutes. The magnitude of blood pressure rise and tachycardia is greatest in those patients who have prior hypertensive disease (even when they have been properly treated).

In addition to the tachycardia, numerous reports of short runs of ventricular arrhythmias have been reported in conjunction with intubation. Whether these are due to the pressor response or to the transient decrease in arterial oxygen associated with intubation is uncertain.

EKG changes associated with ischemia have been reported in patients who have marked increases in blood pressure.[11][12] Although it is probably prudent to avoid an increase in blood pressure in the unstable patient with acute cardiac disease or atherosclerosis, there is little evidence that this response is of any clinical significance in most patients intubated in an emergency department.

Multiple drugs and drug regimens have been adopted to blunt the pressure response. These drugs have included atropine, lidocaine, fentanyl, barbiturates, beta blockers, and benzodiazepines.[13][14][15][16] Many of these drugs are not appropriate for emergency use since they may require administration more than 5 minutes before intubation for useful effect (Figure 9-5). Lidocaine intravenously has been advocated, but randomized studies show no effect when lidocaine is given by either intravenous or tropical routes.[17] Fentanyl may be appropriate in small doses.

There is little evidence that the suppression of the pressor response is needed, appropriate, or warranted. There are, quite simply, no studies that have connected the pressor response with any clinical deterioration of the patient, even when large patient populations are studied. The prudent intubator will reserve use of drugs designed to blunt the pressor response to those patients where a rise in the blood pressure will be detrimental—such as in an abdominal aortic aneurysm.

Intracranial Pressure Increase

Lidocaine has been shown to blunt the rise in ICP associated with intubation, although this is somewhat controversial.[18] It also decreases the cough reflex and may decrease the incidence of postlaryngoscopy hypertension and tachycardia.[19] Lidocaine may be ineffective in blunting hypertension or tachycardia associated with intubation. The recommended dose of lidocaine is 1.5 mg/kg to 3 mg/kg intravenously. As with atropine, lidocaine must be given at least 2 minutes prior to intubation in order to be effective. Alternatively, lidocaine may be sprayed into the posterior pharynx and trachea. Again, this is somewhat controversial, as spraying lidocaine into the trachea may require almost as much manipulation as intubation itself.

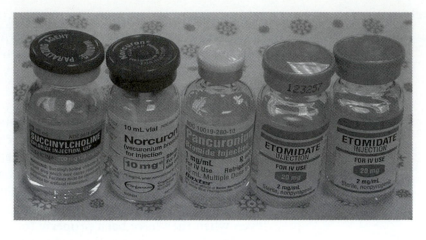

Figure 9-5 Usual RSI drugs
Source: Photo by Charles Stewart and Associates; www.storysmith.net.

Attenuation of adverse CV and ICP responses is certainly optional in moribund and desperate situations.

6. Sedation and Paralysis

Multiple agents have been used for sedation during the process of intubation, including barbiturates, benzodiazepines, opiates, nonbarbiturate sedatives, and dissociative agents. Each of these agents has their proponents, relative indications, contraindications, and detractors. The ideal sedative should induce rapid unconsciousness with short duration and little or no cardiovascular side effects. The ideal agent does not yet exist.

The sedative agent of choice should be given prior to the paralytic agent. Although sedatives and paralytics can be given at the same time, paralysis is such a frightening event that sedation should be assured prior to the onset of paralysis.

Table 9-1 lists commonly used sedatives for RSI. Any of these sedating agents will produce acceptable results in RSI when used at the recommended dose. The choice of sedative agent is based on the clinical state of the patient and effects of medication.

Opiates

The newer synthetic opioid agonists (fentanyl family), which include fentanyl, sufentanil, and alfentanil, are respectively 100, 500 to 1000, and 20 times more potent than morphine.[20] They are fast-acting, having an onset of action of less than 1 minute, and their duration of action is between 15 and 60 minutes.

Fentanyl is a rapid-acting and very potent opiate of relatively short duration. Fentanyl is about 50 to 100 times as potent as morphine. It produces analgesia within 90 seconds with an effective duration of about 30 minutes. Fentanyl results in little or no histamine release, and its cardiovascular effects in the normal host are minimal. Fentanyl has gained widespread popularity in emergency medicine as a fast-acting analgesic and is often used in conscious sedation. For unclear reasons, it has also become used as an induction agent in emergency medicine.[21 22] It has significant problems when used in this role.

TABLE 9-1 RSI DRUGS

Barbiturates and Sedatives

Drug	Dosage	Onset	Duration	Disadvantages
Thiopental	1–5 mg/kg	10–20 seconds	10–30 minutes	Hypotension, Bronchospasm, Porphyria
Methohexital	1–2 mg/kg	<1 minute	5–7 minutes	Hypotension
Propofol	2–3 mg/kg	<1 minute	10–15 minutes	Hypotension
Etomidate	0.2–0.3 mg/kg	<1 minute	1 minute	Cortisol suppression, Vomiting

Thiopental is contraindicated in hypotension, porphyria, and bronchospasm. Thiopental, propofol, and entomidate all decrease intracranial pressure. Thiopental, propofol, and etomidate all decrease the blood pressure. Methohexital may cause seizures in high doses. Thiopental, propofol, and etomidate all exhibit anticonvulsant activity. Propofol is particularly useful for precise sedation. It is titratable as a drip. Propofol is amnestic.

Fentanyl can induce unconsciousness, but it is not an ideal induction agent in the trauma setting. The doses required to induce sedation are extremely variable and if high enough may cause unwanted side effects in the critically ill patient. Depending on the existing state of consciousness and the presence of alcohol or other depressants, the dose necessary to produce unconsciousness can range from 2 μg/kg to 20 μg/kg or more. In one series of patients, many of the patients were able to follow commands and could recall the events surrounding the intubation.[23] A small number of patients were unable to be intubated after receiving 500 micrograms of fentanyl.

The usual recommended dose of fentanyl is 1 μg/kg to 5 μg/kg given 1–3 minutes prior to intubation. A higher dose of 5 μg/kg to 7 μg/kg is indicated to block hypertension and tachycardia and some authorities suggest as much as 25 μg/kg. Neonates appear to be more sensitive to fentanyl, and smaller doses should be used. Administration of large doses of fentanyl is generally impractical for emergency intubation. It is time consuming and may produce a longer period of coma than may be desirable.

Like all opiates, fentanyl causes respiratory depression in a dose-dependent response. The effect of fentanyl on ventilation varies, but doses above 2 μg/kg cause respiratory depression in "normal" subjects. This incidence is even higher when used together with other drugs. This respiratory depression may induce apnea before the patient is paralyzed. Fentanyl induced respiratory depression may be easily reversed with narcotic antagonists such as naloxone.

Fentanyl may cause seizures, chest wall rigidity, and skeletal muscle movements. The muscular rigidity can be prevented with either succinylcholine, a nondepolarizing paralytic, or naloxone. This complication typically occurs when doses greater than 15 μg/kg are used.[24]

Fentanyl has been touted as a valuable preinduction adjunct in intubation of the head-injured patient because of its ability to attentuate the hemodynamic response to intubation. Although effective, when given in sufficient doses to achieve this, increased ICP has been noted. There are other reports of increased ICP in children associated with fentanyl. Fentanyl should be used with caution when ICP is a major factor. This increase in ICP has also been shown with sufentanil and alfentanil administration.[25] Coupled with the tendency to produce premature apnea, the ICP rise makes the use of fentanyl as a sedative agent for RSI controversial.[26]

In addition to its profound sedative and analgesic effects, fentanyl may decrease the tachycardia and hypertension associated with intubation. It appears to be well tolerated hemodynamically with little hypotension in most patients. At higher doses, however, small but potentially significant decreases in blood pressure may occur.

The best role for fentanyl in trauma airway management may be to provide titrated sedation after intubation and analgesia to attenuate hyperdynamic responses from pain and intubation and to make continued intubation and ventilation more tolerable.

Since many of the side effects of fentanyl occur when higher doses of this agent are given, it may be preferable to use a small dose of fentanyl for analgesia, together with both a paralytic agent and a sedative such as midazolam for amnesia. Since other available agents provide both analgesia and amnesia with a single dose, fentanyl is less than optimum for intubation.

Morphine in a dose of 0.1 mg/kg to 0.2 mg/kg has also been used as sedation for RSI. Morphine has both a longer duration of action and a longer onset time than fentanyl. It takes as much as 3–5 minutes for morphine to adequately sedate the patient. In addition, morphine may not blunt the rise in ICP, tachycardia, or hypertension as well as fentanyl. The use of morphine in the management of the trauma airway is discouraged because of its effect on histamine release, which may result in hypotension.

Morphine is not recommended for RSI in the field because of the longer onset time and the failure to blunt tachycardia or hypertension.[27]

Barbiturates and Other Hypnotic Agents
Thiopental (Pentothal) is a short-acting barbiturate with an onset of 10–20 seconds and a duration of 5–10 minutes when given intravenously in a dose of 2 mg/kg to 5 mg/kg. There is abundant emergency and anesthesiology experience with thiopental. Although thiopental is a sedative, there is no analgesic effect.

The barbiturates are central nervous system depressants and are capable of producing the full range of CNS effects, from mild sedation through deep coma. They cause a concomitant decrease in intracranial pressure, intracerebral blood flow, and cerebral oxygen consumption. For this reason, the barbiturates are often considered the agent of choice for anesthesia induction in the patient with elevated intracranial pressure.

Unfortunately, thiopental has significant adverse hemodynamic effects and should not be used when the patient's volume status is unknown. It is a potent myocardial depressant and a strong vasodilator. These effects combine to produce marked hypotension when the patient is volume depleted. In fact, thiopental may induce profound hypotension in a patient who has otherwise compensated for a marginal amount of hypotension. Like all sedatives, thiopental causes respiratory depression.

As noted, thiopental is considered most useful in the patient with increased ICP (head trauma, meningitis) as it does not increase the intracranial pressure.

Unfortunately, if the patient is hypotensive, cerebral blood flow is compromised. This decreases the usefulness of thiopental in trauma intubations.

Thiopental also should not be used for patients with asthma as it may cause additional bronchospasm by release of histamine.

The side effects of hypotension and bronchospasm limit the usefulness of the barbiturates in the prehospital arena. These agents should probably be reserved for ED intubation, and then only when significant clinical information is known about the patient.

The usual dose of thiopental is 5 mg/kg, although authors that suggest using it for RSI also recommend lowering the dose to 1 mg/kg–3 mg/kg in patients with suspected hypovolemia or tenuous cardiac reserves.

Methohexital is a short acting barbiturate with onset in under 1 minute and duration of about 5–7 minutes when given in an intravenous dose of 1–1.5 mg/kg. Methohexital is quite similar to thiopental in action and contraindications. It definitely causes respiratory depression and may cause seizures in high doses.

The side effects of methohexital and thiopental limit their usefulness in prehospital care.

Etomidate is an ultrashort-acting, carboxylated imidazole, nonbarbiturate hypnotic agent that has been used as an induction agent for anesthesia for years.[28] The usual dose is 0.2–0.4 mg/kg intravenously. It is rapidly effective within the arm to brain circulation time. It is ideally suited to be used with succinylcholine as the onset of action and duration of action are essentially the same. It is probably the best all-around choice as an induction agent for RSI and can be used in the overwhelming majority of ED patients.[29]

Etomidate has minimal hemodynamic effects and may be the drug of choice in a hypotensive or trauma patient.[30] It causes less cardiovascular depression than either the barbiturates or propofol.[31] Etomidate has been shown to decrease intracranial pressure, cerebral blood flow, and cerebral oxygen metabolism.[32]

Etomidate may decrease cortisol synthesis somewhat with a single dose, but this effect is more marked when the drug is used for an extended period of time.[33][34] This appears to be of little clinical significance. In appropriate patients, steroid replacement may be used to offset this action.

A significant advantage of etomidate is that it is a noncontrolled substance and does not need to be locked up with the narcotics. This is of significant utility to the prehospital provider. It also comes in preloaded syringes, making rapid administration easily accomplished. For these reasons, etomidate is probably the sedative drug of choice for prehospital RSI.

Propofol is a relatively new anesthetic induction and sedative agent. It has an extremely rapid induction time, within 10 to 20 seconds, and a short duration of action, 10–15 minutes, when given in a dose of 1–3 mg/kg intravenously. It is a modified phenol, which has profound solubility in lipids but not in water. Because of the high lipid solubility, the drug is prepared as an emulsion in lethicin. It is a milky white infusion.

The lipid solubility accounts for much of the drug's mechanism of action. Lipid soluble drugs rapidly cross the blood-brain barrier and are distributed through the entire central nervous system. The onset of action is generally one circulation time between heart and brain. Propofol appears to exert its action by infiltrating the lipid bilayer of the nerve cell membrane and disrupting nerve conduction. Unfortunately, the drug will move out of the central nervous system equally quickly. As the drug is redistributed through the body, it is dissolved in adipose tissue and the concentration in the CNS rapidly drops.[35][36]

Although RSI is well described with this agent, it is unlikely that propofol will be carried by most EMS services. The apnea produced by rapid injection of propofol is a profound limiting factor in prehospital use.[37]

Propofol decreases intracranial pressure and cerebral metabolism.[38] It may cause significant hypotension, which limits usefulness in trauma patients. It does not cause myocardial depression. Propofol's hypotension seems to be a complex interaction with the entire cardiovascular system. Lower doses can be used for patients with unstable blood pressure.

Propofol is an anticonvulsant and may be a drug of choice for status epilepticus.[39] Unlike many other sedatives, propofol is also an antiemetic.

Unlike other agents, propofol can be used as a drip for continued sedation after the procedure. The continued sedation dose is 0.15–0.75 mg/kg/min.

Benzodiazepines

Benzodiazepines (diazepam and midazolam) have been used alone and in combination with narcotics, as RSI sedative agents. The benzodiazepines provide good anxiolysis and amnesia for the procedure. Unfortunately, large doses of benzodiazepines are usually needed to produce adequate sedation. No analgesia is provided by the benzodiazepines.

The effects of the benzodiazepines are generally not as reliable for RSI as the hypnotic agents. Even at doses of 0.3 mg/kg, induction with midazolam is not always predictable. Benzodiazepines are most useful as an adjunct to provide retrograde amnesia of the procedure in the previously awake patient or as agents in the patient with ongoing seizures. Benzodiazepines have little effect on the intracerebral pressure.

All of the benzodiazepines are reversible with flumazenil. This may be particularly dangerous to do if there is any history of seizures or seizure-prone injury, disease, or overdose. The wise practitioner who uses flumazenil al-

TABLE 9-2

Benzodiazepines

Drug	Dosage	Onset	Duration	Disadvantages
Midazolam	0.1–0.3 mg/kg	1–2 minutes	30–60 minutes	Slow onset, wildly variable dosage range
Diazepam	0.25–0.4 mg/kg	2–4 minutes	30–90 minutes	Variable dosage range

Both midazolam and diazepam are amnestic, have excellent anticonvulsant activity, and are reversible with flumazenil. Neither agent has any analgesic effect. Both can be irritating as intravenous injections. Hypotension is rare with both. There is little effect on the ICP with either agent.

ways remembers that the half-life of flumazenil is considerably shorter than most benzodiazepines.

Benzodiazepines should not be used as the sedative for EMS intubation as the effects are both relatively unpredictable and better agents can be found. Benzodiazepines may be effectively used in field RSI for their amnestic effects after the patient has been successfully intubated.

Diazepam is a moderately long-acting benzodiazepine (30–90 minutes) with slow onset (2–4 minutes). The usual dose is 0.2–1.0 mg/kg given intravenously. Effectively a dose of 5–15 mg in the adult will usually provide adequate sedation for intubation.

As with all of the benzodiazepines, hypotension is a real problem, but diazepam may be the worst of the three presented here. It usually causes less cardiovascular and respiratory depression than the barbiturates. If alcohol is present, the respiratory depression of diazepam is augmented.

Diazepam must be titrated, as the effective induction dose is quite variable. Diazepam is more useful as a long-term sedative agent for the intubated patient after the procedure. Diazepam has significant amnestic effects.

Diazepam is irritating to veins and may cause localized thrombosis. Do not use diazepam in a patient with glaucoma.

Lorazepam (0.1–0.4 mg/kg) is a long-acting benzodiazepine. The maximal onset of sedation occurs 15–20 minutes after injection, so it has little use as sedation for RSI unless the intubation can be planned well in advance. It is the most useful drug for long-term sedation of the intubated patient.

Blood pressure effects of lorazepam are minimal. Smaller doses should be used in the elderly.

Midazolam (0.1–0.4 mg/kg IV) is a rapid onset and short-acting benzodiazepine (30–60 min) with potent amnestic effects. Midazolam is the most commonly used benzodiazepine for airway management and is two to four times as potent as diazepam.

Midazolam is faster in onset, shorter in action, and has a narrower dose range than either lorazepam or diazepam. An induction dose of midazolam takes effect within 1 to 2 minutes and has a duration of action of between 30 and 60 minutes. Midazolam may require 3 to 5 minutes for complete effect. The typical RSI dose is much higher than a dose used for sedation and still may not be reliably effective in 0.3 mg/kg dose. It is slower in onset than the hypnotic agents and should be administered at least 2 minutes before intubation is attempted. This limits its use in many emergency intubation situations.

Midazolam causes respiratory and cardiovascular depression, even in the recommended RSI dose.[40] The recommended RSI dose can be accompanied by side effects such as severe respiratory depression (even more than equivalent doses of thiopental). Significant decreases in blood pressure and cardiac contractility can occur, especially in patients with hypovolemia or heart disease. All these effects are more pronounced when opioids are given simultaneously.

Midazolam does not increase ICP and may provide some small decrease in cerebral blood flow.

Neuroleptic Agents

Ketamine The only neuroleptic agent that is useful in intubation is ketamine, closely related to the illicit drug PCP (phencyclidine).[41] Ketamine is often described as a dissociative anesthetic, where the patient may appear to be awake but is amnestic and unresponsive to pain.

Its onset of action is within 1 minute when given intravenously, and its duration of action ranges from 5 to 15 minutes.[42 43] Unless given rapidly, apnea does not occur. It is slower in action when given intramuscularly and will last slightly longer. This is advantageous when rapid control of the patient without venous access is needed. The IV dose of ketamine for RSI in children is 2 mg/kg. Some authorities feel that children who are sedated with ketamine should be also treated with atropine to reduce the secretions, but this opinion is not universal.

In contrast to the other sedative agents, ketamine increases the cardiac output, pulse rate, blood pressure, myocardial oxygen consumption, cerebral blood flow, intraocular pressure, and possibly intracranial pressure.[44] Although it is a direct myocardial depressant, it causes a release of endogenous catecholamines resulting in the positive overall effects. Heart rate and blood pressure are usually maintained or increased because of centrally mediated sympathetic stimulation. Indeed, ketamine may cause hypertension. This effect is enhanced when other adrenergic agents are given, or the patient has been using cocaine.

There are two major advantages to the use of ketamine. First, ketamine's release of endogenous catecholamines relaxes bronchial smooth muscle. This makes ketamine ideal for intubation of the COPD or asthmatic patient, as both a bronchodilator and a sedative. It is the sedative choice in the asthmatic patient with respiratory failure.[45 46] The other major advantage of ketamine is in the setting of the hypovolemic patient, especially when the heart is directly involved, such as in pericardial tamponade or cardiogenic shock. Ketamine provides the most cardiovascular and respiratory support of any agent.

TABLE 9-3

Opiates				
Drug	Dosage	Onset	Duration	Disadvantages
Morphine	0.1–0.2 mg/kg	2–5 minutes	4–6 hours	Histamine reaction
Fentanyl	2–10 mcg/kg	<1 minute	30–60 minutes	Variable effect on ICP, chest wall rigidity
Alfentanyl	10–20 mcg/kg	<1 minute	~1 hour	? increased ICP

Fentanyl can produce sedation in the 2–3 μg/kg dose but to block sympathetic responses a dose of 5–7 μg/kg is required. The action of fentanyl on ICP is controversial, and there are conflicting studies in the literature. They do seem to indicate that fentanyl may increase ICP. Morphine is not as effective in blunting the sympathetic response to intubation.

TABLE 9-4				
Neuroleptic Agents				
Drug	**Dosage**	**Onset**	**Duration**	
Ketamine	1–4 mg/kg	<1 minute	10–20 minutes	Increases ICP, increases secretions

Ketamine is amnestic and hallucinogenic. A bronchodilator, it is particularly useful in the asthmatic patient. Atropine is often used with this agent. It is useful in hypotension because sympathetic stimulation will increase blood pressure. Ketamine should not be used in the presence of increased intracranial pressure, hypertension, glaucoma, and open eye injuries.

It should be readily available for the EMS provider who performs rapid sequence intubation.

Ketamine also increases salivary and bronchial secretions.[47] Secretions can be decreased with atropine 0.01 mg/kg or glycopyrrolate 0.005 mg/kg. A usual dose of glycopyrrolate is 0.2 mg or 0.4 mg.

Ketamine causes awakening (emergence) hallucinations that many adults find unpleasant.[48] These emergence reactions occur in up to 50 percent of adults but are rare in children under 10 years of age.[49] They may be readily abolished with concomitant use of a benzodiazepine. If the drug is being used as a pure sedative as an adjunct for a painful procedure, this may be of some concern. When ketamine is used for RSI, it may be followed with a longer-acting sedative such as lorazepam, which will prevent an emergence reaction.

The disadvantages of ketamine are few. It may result in worsening hypotension if given to patients who are either sympathetically depleted or those who have severe coronary artery disease and may not tolerate increased myocardial oxygen consumption. Administration of any sedative agent in this setting is hazardous.

Ketamine increases upper airway secretions. This effect is easily controlled by administration of a single dose of atropine (0.02 mg/kg, minimum dose 0.15 mg) prior to the use of ketamine.

The biggest concern over the use of ketamine is its potential to affect ICP secondary to its ability to increase cerebral blood flow by 30 percent to 60 percent. It is currently contraindicated in head injury due to both increased oxygen consumption and increased intracranial pressure associated with ketamine.[50] It should be used with extreme caution in hypertensive patients (increases blood pressure) and those with open eye injuries and glaucoma (due to increased intraocular pressure). Ketamine may be an appropriate drug for the hypotensive unstable patient, however.

Even though the cerebral metabolic rate is increased with ketamine, cerebral blood flow is probably sufficient to meet demand. Evidence is accumulating that this increase in cerebral blood flow does not increase ICP.[51] In fact, there is growing evidence that ketamine is neuroprotective in head trauma.[52] As noted, there is reluctance to use ketamine when the patient has head injury. Ketamine may be useful when induction is needed in a profoundly hypotensive patient: Any reduction in mean arterial pressure is more likely to worsen cerebral ischemia than will a transient rise in ICP.

Depolarizing Neuromuscular Blocking Agents

The perfect paralytic agent would have an extremely rapid onset, a duration that is proportional to the dose used, have sedative, analgesic, and amnestic properties, be safe from age 1 hour to over 100 years, have minimal side effects, and not require any special storage. This agent does not yet exist. Current neuromuscular blocking agents may be either a depolarizing agent such as succinylcholine or a nondepolarizing agent such as pancuronium, rocuronium, or curare (very dated). None of these have sedative properties.

Use of neuromuscular blocking agents is controversial, with anesthesiologists fearing increased morbidity and mortality when nonanesthesiologists use these agents. The largest study to date in a community hospital with emergency physician intubation with these agents has not validated these concerns.[53] The only absolute contraindication to use of a neuromuscular blocking agent would be inability to manage the airway after making the patient apneic.

Succinylcholine is considered an ideal paralytic agent because of the rapid onset of action (within 45 seconds) and the short duration of the drug (4–10 minutes). Succinylcholine binds to acetylcholine receptors at the neuromuscular junction and stimulates depolarization of the muscle cell. The depolarization at the muscle can be witnessed by clinically visible muscle fasciculations. Unlike acetylcholine, succinylcholine produces continuous stimulation of the muscle cell. The muscle cell is unable to return to its resting state and paralysis occurs. The paralysis will wane when the succinylcholine is hydrolyzed by pseudocholinesterase.

TABLE 9-5

Neuromuscular Blocking Agents

Drug	Priming Dose	Effective Dose	Onset	Duration
Succinylcholine	.1 mg/kg	1.5 mg/kg IV	15–30 seconds	5–12 minutes
Vecuronium	0.01 mg/kg	.1–0.2 mg/kg	1–4 minutes	20–60 minutes
Mivacurium		.15–3 mg/kg	75–120 seconds	10–30 minutes
Rocuronium		.6–1.0 mg/kg	30–60 seconds	30–60 minutes
Pancuronium	0.01 mg/kg IV	0.1–0.2 mg/kg	120 seconds	45–90 minutes
Cisatracurium		0.15–0.2 mg/kg	90–120 seconds	60 minutes
Curare		0.6 mg/kg	2–6 minutes	45–90 minutes

Succinylcholine has multiple side effects. Curare has no vagolytic effects and may cause a histamine release. Vecuronium has no vagolytic effect or histamine release. It may have the fewest cardiovascular side effects. Consider use in open eye injuries. It has a very slow onset. Pancuronium causes increased heart rate, increased blood pressure, and is vagolytic. Rocuronium causes increased heart rate but few other cardiovascular effects. Mivacurium causes histamine release. Rocuronium and mivacurium are the fastest acting nondepolarizing agents. Duration of action of nondepolarizing agent is directly proportional to the dose used, with the exception of cisatracurium. Cisatracurium degrades with a set dose per minute (first order Hoffman pharmacokinetics). Cisatracurium is independent of liver and renal function.

Unfortunately, succinylcholine has significant side effects, largely related to the depolarization of the muscle cell.

Succinylcholine first will paralyze muscles that are easily fatigued, such as the eyelids. Loss of the blink reflex indicates that the succinylcholine is working properly. Unfortunately, the diaphragm is about the last muscle to be affected. This is important because the diaphragm is the major muscle involved in involuntary retching. Intubation conditions are predictable by paralysis of the jaw muscles, so check for jaw laxity before proceeding with intubation.

Contraindications to Succinylcholine

- Crush injury (more than three days following trauma)
- Burn (more than three days following trauma)
- Spinal trauma (more than three days following trauma)
- Paraplegia
- History or family history of malignant hyperthermia
- Pseudocholinesterase disease
- History or family history of neuromuscular disease
- Muscular dystrophy
- Myotonia
- Polyneuropathy
- Disuse atrophy
- Metastatic rhabdomyosarcoma
- Hyperkalemia
- Glaucoma (relative)
- Penetrating eye injuries (relative)
- Purpura fulminans
- Parkinson's disease (relative)

Complications from succinylcholine fall into three major categories: malignant hyperthermia, hyperkalemia, and extended paralysis. Potential ICP increases and penetrating eye injuries are not absolute contraindications for use of succinylcholine, but the operator should be well aware of these potential complications.

Hyperkalemia Perhaps the most clinically significant complication of succinylcholine is hyperkalemia. Although the effect has been documented for over 30 years, the precise mechanism of hyperkalemia is not yet known. It is currently thought to be due to an increased number of acetylcholine receptors in these patients. The acetylcholine receptors are found within the muscle membrane, not just at the neuromuscular junction. The increase in acetylcholine receptor sites occurs within 5 to 20 days after the development of the disease or injury. Succinylcholine can cause lethal hyperkalemia in patients with burns, crush injuries, abdominal infections, tetanus, muscle disorders, and denervation disorders.[54][55][56] Succinylcholine can be safely used in massive trauma, burns, spinal cord injuries, etc., if used within this five-day grace period.

This rise in potassium occurs to a lesser extent in normal patients. Usually, the elevation in potassium is on the order of 0.5 mEq/liter and is of no clinical significance. Obviously, patients with underlying hyperkalemia, such as renal failure patients, should not be given succinylcholine. Succinylcholine is best avoided in the patient with known renal failure unless the potassium has been measured and is known to be in the normal range.

Prolonged paralysis Succinylcholine can cause prolonged paralysis in patients who have a deficiency of pseudocholinesterase or an atypical pseudocholinesterase.[57] Several drugs have also been associated with prolonged paralysis including magnesium, lithium, and quindine.[58] Patients who are intoxicated with cocaine may have prolonged paralysis when given succinylcholine because cocaine is competitively metabolized by cholinesterase. The net effect of any disturbance in metabolism of succinylcholine is to prolong paralysis from 5–10 minutes to several hours. Although known pseudocholinesterase deficiency is a contraindication, the only complication would be prolongation of the paralysis.

Malignant hyperthermia Malignant hyperthermia is thought to occur from excessive calcium influx through open channels.[59] Since this condition occurs most frequently in a rare genetic disorder, succinylcholine should be avoided in any patient with a personal or family history of malignant hyperthermia. It is associated with markedly increased temperatures, metabolic acidosis, rhabdomyolysis, and disseminated intravascular coagulopathy. It is thought to occur once in every 15,000 patients given succinylcholine.[60] This problem has prompted the FDA to ban the use of succinylcholine in infants and children except in emergency situations.[61] If one suspects malignant hyperthermia after use of succinylcholine, then dantrolene 1 mg/kg should be given every 1–3 minutes up to 10 mg/kg. The patient must be adequately cooled with whatever means are available and appropriate. The patient requires high-flow oxygen therapy because of the increased metabolism caused by hyperthermia.

Increased intraocular pressure Succinylcholine causes a transient rise in intraocular pressure. Theoretically, this increased intraocular pressure could cause expulsion of the vitreous in an open eye injury. There has never been a documented case of this complication despite a widespread use in open eye surgery.[62] The prudent practitioner will use a nondepolarizing agent in penetrating eye injuries if readily available.

Increased intracranial pressure The significance of the rise in intracranial pressure that accompanies succinylcholine is controversial. The drug has been used widely and successfully in this setting. The rise in intracranial pressure is transient, and the overall benefit of the drug appears to outweigh the small transient rise in ICP.

The transient rise in pressure may be due to a direct effect of fasciculations, increased cerebral blood flow, or sympathetic stimulation. Pretreatment with a nondepolarizing agent will blunt this response.[63] Pretreatment may not be practical when intubation is urgent.

Muscle fasciculations Fasciculations are synchronous contractions of every muscle fiber. These fasciculations occur until paralysis sets in. Diffuse muscle pain is a common complaint after the use of succinylcholine. During fasciculations, gastric pressure increases, enhancing the risk of aspiration.[64] Fasciculations can be prevented by pretreatment with a small dose of a nondepolarizing agent, such as vecuronium, prior to the administration of succinylcholine.[65]

If intubation is not successful during the initial paralysis, a second dose of succinylcholine can be used in adolescents and adults. A repeated dose of succinylcholine in infants and small children may cause bradycardia and even asystole and should not be used.[66] Atropine should be available at the bedside whenever succinylcholine is administered.

Succinylcholine requires refrigeration. In an ambulance, this can be easily provided with a small, portable, electric-powered refrigerator stored in the back of the ambulance. The refrigerator can also be used to store other drugs that are sensitive to the heat.

Succinylcholine should be available to every EMS provider who uses RSI. This may change, as newer nondepolarizing agents become readily available.

Nondepolarizing Neuromuscular Blocking Agents

The nondepolarizing neuromuscular blocking agents bind in a competitive nonstimulatory fashion to the α-submit of the acetylcholine receptor. Because there is no muscle stimulation prior to paralysis, these agents do not produce fasciculations. Three types of nondepolarizing drugs are available: benzylisoquinoliniums, aminosteroids, and quaternary amines. Of these, only the benzylisoquinoliniums and aminosteroids are used in RSI.

Although usually not needed in the emergency department, nondepolarizing agents can be reversed by use of an anticholinesterase agent, such as edrophonium or neostigmine. Reversal may take several minutes. The wise emergency provider should not depend on reversal in the "can't intubate, can't ventilate" scenario.

> *Drugs that last a long time tend to last far longer when you really want (or need) the patient to breathe on her or his own.*

The newer nondepolarizing agents (vecuronium, rocuronium, and mivacurium) can induce intubating paralysis in a time frame comparable with succinylcholine.[67] Unfortunately, even the shortest duration nondepolarizing agent has duration twice that of succinylcholine. Onset time of paralysis of the nondepolarizing agents is inversely related to the potency of the agent.

None of the nondepolarizing agent should be used in patients with myasthenia gravis.

Some patients have significant release of histamine associated with use of some of the nondepolarizing muscle relaxants.[68] Histamine release can transiently dilate the cerebral vessels, elevate the intracranial pressure, and decrease both systemic blood pressure and cerebral perfusion pressure. These symptoms can be avoided with slower infusion of the agent, but this may not be an option during intubation. Unlike many other nondepolarizing agents such as d-turbocuranine and atracurium, vecuronium and rocuronium do not release histamine.

Vecuronium Vecuronium (Norcuron) is an aminosteroid nondepolarizing agent. It has an intermediate duration of action of 30–60 minutes with an initial dose of about 0.1 mg/kg. It produces clinical effects in 30 seconds and optimal intubation paralysis in 1–4 minutes. Complete recovery will take 45–60 minutes. Since vecuronium is metabolized in the liver, liver failure or cirrhosis may double the recovery time. Concerns of arrhythmias in children associated with succinylcholine use have made high dose vecuronium (0.28 mg/kg) a popular choice for emergent pediatric airways.[69]

Vecuronium has been associated with a myopathy of critical illness in children who have concomitantly received high doses of steroids. The exact mechanism of the myopathy is not known. It is associated with use of other aminosteroid neuromuscular blocking agents. It is unlikely that single use of these agents will be associated with this myopathy, but caution should be used in children receiving high doses of steroids.

Two techniques can be used to hasten the onset of vecuronium paralysis:

a. **High Dose Vecuronium:** Using double or triple the usual paralyzing dose of vecuronium will shorten the onset of action. About 0.3 mg/kg of vecuronium by rapid IV push will decrease the onset of paralysis to about 90 seconds. Unfortunately, this will also result in quite long paralysis, up to two hours in duration.
b. **The Priming Principle:** This technique involves the administration of a small subparalytic dose of vecuronium (about 1/10 of the intubating dose) 3 minutes before the full paralytic dose. The paralytic dose is then increased to 0.15 mg/kg. This will decrease the onset time of paralysis to about 90 seconds.

Rocuronium Rocuronium is an aminosteroid nondepolarizing agent similar to vecuronium with a very rapid onset of action. The onset of action is almost as quick as that of succinylcholine. A dose of 0.8 mg/kg will produce paralysis in infants and children in 30 seconds or less.[70] Adults may take as much as 45 seconds. Recovery time from paralysis is between 30–45 minutes.

The duration of action of rocuronium is significantly longer than that of succinylcholine. The typical paralytic dose of 0.6 to 1.2 mg/k will last between 25 and 60 minutes.[71] This agent may be used quite successfully as a replacement for succinylcholine, if the extended recovery time is tolerable. Rocuronium is a liquid that does not require reconstitution before use. It should be available in the RSI kit for the paramedic.

Mivacurium Mivacurium is another neuromuscular blocking agent with a clinical onset similar to that of vecuronium. Although this agent is slower than rocuronium, the major advantage of mivacurium is that it has a relatively brief duration of action.[72]

Mivacurium is a short-acting nondepolarizing benzylisoquinolinium muscle relaxant. It has a short onset of action (30–60 seconds), producing intubation conditions within 75–120 seconds.[73] It lasts only about 15 to 20 minutes at the lower dosing. The typical RSI dose is about 0.15–0.3 mg/kg.

Mivacurium is metabolized by plasma cholinesterase, and children recover from blockade much quicker than adults do.[74 75]

Another advantage of mivacurium is that it is a benzyoisoquinolinium and not an aminosteroid like most of the other nondepolarizing agents. Aminosteroids have been linked to a myotonia-like syndrome in patients who are on chronic steroids (such as asthmatics).[76][77] Mivacurium is a good alternative for the RSI kit.

Cisatracurium Cisatracurium is one of 10 isomers of atracurium besylate and has similar pharmacologic properties. It has a relatively slower onset of action than rocuronium. It will produce intubation conditions within 90 to 120 seconds. Unlike the parent compound, it does not cause histamine release. The drug metabolism is not dependent on kidney or hepatic function, making it ideal for use in liver and renal failure patients.

Degradation of cisatracurium is unlike most of the other nondepolarizing agents. It will metabolize by first order kinetics so a set amount of the drug is metabolized every minute. This leads to a very predictable return of the patient's muscle function.

The typical dose of cisatracurium is 0.15 mg/kg to 0.20 mg/kg. This will usually last 60 minutes in the adult and slightly shorter duration in the child.

Rapacuronium Rapacuronium is the first nondepolarizing muscle relaxant that combines the desirable characteristics of rapid onset of paralysis and a short to intermediate duration of action.[78]

Pancuronium Pancuronium (Pavulon) is another aminosteroid neuromuscular blocking agent that will provide acceptable conditions for intubation in 90–120 seconds with paralysis that lasts from 45 to 90 minutes. It is classified as a long-acting agent with a slow onset. The slow onset limits usefulness in the EMS setting. It may be an appropriate agent when paralysis will be required for long periods of mechanical ventilation.

Pancuronium will frequently result in tachycardia. Pancuronium is primarily excreted in the urine, so reduced renal function or urinary output will increase the duration of effect. Pancuronium can also cause histamine reactions.

7. Sellick's Maneuver

Sellick's maneuver or cricoid pressure will decrease the chances of regurgitation by pressing the cricoid cartilage firmly against the esophagus.[79] The relatively soft yielding esophagus will be compressed between the cricoid cartilage and the vertebral column. Don't release cricoid cartilage pressure until you are certain that the tube is in the trachea. Since Sellick's maneuver is not certain protection against regurgitation, inflate the cuff of the tube as soon as possible.

8. Intubate the Patient

Intubation is performed after there is full relaxation of the airway muscles. This usually occurs about 45 seconds after the administration of succinylcholine. Cricoid pressure should be maintained until the cuff is inflated and the tube position verified.

If intubation fails, cricoid pressure should be maintained and the patient ventilated with a bag-valve-mask for 60–90 seconds. It is much more prudent at this point to withdraw the laryngoscope, provide assisted ventilations to maintain oxygen saturation, and then re-attempt intubation. After the patient is reoxygenated, then either another intubation with other equipment, or better positioning should be attempted, or an alternative airway technique employed. If an additional dose of sedative or paralytic agent is required, then it should be employed about 5 minutes after the first.

9. Verify Placement

After rapid sequence intubation, the tube must be confirmed to be in the trachea. This verification is more important than the intubation itself, since the patient is now paralyzed. The benefits of endotracheal intubation are confined to the group of patients in which the endotracheal tube is correctly placed in the trachea. The stomach does not exchange gas with the blood stream and ventilating the stomach will quickly lead to hypoxia and death. Accordingly, the operator must be certain that the endotracheal tube is in the trachea.

10. Secure the Tube

Security of the tube includes sedation so that the patient will not move and ensuring that the patient's head does not move during transport after intubation. After each movement of the patient, the oxygen saturation should be carefully monitored. A falling saturation should prompt the astute clinician to reassess the placement of the endotracheal tube.

The risk of inadvertent dislodgment of the ETT or mainstem bronchus intubation is much higher in the small child than in the adult due to the shorter trachea and bronchus. The trachea is about 12–15 cm long in the adult and only 4 cm long in the newborn. The endotracheal tube must protrude only 3–4 cm past the cords in order to avoid a right mainstem bronchus intubation. Since the child's neck is much more flexible than the adult's, motion of the neck can dislodge an ETT in a child. This is not true in the child.

Complications of Rapid Sequence Intubation

- Failed intubation
- Hypoxemia
- Hypotension
- Dysrhythmia
- Pressor response
- Intracranial hypertension

Intradepartmental resistance

Although this is not readily a patient-related complication, it is certainly a complication that providers at all levels must deal with. Administration of neuromuscular blocking agents by the nonanesthesiologist is not accepted in some centers. Literature-based evidence supports the use of RSI in the emergency department and in the field setting since 1982 and 1988 respectively.[80][81][82][83][84][85][86][87] Indeed, field studies have shown that the introduction of RSI increases the success rate of intubation on the order of about 20 percent over non-RSI intubation rates.[88]

Trauma surgeons have advocated the use of RSI for years because it is both useful and safe.

Alternative Intubation Techniques and the Failed Intubation

Any emergency practitioner attempting to intubate a paralyzed patient must be prepared to handle the failed intubation. After the patient has been paralyzed, the intubation may be attempted as long as the patient is oxygenated. This can be determined easily by continuous pulse oximetry. Depending on the clinical situation, this may be less than a minute to over four minutes.

> **ALWAYS HAVE A CONTINGENCY PLAN . . .**
> Always, Always, Always

Bag-valve-mask ventilation may be used while Sellick's maneuver is maintained to decrease the incidence of gastric insufflation and increased risk of aspiration. After the patient is reoxygenated, the intubation attempt may be repeated. Caution should be used when giving additional succinylcholine. Repeat doses of succinylcholine can cause marked vagal effects in infants and small children. A nondepolarizing agent may be more reasonable at this point.

At times, visualized oral or nasal intubation is either not feasible or is contraindicated. In these cases, alternative airway management techniques may be appropriate. These methods include laryngeal mask airway, blind nasal intubation, fiberoptic laryngoscopic intubation, retrograde intubation, lighted stylet intubation, and digital orotracheal intubation. The techniques

TABLE 9-6

Miscellaneous Useful Agents		
Drug	Dosage	Comment
Atropine	0.01–.02 mg/kg	Minimum dose 0.15 mg/kg. Atropine is used routinely by some clinicians for children, particularly when succinylcholine is used.
Lidocaine	0.5 mg/kg	Lowers the intracranial pressure and suppresses cough reflexes. May blunt hypertension and tachycardia associated with laryngoscopy.
Esmolol	1.5 mg/kg over 30 seconds	Postintubation hypertension and tachycardia can be managed with beta blockers. This is particularly important in the head-injured patient. Beta blockers must not be used in the patient with shock.
Labetalol	0.25 mg/kg over 2 min	See note above.
Nitrates	Small doses of nitrates have been used to control the cardiovascular response to intubation. Cerebral vasodilation will lead to increased cerebral blood flow and intracranial blood pressure. There is no significant literature to recommend this practice.	

TABLE 9-7

Clinical Situations

Situation	Sedative Options		
Isolated respiratory failure	Etomidate	Midazolam	Thiopental
Status asthmaticus	Ketamine	Etomidate	Midazolam
Combative patient	Etomidate	Midazolam	Propofol
Status epilepticus	Midazolam	Thiopental	Etomidate
Isolated head injury	Etomidate	Midazolam	Propofol
Hypotensive trauma—no head injury	Etomidate	Ketamine?	Midazolam
Trauma—no head injury	Etomidate	Midazolam?	Propofol
Nontraumatic intracranial process	Etomidate	Propofol	Thiopental

of blind nasal intubation, fiberoptic intubation, lighted stylet intubation and digital intubation are well described in this publication.

END NOTES

[1] Tayal, V. S., Riggs, R. W., Marx, J. A., et al. "Rapid-sequence intubation at an emergency medicine residency: Success rate and adverse events during a two-year period," *Acad Emerg Med* 1999;6:31–37.

[2] Thibodeau, L. G., Verdile, V. G., and Bartfield, J. M. "Incidence of aspiration after urgent intubation," in *Am J Emerg Med* 1997;15:562–565.

[3] Bernhard, W. N., Cottrell, J. E., Sivakumaran, C., et al. "Adjustment of intracuff pressure to prevent aspiration," in *Anesthesiology* 1979;50: 363–364.

[4] Dines, D. E., Titus, J. L., and Sessler, A. D. "Aspiration pneumonitis," in *Mayo Clin Proc* 1970;45:347–360.

[5] Gerardi, M. J., Sacchetti, A. D., Cantor, R. M., et al. "Rapid sequence intubation of the pediatric patient," in *Ann Emerg Med* 1996;28:55–74.

[6] Roberts, D. J., Clinton, J. E., and Ruiz, E. "Neuromuscular blockade for critical patients in the emergency department," in *Ann Emerg Med* 1986; 15:152–156.

[7] McBrien, M. E., Pollock, A. J., and Steedman, D. J. "Advanced airway control in trauma resuscitation," in *Arch Emerg Med* 1992;9:177–180.

[8] Zink, B. J., Snyder, H. S., and Raccio-Borak, N. "Lack of a hyperkalemic response in emergency department patients receiving succinylcholine," in *Acad. Emerg Med* 1995;2:974–978.

[9] Yamamoto, L. G. "Rapid sequence anesthesia induction and advanced airway management in pediatric patients," in *Emerg Clin N America* 1991; 9:611–638.

[10] Yamamoto, L. G., Yim, G. K., and Britten, A. G. "Rapid sequence anesthesia induction for emergency intubation," in *Ped Emerg Care* 1990; 6:200–213.

[11] Prys-Roberts, C., Meloche, R., and Foex, P. "Studies of anaesthesia in relation to hypertension I: Cardiovascular responses of treated and untreated patients," in *Br J Anaesth* 1971;43:122.

[12] Prys-Roberts, C., Greene, L. T., Meloche, R., et al. "Studies of anaesthesia in relation to hypertension II: Haemodynamic consequences of induction and endotracheal intubation," in *Br J Anaesth* 1971;43:531.

[13] Forbes, A. M., and Dally, F. G. "Acute hypertension during induction of anaesthesia and endotracheal intubation in normotensive man," in *Br J Anaesth* 1970;42:618.

[14] Fassoulaki, A., and Kanaris, P. "Does atropine premedication affect the cardiovascular response to laryngoscopy and intubation?," in *Br J Anaesth* 1982;54:1065.

[15] Boralessa, H., Senior, D. F., and Whitman, J. G. "Cardiovascular response to intubation," in *Anaesthesia* 1983;38:623.

[16] Martin, D. E., Rosenberg, H., Aukburg, S. J., et al. "Low-dose fentanyl blunts circulatory response to tracheal intubation," in *Anesth Analg* 1982; 61:680.

[17] Laurito, C. E., Baughman, V. L., Becker, G. L., et al. "Effects of aerosolized and/or intravenous lidocaine on hemodynamic responses to rapid sequence induction of general anesthesia. A double blind controlled clinical trial," in *Anesth Analg* 1965;65:1037.

[18] Yamamoto, L. G., Yim, G. K., and Britten, A. G. "Rapid sequence anesthesia induction for emergency intubation," in *Ped Emerg Care* 1990; 6:200–213.

[19] Morris, I. "Pharmacologic aids to intubation and the rapid sequence induction," in *Emerg Med Clin North America* 1988;6:753–768.

[20] Stoelting, R. K. "Opioid agonist and antagonist," in Stoelting, R. K., ed., *Pharmacology and Physiology in Anesthetic Practice,* 2nd ed. Philadelphia, PA: JB Lippincott, 1991, p. 70.

[21] Vilke, G. M., Hoyt, D. B., Epperson, M., et al. "Intubation techniques in the helicopter," in *J Emerg Med* 1994;12:217.

[22] Dronen, S. C. "Pharmacologic adjuncts to intubation," in Roberts, J. R., and Hedges, J. R., eds., *Clinical Procedures in Emergency Medicine,* 2nd ed. Philadelphia, PA: WB Saunders, 1991, p. 29.

[23] Mostert, J. W., Trudnowskin, R. J., Seniff, A. M., et al. "Clinical comparison of fentanyl with meperidine," in *J Clin Pharmacol* 1968;8:382.

[24] Mostert, J. W., Trudnowskin, R. J., Seniff, A. M., et al. "Clinical comparison of fentanyl with meperidine," in *J Clin Pharmacol* 1968;8:382.

[25] Moss, E. "Alfentanil increases intracranial pressure when intracranial compliance is low," in *Anesthesia* 1992;47:134.

[26] Walls, R. M. "Rapid sequence intubation in head trauma," in *Ann Emerg Med* 1993;22:1008.

[27] Stoelting, R. K. "Opioid agonist and antagonist," in Stoelting, R. K., ed., p. 70.

[28] Giese, J. L., and Stanley, T. H. "Etomidate: A new intravenous anesthetic induction agent," in *Pharmacotherapy* 1983;3:251–258.

[29] Johnson, D. M., King, R. W., and Bohnett, M. "The safety and efficacy of etomidate as an adjunct to endotracheal intubation in the ED," in *Acad Emerg Med* 1994;1:318.

[30] Plewa, M. C., King, R., Johnson, D., et al. "Etomidate used during emergency intubation of trauma patients," in *Am J Emerg Med.* 1997; 15:98–100.

[31] Dearden, N. M., and McDowald, D. G. "Comparison of etomidate and althesin in the reduction of increased intracranial pressure after head injury," in *Br J Anesthesia* 1985;57:61–368.

[32] Watson, J. C., Drummond, J. C., Patel, P. M., et al. "An assessment of the cerebral protective effects of etomidate in a model of incomplete forebrain ischemia in the rat," in *Neurosurgery* 1992;30:540–544.

[33] Wagner, R. L., and White, P. F. "Etomidate inhibits adrenocortical function in surgical patients," in *Anesthesiology* 1984;61: 647–651.

[34] Fragen, R. J., Shanks, C. A., Molteni, A., et al. "Effects of etomidate on hormonal response to surgical stress," in *Anesthesiology* 1988;69: 652–656.

[35] Harris, C. E., Murray, A. M., Anderson, J. M., et al. "Effects of thiopentone, etomidate, and propofol on the haemodynamic response to tracheal intubation," in *Anaesthesia.* 1988;43(suppl):32–36.

[36] Gold, M. I., Abraham, E. C., and Herrington, C. "A controlled investigation of propofol, thiopentone, and methohexitone," in *Can J Anaesth* 1987;34:478–483.

[37] Smith, I., White, P. F., Nathanson, M., et al. "Propofol: An update for its clinical use," in *Anesthesiology* 1994;81:1005–1043.

[38] Pnaud, M., Lelasque, J. N., Chetanneau, A., et al. "The effects of propofol on cerebral hemodynamics and metabolism in patients with brain trauma," in *J Neurosurg* 1991;73:404–409.

[39] Shepard, S. "Management of status epilepticus," in *Emerg Med Clin NA* 1994;12:951–961.

[40] Adams, P., Gelman, S., Reves, J. G., et al. "Midazolam: pharmacodynamics and pharmacokinetics during acute hypovolemia," in *Anesthesiology* 1985;63:140.

[41] Stoelting, R. K. "Nonbarbiturate induction agents," in Stoelting, R. K., ed., p. 134.

[42] L'Hommedieu, C. S. "The use of ketamine for the emergency intubation of patients with status asthmaticus," in *Ann Emerg Med* 1987;16:568–571.

[43] White, P. F., Way, W. L., and Trevor, A. J. "Ketamine: Its pharmacology and therapeutic uses," in *Anesthesiology* 1982;56:119–136.

[44] Green, L. M., Nakamura, R., and Johnson, N. E. "Ketamine sedation for pediatric procedures: Parts I and II," in *Ann Emerg Med* 1990;19: 1024–1046.

[45] Tobias, J. D. "Airway management for pediatric emergencies," in *Pediatric Ann* 1996;25:317–328.

[46] Nichols, D. G. "Emergency management of status asthmaticus in children," in *Ped Annals* 1996;25:394–403.

[47] Epstein, F. B. "Ketamine dissociative sedation in pediatric emergency medical practice," in *Am J Emerg Med* 1993;11:180–182.

[48] Cartwright, P. D., and Pingel, S. M. "Midazolam and diazepam in ketamine anesthesia," in *Anaesthesia* 1984;59:439.

[49] Jankiewizc, A. M., and Nowakowski, P. "Ketamine and succinylcholine for emergency intubation of pediatric patients," in *DICP* 1991;25:475–476.

[50] Hougaard, K., Hansen, A., and Brodersen, P. "The effect of ketamine on regional cerebral blood flow in man," in *Anesthesiology* 1974;41:562–567.

[51] Rodriguez, A., and Sanchez, L. "Intravenous ketamine does not increase intracranial pressure in neurosurgical patients with normal or increased ICP [abstract]," in *Crit Care Med* 1994;24:A57.

[52] Smith, D. H., Okiyama, K., Gennarelli, T. A., et al. "Magnesium and ketamine attenuate cognitive dysfunction following experimental brain injury," in *Neurosci Lett* 1993;157:211.

[53] Dufour, D. G., Larose, D. L., and Clement, S. C. "Rapid sequence intubation in the emergency department," in *J Emerge Med* 1995;13:705–710.

[54] Zink, B. J., Snyder, H. S., and Raccio-Robak, N. "Lack of a hyperkalemic response in emergency department patients receiving succinylcholine," in *Acad Emerge Med* 1995;2:974.

[55] Smith, R. B., and Grenvik, A. "Cardiac arrest following succinylcholine use in patients with central nervous system injuries," in *Anesthesiology* 1970; 33:558.

[56] Tomie, J. D., Joyce, T. H., and Mitchell, G. D. "Succinylcholine danger in the burned patient," in *Anesthesiology* 1969;31:540.

[57] McStravog, L. J. "Dangers of succinylcholine in anesthesia," in *Laryngoscope* 1974;84:929.

[58] Morris, I. R. "Pharmacologic aids to intubation and the rapid sequence induction," in *Emerg Med Clin North Amer* 1988;6:753–768.

[59] Gronert, G. A., and Antognini, J. F. "Malignant hyperthermia," in Miller, R. D., ed., *Anesthesia,* 4th ed., Vol. 1. New York: Churchill Livingstone, 1994,pp. 1075–1093.

[60] Ording, H. "Incidence of malignant hyperthermia in Denmark," in *Anesth Analg* 1985;64:700–704.

[61] *Physician's Desk Reference,* 50th ed. Montvale, NJ: Medical Economics, 1996,pp. 1073–1075.

[62] Libonati, M. M., Leahy, J. J., and Ellison, N. "The use of succinylcholine in open eye surgery," in *Anesthesiology* 1985;63:727.

[63] Saverese, J. J., Miller, R. D., Lien, C. A., et al. "Pharmacology of muscle relaxants and their antagonists," in Miller, R. D., ed., *Anesthesia,* 4th ed., Vol. 1. New York: Churchill Livingstone, 1994, pp. 417–487.

[64] Kharasch, M., and Graff, J. "Emergency management of the airway," in *Crit Care Clinics N Amer* 1995;11:53–66.

[65] Saverese, J. J., Miller, R. D., Lien, C. A., et al. "Pharmacology of muscle relaxants and their antagonists," in Miller, R. D., ed., *Anesthesia,* 4th ed., Vol. 1. New York: Churchill Livingstone, 1994,pp. 417–487.

66 Rosenburg, H., and Gronert, G. A. "Intractable cardiac arrest in children given succinylcholine [letter]," in *Anesthesiology* 1992;77:1054.

67 Crul, J. F., Vangelleghem, V., Buyse, L., et al. "Rocuronium with alfentanyl and propofol allows intubation within 45 seconds," in *Europ J Anaesthes* 1995;12(suppl 11):111–112.

68 Sarner, J. B., Brandom, D. W., Woelfel, S. K., et al. "Clinical pharmacology of mivacurium chloride in children during nitrous oxide-halothane and nitrous oxide-narcotic anesthesia," in *Anesth Analg* 1989;68:116–121.

69 Wright, J. L., and Patterson, M. D. "Resuscitating the pediatric patient," in *Emerg Clin N Amer* 1996;14:219–231.

70 O'Kelly, B., Fiset, P., Weistelman, C., et al. "Pharmacokinetics of rocuronium in pediatric patients during N_2O-halothane anesthesia," in *Can J Anesth* 1991;38:490–495.

71 Gerardi, M. J., Sacchetti, A. D., Cantor, R. M., et al. "Rapid sequence intubation in the pediatric patient," in *Ann Emerg Med* 1996;28:55–74.

72 Gerardi, M. J., Sacchetti, A. D., Cantor, R. M., et al. "Rapid sequence intubation in the pediatric patient," in *Ann Emerg Med* 1996;28:55–74.

73 Bartkowski, R. R., Witkowski, T. A., Azad, S., et al. "Rocuronium onset of action: A comparison with atracurium and vecuronium," in *Anesth Analg* 1993;77:574–578.

74 Goudsouzian, N. G., Denman, W., Schwartz, A., et al. "Pharmacodynamic and hemodynamic effects of mivacurium in infants anesthetized with halothane and nitrous oxide," in *Anesthesiology* 1993;79:919–925.

75 Goudsouzian N. G., Denman W., Schwartz A., et al. "Pharmacodynamic and hemodynamic effects of mivacurium in infants anesthetized with halothane and nitrous oxide," in *Anesthesiology* 1993;79:919–925.

76 Douglas, J. A., Tuxen, D. V., Horne, M., et al. "Myopathy in severe asthma," in *Am Rev Respir Dis* 1992;146:517–519.

77 Garohn, R. J., Jackson, C. E., Rogers, S. J., et al. "Prolonged paralysis due to nondepolarizing neuromuscular blocking agents and corticosteroids," in *Muscle and Nerve* 1994;17:647–654.

78 Schiere, S., Proost, J. H., Shuringa, M., et al. "Pharmacokinetics and pharmacokinetic-dynamic relationship between rapacuronium (ORG 9487) and its 3-desacetyl metabolite (ORG 9488)." *Anesth Analg* 1999;88:640–647.

79 Sellick, B. A. "Cricoid pressure to control regurgitation of stomach contents during induction of anesthesia," in *Lancet* 1961;2:404–406.

80 Ross, W. D., Anderson, L. D., and Edmond, S. A. "Analysis of intubations: Before and after establishment of a rapid sequence intubation protocol for air medical use," in *Air Medical J* 1994;13:475–478.

81 Syverud, S. A., Borron, S. W., Storer, D. L., et al. "Prehospital use of neuromuscular blocking agents in a helicopter ambulance program," in *Ann Emerg Med* 1988;17:236–242.

82 Rhee, K. J., and O'Malley, R. J. "Neuromuscular blockade-assisted oral intubation versus nasotracheal intubation in the prehospital care of injured patients," in *Ann Emerg Med* 1994;23:38–42.

83 Vilke, G. M., Hoyt, D. B., Epperson, M., et al. "Intubation techniques in the helicopter," in *J Emerg Med* 1994;12:217–224.

[84] Falcone, R. E., Herron, H., Dean, B., et al. "Emergency scene endotracheal intubation before and after the introduction of a rapid sequence induction protocol," in *Air Medical J* 1996;15:163–166.

[85] Hedges, J. R., Dronen, S. C., Feero, S., et al. "Succinylcholine-assisted intubations in prehospital care," in *Ann Emerg Med* 1996;3:41–45.

[86] Murphy-Macabby, M., Marshal, W. J., Schneider, C., et al. "Neuromuscular blockade in aeromedical airway management," in *Ann Emerg Med* 1992;21:664–668.

[87] Sing, R. F., Reilly, P. M., Rotondo, M. F., et al. "Out-of-hospital rapid sequence induction for intubation of the pediatric patient," in *Acad Emerg Med* 1996;3:41–45.

[88] Slater, E. A., Weiss, S. J., Earnst, A. A., et al. "Preflight versus en route success and complications of rapid sequence intubation in an air medical service," in *J Trauma* 1998;45:588–592.

Chapter **Ten**

Pediatric Airway Management

The agitated or unconscious child or infant with a comprised airway is a challenging, anxiety provoking clinical problem that may be faced by every EMS provider from BLS to emergency physician. The ability to handle this child's airway is one of the most important lifesaving skills that an EMS provider can possess.

Unfortunately, adult intubation techniques, tools, and skills do not easily transfer to children. This does not mean that intubation of the pediatric airway is any more difficult, just that different skills and tools are required of the operator. Both fortunately and unfortunately, far fewer children than adults require prehospital or emergent intubation. Fortunately, children account for only about 10 percent of all ambulance transports and only 1 percent of critically ill patients who are transported are children.[1] Unfortunately, the very operators who must intubate the critically ill patient often have had little real experience and do not retain those skills as well as for the more common adult intubation. Also, adult techniques that may be quite usable in older children and adolescents may be very different or dangerous in infants and smaller children.

Recognition of the paucity of experience has led to the co-development of the Pediatric Advanced Life Support course (PALS) by the American Academy of Pediatrics and the American Heart Association. The emphasis in this course is recognition of the critically ill child prior to cardiorespiratory failure. By early identification of these children at risk, the physician can better prevent a poor outcome.

When the patient has risk factors for a difficult intubation, the clinician may choose to delay rather than risk a failed intubation. This delay may be to the patient's detriment. At normal body temperature, irreversible brain damage begins after 4 to 6 minutes of anoxia. On arrival, the patient may range from frankly moribund to simply "running out of steam," so 4 to 6 minutes may represent a very optimistic limit when the pediatric patient finally ceases to breathe.

If the pediatric patient has trauma, there is a significant chance that head trauma will be involved and the airway compromised.[2] Airway obstruction, aspiration and apnea are major hazards to the pediatric patient with a head injury. These factors increase the risks of hypoxia and secondary brain injury. Rapid endotracheal intubation assures optimal gas exchange.

Anatomical Differences

The upper airway can be divided into three distinct segments: the oropharynx, the hypopharynx, and the larynx. The oropharynx includes the tongue and soft palate. The hypopharynx includes the epiglottis, the vallecula, aryepiglottic folds, and the retropharyngeal area. The larynx is the entrance to the airway and includes both the true and false vocal cords. The cricoid cartilage separates the larynx from the trachea and is completely composed of cartilage.

The airway of the one- to two-year-old is very different from that of the older child or adult, and these pediatric features are usually present until about age eight or nine (Figure 10-1). After this age, the airway becomes more adultlike in configuration and the generalist emergency physician is on more familiar ground.

Neck

The child's neck is much shorter with a more anterior and cephalad larynx. Indeed, the larynx is so anterior that Sellick's maneuver is often required not only to occlude the esophagus, but also to bring the vocal cords into view. Another maneuver is to get lower than the patient and look up at a 45 degree or greater angle when intubating. In very small children it may be worthwhile to place the small finger of the left (laryngoscope) hand on the thyroid cartilage to help with this posterior displacement. An assistant is more likely to be useful in intubating smaller children.

The larger mass of adenoidal tissues may make nasotracheal intubation more difficult. Nasopharyngeal airways are more difficult to pass in infants less than 1 year of age.

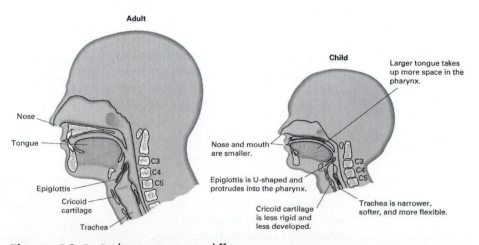

Figure 10-1 Pediatric anatomic differences.

The epiglottis is flaccid, high, long, and narrow in the small child. It is also angled away from the long axis of the trachea. This makes direct laryngoscopy more difficult as the angle between the base of the tongue and the glottic opening is more acute. The epiglottis in an infant and young child up to about 8 years of age is more easily picked up by a straight (Miller or similar) blade to facilitate intubation.

The risk of mainstem bronchus intubation is much higher in the small child due to the shorter trachea and bronchus. The trachea is about 12–15 cm long in the adult and only about 4 cm long in the newborn. The endotracheal tube must protrude only 3 to 4 cm past the cords in order to avoid a right mainstem bronchus intubation.

The narrow tracheal diameter and the shortened distance between tracheal rings makes tracheostomy technically more difficult (Figure 10-2). The American Heart Association recommends a needle crichothyrotomy in children rather than an open cricothyrotomy for this reason.

The child's head and occiput are proportionately larger than in an adult. This will cause neck flexion and possible airway obstruction when the child is supine. The proper position of the child's airway should be the sniffing position. A roll may be placed under the occiput, rather than under the neck to better achieve this position.

Finally, the tongue is large compared with an adult's. This result is less oral space for intubation. Decreased muscle tone will increase the likelihood of passive airway obstruction by the tongue. Indeed, this is the most common cause of airway obstruction in children. Obstruction from tongue displacement may usually be helped with better head positioning or with the use of an airway adjunct such as an oropharangeal or nasopharyngeal airway.

Airway Size

The diameter of the pediatric airway is much smaller than the adult airway. This means that it is far more vulnerable to obstruction by either foreign objects or edema than in the adult. Minor narrowing from respiratory infections or bronchospasm may result in profound airway difficulties.

Airflow through a pipe like the bronchi is described by Poisson's equations. Airflow in the narrowed airway meets resistance that is described by an inverse proportion to the fourth power of the radius of the airway for laminar airflow and the fifth power for turbulent airflow.[3]

$$R_{resistance} = 1/radius^4$$

This relationship means that 1 mm of circumferential edema in an infant's airway will decrease the cross sectional area by 75 percent and increase

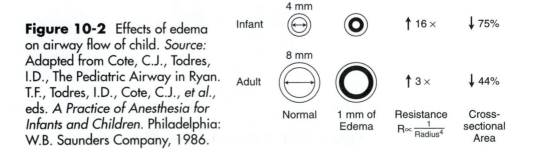

Figure 10-2 Effects of edema on airway flow of child. *Source: Adapted from Cote, C.J., Todres, I.D., The Pediatric Airway in Ryan. T.F., Todres, I.D., Cote, C.J., et al., eds. A Practice of Anesthesia for Infants and Children.* Philadelphia: W.B. Saunders Company, 1986.

the resistance to airflow 16-fold. Turbulent airflow, such as in a crying child, would increase the work of breathing 32-fold.

In adults, the thickness of cuff and material of the tube offer little resistance to flow through the tube. In a child, the very thickness of the tube becomes a detriment to effective airflow through the tube. Likewise, in the adult, if the wrong tube size is chosen, inflating the cuff will compensate. In the child, the uncuffed tube requires that the correct size of tube be used to prevent air leaks and aspiration.

Cuffed tubes further decrease the size of the airway and limit effective ventilation in smaller children.[4] The narrowest part of the pediatric airway is in the subglottic area, rather than at the cords (as in adults). In children, cuffed tubes will add little to prevention of aspiration and the smaller size of the tube will markedly decrease the airflow.[5] Infants ventilated through small endotracheal tubes will have prolonged inspiration and expiration leading to smaller delivered tidal volumes and a positive end expiratory pressure during ventilatory support.[6]

Mechanics of Ventilation

The child's chest wall is more compliant than the adult's because it has more cartilage than bone. The diaphragm is higher because of the relatively larger size of the abdominal contents and the smaller lung volumes of the child. Unfortunately, the child's lungs are also small in relationship to the child's metabolic needs, so there is little margin.

Physiologic Responses

The infant is a nose breather until approximately 3–6 months of age. Obligate nose breathing means that even a stuffy nose can lead to some obstructive apnea.

Higher metabolic rates, small lung volumes, and a small functional residual capacity in relation to the infant's metabolic needs means that the infant has significantly less reserve and apnea. Even with adequate preoxygenation, the child will rapidly desaturate with subsequent cyanosis.

The infant and small child are at further risk of respiratory problems because of immature physiologic responses. The infant will become apneic and bradycardic in response to a hypoxic challenge instead of increasing the respiratory effort and heart rate.

Behavioral immaturity can increase the risk of respiratory problems. The child is unable to talk and tell us that he or she is starting to wear out. The child is also prone to dangerous behavior without realizing the danger (example, aspiration of foreign bodies).

Choosing a Pediatric Tube Size

An uncuffed tube that is too large will cause mucosal ulceration, tracheal swelling, and postextubation croup. A tube that is too small will allow aspiration and make positive pressure ventilation more difficult. An uncuffed tube should be large enough to fit the subglottic area and leak at about 25–30 mm Hg of inspiratory pressure. If the tube is so large that it does not leak at all, then the child should be reintubated with the next smaller size tube.

There are many charts and tables to aid in tube size and selection, but these are rarely available when needed. A superior and often readily available written aid to tube size and doses of resuscitation drugs is the Broselow tape. This body tape converts body length into appropriate sizes for tubes, blades, length of tube to be inserted, size of laryngoscope blades to be used, and doses of drugs.

Remember in the child that you must not only select the proper size tube, you must put it into the larynx to the proper depth. Usually the depth of the tube in centimeters can be calculated as three times the size of the tube. A lighted endotracheal tube can be visualized in the child's neck, giving an appropriate depth. Alternatively, the Broselow tape gives the proper depth of insertion.

The cogent and prepared emergency practitioner should also copy a few rules to cerebral wetware. Make sure that you have both a half size larger and smaller than your predicted choice readily available when you use these rules (Figures 10-3–10-7).

Cerebral Wetware Rules:

1. If in doubt, use a tube that fits through the nose.
2. Alternatively, use a tube about the size of the patient's little finger.
3. For children the formula

$$\frac{\text{Age (years)}}{4} + 4 = \text{tube size}$$

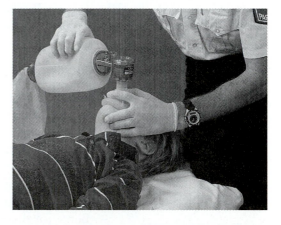

Figure 10-3 Preventilation and oxygenating prior to intubation attempt.

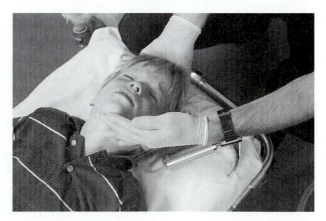

Figure 10-4 Positioning airway for intubation.

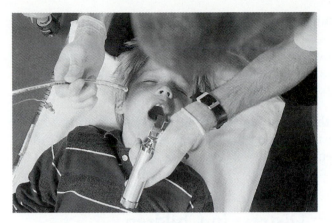

Figure 10-5 Visualization with laryngoscope.

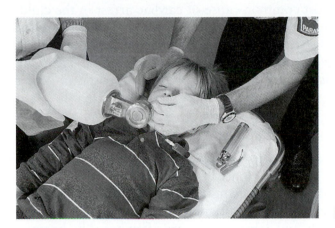

Figure 10-6 Ventilation.

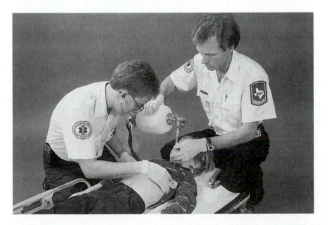

Figure 10-7 Verification of tube placement.

Since the smallest easily available tube size is 3.0 mm, this is appropriate for the premature newborn, while the newborn should get a 3.5 mm tube and the 1-year-old should get about a 4.0 mm ID tube.

4. A useful formula for oral tube length (tube insertion depth) is:

$$\frac{\text{Age (years)}}{2} + 12 = \text{tube length}$$

Nasal tubes should be about 3 cm longer than the oral tube.

5. Remember to use uncuffed tubes when intubating with a 5.0 or smaller ET tube.
6. Remember that the most common pitfall in pediatric intubation is inserting the scope too far. This means that inability to see the cords may be because the laryngoscope is already past the cricoid membrane!

After the intubation the child will require meticulous attention to tube placement and securing the tube to prevent movement. With the smaller tubes used in infants and children, fastidious maintenance of tube patency and security is essential.

Signs of Respiratory Distress in Children

Respiratory failure is the most common cause of cardiac arrest in the child. Respiratory failure can result from disease of the upper or lower airway or may be the end result of other disease processes. In most cases, the respiratory failure is preceded by a period of respiratory distress. The signs and symptoms of respiratory distress in children may be quite obvious or rather subtle.

History

Most commonly, a child in respiratory distress will have a history of "trouble breathing." The parents may note some coughing, rapid or noisy breathing, or some change in behavior. In neonates and young infants, tachypnea may alternate with bradypnea or apnea. Difficulty breathing, exhaustion, decreased activity and/or feeding, and color changes are often noted by parents. Small infants may have difficulty drinking from a bottle because of the mechanics of breathing through the nose while drinking and because drinking increases the work of breathing. Parents of older children may note wheezing or decrease in physical activity.

The past medical history is important, even in very small children, in determination of the acute problem. The examiner should note as a minimum whether the child was premature, product of a normal or abnormal birth, and whether the child went home with mother. The parents of the asthmatic child should be questioned about past hospitalizations, exacerbations, and intubations. A child with chronic cough or multiple episodes of pneumonia may be harboring a foreign body, may have undiagnosed cystic fibrosis, or have reactive airway disease.

In older children, the examiner should remember that tachypnea may be due to hypovolemia, diabetic ketoacidosis, and/or sepsis.

Examination of the Child

Simply observing the patient is an important part of the physical examination. Is this child alert, cooperative and playful or listless, responding only to painful stimuli? An alert, awake, and playing child is simply not in respiratory distress. The child with early respiratory distress is often irritable and anxious. They may not be able to assume a comfortable position, even in the mother's arms (Figure 10-8). Early respiratory failure will be marked by agitation and finally by lethargy, listlessness, and somnolence (Figure 10-9).

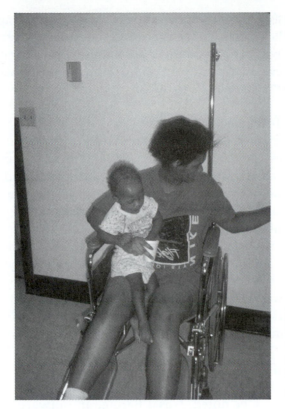

Figure 10-8 Child with foreign body in airway (sometimes it's just plain hard to tell) (the child did have tachypnea!). *Source:* Photo by Charles Stewart and Associates; www.storysmith.net.

Tachypnea

The child in respiratory difficulty will almost always have tachypnea. Tachypnea is the most common response to an increased respiratory demand. Remember that tachypnea may also be noted as a response to metabolic acidosis, sepsis, pain, or central nervous system disease or injury.

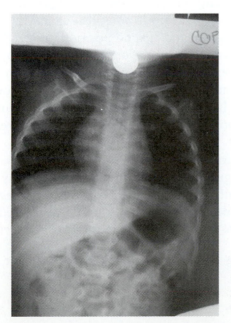

Figure 10-9 X-ray of above child showing coin in airway. *Source:* Photo by Charles Stewart and Associates; www.storysmith.net.

Since the normal respiratory rate varies with the age of the child, tachypnea must be assessed in the context of the patient's overall milieu. Newborns normally breathe 40 to 50 times per minute. By 1 year of age, the respiratory rate is around 30 to 35; by 4 years, 20 to 25; and by age 8 to 10 years it is at the usual adult rate of 12 to 15.

Use of Accessory Muscles

Inspection of the chest wall and neck may reveal retractions, as accessory muscles are recruited to help the child breathe. Retractions may be seen in the supraclavicular, infraclavicular, subcostal, and intercostal areas. If severe disease is present, the entire sternum may retract on inspiration. Retractions imply a significant amount of respiratory distress. They should never be ignored.

Patients who are struggling to breathe and not moving air or have limited air exchange are in imminent danger of respiratory arrest. These children should never be left alone, even for a moment.

Most respiratory dysfunction originates in the airway and/or lungs; however, respiratory distress may be due to impaired diaphragmatic excursion (abdominal or gastric distension) or metabolic or CNS abnormalities.

Nasal Flare

When the child has increasing difficulty with the work of breathing, nasal flare may be noted. Nasal flaring, an outward and upward flaring of the nares on inspiration, is thought to be a primitive reflex seen in young infants, who are obligate nose breathers for the first 2 to 3 months of life. It probably is an attempt to decrease the airway resistance at the nares in the young infant. Again, this finding cannot be ignored.

Tripod Position

The first position that the child will assume with respiratory distress is a "position of comfort." This usually will be upright, leaning slightly forward, open mouth, and with head, neck, and jaw thrust forward to aggressively open the airway. This position is also called the "sniffing position."

Patients may assume the "tripod position" when they are in severe respiratory distress. This consists of the upright posture, leaning forward and supporting the upper body with the arms placed either on the thighs or the bed. This position enhances the full use of the thoracoabdominal muscles for the work of breathing. It represents the final stage in recruitment of the accessory muscles of respiration. This patient is about to have a respiratory arrest.

Altered Respiratory Sounds

Listening to grossly audible breath sounds may help to localize the pathology or to confirm the patient's respiratory distress. Auscultation of the chest may reveal decreased breath sounds, decreased air movement, and slowing respirations as the child progresses towards respiratory arrest.

Drooling Drooling implies pooled secretions and at least a partially obstructed airway.

Grunting Respirations Grunting is an ominous sign of impending respiratory failure. It is produced by partial closure of the glottis on the end of expiration. Grunting seems to provide an increased end-expiratory pressure and keep the terminal airways open.[7] Grunting may be seen in primary lung disease or from systemic illnesses such as sepsis. Observations of neonates who grunted led to the development of continuous positive airway pressure (CPAP) and positive end-expiratory pressure (PEEP) in the treatment of neonatal hyaline membrane disease. Grunting localizes the respiratory disease to the lower respiratory tract. That is, patients who grunt have pneumonia, asthma, or bronchiolitis and not upper respiratory obstruction.

Stridor Stridor is a harsh, high-pitched respiratory noise caused by turbulent airflow through a narrowed upper airway. Stridor may be heard on both inspiration and expiration. In the child, stridor implies at least a 50 percent narrowing of the upper airway. Stridor may indicate severe upper airway pathology, such as include croup, epiglottitis, or foreign bodies in the airway. A less common cause is a congenital or iatrogenic narrowing of the glottic area.

Any examination of the upper airway should be done with extreme caution in the patient who has stridor. Any maneuvers that agitate the patient should be avoided, including separation from the parents, alteration of the patient's posture, rectal temperatures, blood draws, intravenous lines, and examination of the oral cavity.

Grossly audible wheezing represents some obstruction at the level of the lower airways.

Rales The presence of rales requires a significant accumulation of alveolar fluid. Rales in a previously healthy child with cough and fever usually indicates pneumonia or reactive airway disease (asthma or bronchiolitis). In cardiac disease, nephrosis, and severe malnutrition, rales indicate significant pulmonary edema or congestive heart failure.

Poor Perfusion

Ominous signs of poor perfusion and oxygenation in the child or infant include pallor or cyanosis. Cyanosis is most easily noted circumorally in the child. The child's cyanosis will be central and will often be associated with somnolence.

Cyanosis, while the most dramatic sign, has significant limitations as a field diagnostic tool. It depends on the amount of the hemoglobin in the blood and the status of the peripheral circulation. A child with severe anemia, for example, may have significant hypoxia without any visible cyanosis. Conversely, a very young infant whose hemoglobin has not yet fallen from the high levels found at birth may have peripheral cyanosis despite a normal PO_2. Detection of cyanosis is quite difficult in poor light and in children with dark skin, such as blacks and some Asians. Finally, even when present, cyanosis is a late development in respiratory diseases.

Early Management of the Infant's Airway

The prominence of the occiput, the small neck, and the narrow thorax means that the position of the child to avoid airway obstruction is different than that of the adult. The child should have a pad or folded sheet under the chest to lift the chest and compensate for the large occiput. This will allow the neck to assume a neutral position.

Hyperextension of the neck may occlude the child's airway. The child's larger tongue may require a jaw-thrust or chin-lift in order to open the airway.

Oral airways in children can maintain a patent airway or eliminate the pharyngeal obstruction by the tongue. This airway must be properly measured before use. An oral airway that is too large can cause pharyngeal and glottic trauma. An airway that is too small can push the tongue down and actually worsen the occlusion.

Nasal trumpets are useful for older children and adolescents. They are not available for small children and infants. Insertion techniques, complications, and contraindications are unchanged from those used in adults.

Bag-valve-mask ventilation is unchanged from that used in adults. In children, the size of the mask is critical. The mask must fit over the nose, cheeks, and chin. Using a bag that is too small will result in inadequate ventilation. Small volume self-inflating bags do not deliver an adequate tidal volume to the infant with poorly compliant lungs. Child size and adult size self-inflating bags may be used for the entire range of infants and children without fear of overinflation or barotrauma.[8] All bag-valve-mask systems require a reservoir to ensure that 100 percent oxygen is delivered.

Pediatric bag-valve-mask devices are usually fitted with pop-off valves set at about 30–35 cm H_2O pressure. This pressure cut off was based on an experimental study involving newborn lungs and cannot be well extrapolated to the clinical picture. In the clinical model, increased airway resistance and decreased lung compliance may require ventilatory pressures well in excess of 30 cm H_2O.[9] Activation of the pop-off valve may lead to inadequate delivery of needed volume, particularly in the presence of reduced lung compliance or increased airway resistance.[10]

When using the BVM to ventilate the patient, it is important to ensure that the child has a clear airway and that the chest rises while using the bag. Effective ventilation will move the child's chest about the same amount as when a child takes a deep breath. If there is no chest movement, there is no ventilation. If the ventilation is ineffective, both the airway and the ventilation efforts need to be promptly reassessed.

The optimal position for the operator is usually behind the patient's head. Cricoid pressure should be used when the child is at risk for aspiration or vomiting.

Mouth-to-mask resuscitation is effective in children and infants and may be more effective than BVM.

RSI in Children

Ten-Step RSI Protocol in Children

- Assess the risks
- Get equipment ready

- Monitor the patient
- Preoxygenate the patient
- Medicate the patient
- Sedation/paralysis
- Sellick's maneuver
- Intubate the patient
- Verify placement
- Secure the tube

Airway obstruction, apnea, and circulatory arrest demand immediate endotracheal intubation without any preparatory medications. Fortunately, such situations are relatively rare, even in a "children's" emergency department.[11] Multiple clinical studies have demonstrated that RSI, for pediatric patients, can be performed safely and effectively in the field by properly trained providers.[12] These reports encompass patients with a wide range of ages and clinical presentations.

Assess the Risks

As in adults, ensure that at least the AMPLE history is available, if possible (Allergies, Medications, Past medical history, Last meal, Existing circumstances). The intubating clinician should personally examine the neck, face, head, nose, throat and chest, even when a full surgical team approach is used for resuscitation.

Get Equipment Ready

In many emergency departments, equipment for pediatric emergency intubation is not kept in the same working area where it will be needed. The operator should ensure that all needed equipment is opened, laid out, and fully functional before any medications are given to the patient.

Generally a straight blade is used for pediatric intubation, particularly for infants under a year old. The more anterior airway and the floppy epiglottis of the child and infant may make the straight blade more appropriate for the child from 12 months to 6 years of age. For a child older than 6–8 years of age, the operator's preference is appropriate. Both Macintosh and straight blades are appropriate in this age group.

Minimum Immediately Available Equipment Includes

- Appropriately sized bag-valve-mask with reservoir
- Suction (fully hooked up and working)
- Oxygen (hooked up to a bag-valve-mask)
- Laryngoscope with appropriately sized blades and functioning lights
- Appropriately sized endotracheal tubes (as noted previously, get at least one size above and below the predicted size)
- Stylet for the endotracheal tube
- All pharmaceutical agents to be used in the procedure in the room where intubation is planned
- Alternative airway equipment in the location where intubation is planned

Equipment for an alternative airway should always be readily available in the room where the intubation is proposed. For the field EMS provider, this means that the airway control kit always has the tools to rescue the airway. In the pediatric population, this should include both cricothyrotomy and jet ventilation equipment. Depending on the experience of the operator, an appropriately sized laryngeal mask airway could also be used.

Monitor the Patient

Cardiorespiratory monitoring is essential for all patients who are ill enough to need intubating. The child should be no exception. Heart monitoring, pulse oximetry, and automated blood pressure monitoring should be readily available in every emergency department. These monitors should be used as a routine measure in every patient where intubation is even considered as a possible procedure.

Cardiac monitoring may alert the operator to bradycardia, tachycardia, or dysrhythmia in apneic patients. Pulse oximetry is the best monitoring to show the operator if the patient develops hypoxia during an intubation attempt. Unsuspected hypotension may be revealed with automated blood pressure monitoring.

After intubation in an emergency department, the proper endotracheal tube position must be confirmed with physical examination, chest x-ray, and a nonauscultatory procedure.

Preoxygenate the Patient

Preoxygenation replaces the patient's functional residual capacity of the lung with oxygen. If the patient is placed on 100 percent oxygen as soon as intubation is considered, then the patient has already been preoxygenated prior to the intubation.

In adults, preoxygenation will permit as much as 3–4 minutes of apnea before hypoxia develops. The child may not be able to tolerate apnea as long due to the smaller functional residual capacity and the higher basal oxygen consumption of the child. This gives only limited security if the patient is apneic during the RSI sequence.

Rise of the $PaCO_2$ in apnea is not usually a significant concern unless the patient has a head injury or is severely compromised prior to the intubation. $PaCO_2$ will rise at about 3 mm Hg/min when the patient is apneic.

Ordinarily, a bag and mask should not be used to artificially ventilate the patient. The risk of gastric insufflation and subsequent regurgitation is reduced if bagging is not used. When the patient is adequately preoxygenated, there is no need to ventilate the patient prior to intubation. Ventilations may be assisted in synchrony with natural respirations while the patient is still breathing. If bagging is necessary because of a failed intubation, then cricoid pressure should be continued at all times.

Medicate the Patient

These medications are discussed in significantly greater detail in the section on adult rapid sequence intubation.

The first medications given in RSI should reduce the physiologic responses of the patient to the subsequent intubation. These responses include bradycardia, tachycardia, hypertension, hypoxia, increased intracranial pressure, increased intraocular pressure, and cough and gag reflexes.

Infants and young children can develop profound bradycardia during intubation from medication effects, vagal stimulation, and hypoxia. Vagal stimulation and subsequent bradycardia may occur from stimulation of the oropharynx by the laryngoscope blade. Succinylcholine can also produce profound bradycardia in the infant. Hypoxia, of course, can rapidly cause profound bradycardia.

Atropine blocks the reflex bradycardia that is associated with the use of succinylcholine and laryngoscopy. In children under the age of 5, this reflex is more pronounced. Pretreating these pediatric patients with atropine can minimize vagal effects.[13][14] The appropriate dose is 0.02 mg/kg to a maximum of 0.5 mg in the child and 1 milligram in the adolescent. A minimum dose of atropine should be 0.15 mg. For effect at the time of intubation, atropine should be administered at least 2 minutes prior to intubation.

Lidocaine has been shown to blunt the rise in ICP associated with intubation, although this is somewhat controversial.[15] It also decreases the cough reflex and may decrease the incidence of postlaryngoscopy hypertension and tachycardia.[16] Lidocaine may be ineffective in blunting hypertension or tachycardia associated with intubation. The recommended dose of lidocaine is 1.5 to 3 mg/kg intravenously. As with atropine, lidocaine must be given at least 2 minutes prior to intubation in order to be effective. Alternatively, lidocaine may be sprayed into the posterior pharynx and trachea. Again, this is somewhat controversial as spraying lidocaine into the trachea may require almost as much manipulation as intubation itself.

Beta blockers such as esmolol 1.5 mg/kg over 30 seconds or Labetalol 0.25 mg/kg may be used in the stable patient. Use of beta blocking agents is dangerous in the patient with cardiovascular instability or the asthmatic patient.

Attenuation of adverse CV and ICP responses is optional in moribund and desperate situations. In these patients, the intubator should proceed directly to paralytic and sedation agents.

Sedation/Paralysis

Multiple agents have been used for sedation during the process of intubation in children, including barbiturates, benzodiazepines, opiates, nonbarbiturate sedatives, and dissociative agents. Each of these agents has their proponents, detractors, relative indications, and contraindications. The ideal sedative should induce rapid unconsciousness in the child with a short duration and little or no cardiovascular side effects. The ideal agent does not exist.

The sedative agent of choice should be given prior to the paralytic agent. Although sedatives and paralytics can be given at the same time, paralysis is such a frightening event that sedation should be assured prior to the onset of paralysis.

Tables 9.3–9.6 list commonly used sedatives for RSI for both adults and children. Any of these sedating agents will produce acceptable results in

RSI when used at the recommended dose. The choice of sedative agent is based on the clinical state of the patient and the effects and side effects of the medication.

> *If the patient has an airway obstruction or a potential obstruction, it is generally safer to let them continue to breathe than to paralyze them.*

Opiates

Fentanyl is a rapid-acting and very potent opiate of relatively short duration. It produces analgesia within 90 seconds with an effective duration of about 30 minutes. In addition to its profound sedative and analgesic effects, fentanyl may decrease tachycardia and hypertension associated with intubation. It appears to be well tolerated hemodynamically with little hypotension in most children. Fentanyl is indicated when hemodynamic control of the patient is critical. Fentanyl may be easily reversed with narcotic antagonists such as naloxone.

The usual recommended dose of fentanyl is 2 to 3 μg/kg, given 1–3 minutes prior to intubation. A higher dose of 5–7 μg/kg is indicated to block hypertension and tachycardia, and some authorities suggest as much as 15 μg/kg. Neonates appear to be more sensitive to fentanyl, and decreased doses should be used.

An alternative narcotic agent is alfentanil 20–30 mg/kg. This agent has similar properties to fentanyl.

All opiates, fentanyl included, cause respiratory depression in a dose dependent response. Fentanyl may also cause seizures, chest wall rigidity, and skeletal muscle movements. There are some reports of increased ICP associated with fentanyl, particularly in children. It should be used with caution when ICP is a major factor.

Morphine is not recommended for use in RSI in children.

Barbiturates and Other Hypnotic Agents

Thiopental (2–5 mg/kg IV) is a short-acting barbiturate with an onset of 10 to 20 seconds and a duration of 5–10 minutes. There is abundant emergency and anesthesiology experience with thiopental. Although thiopental is a sedative, there is no analgesic effect. It causes a decrease in intracranial pressure, intracerebral blood flow, and cerebral oxygen consumption. It is most useful in patients with increased ICP (head trauma, meningitis).

Thiopental should not be used for patients with asthma as it may cause additional bronchospasm by release of histamine. Thiopental may cause hypotension by vasodilation and myocardial depression. It should not be used in the hypotensive or hypovolemic patient. Like all sedatives, thiopental causes respiratory depression

Methohexital (1–1.5 mg/kg IV) is a short-acting barbiturate with an onset under 1 minute and a duration of about 5–7 minutes. Methohexital is quite similar to thiopental in action and contraindications. It definitely causes respiratory depression and may cause seizures in high doses. It has no advantages over thiopental in children.

Etomidate (0.2–0.4 mg/kg IV) is an ultrashort-acting, nonbarbiturate hypnotic agent that has been used as an induction agent for anesthesia for years in both children and adults.[17]

Etomidate has minimal hemodynamic effects and may be the drug of choice in a hypotensive or trauma patient.[18] It causes less cardiovascular depression than either the barbiturates or propofol. Etomidate has also been shown to decrease intracranial pressure, cerebral blood flow, and cerebral oxygen metabolism.

Propofol (1–3 mg/kg IV) is a relatively new anesthetic induction and sedative agent. It has an extremely rapid induction time, within 10 to 20 seconds, and a short duration of action 10 to 15 minutes.

Propofol decreases intracranial pressure and cerebral metabolism. It may cause significant hypotension, which limits usefulness in trauma patients. Lower doses can be used for patients with unstable blood pressure.

Unlike other agents, propofol can be used as a drip for continued sedation after the procedure. The continued sedation dose is 0.75 to 0.15 mg/kg minute.

Benzodiazepines

Diazepam (0.2–1.0 mg/kg IV) is a moderately long-acting benzodiazepine (30–90 minutes) with a slow onset (2–4 minutes). It causes less cardiovascular and respiratory depression than the barbiturates. If alcohol is present, the respiratory depression of diazepam is augmented.

Diazepam must be titrated as the effective induction dose is quite variable. Diazepam is more useful as a long term sedative agent for the intubated patient after the procedure. Diazepam has significant amnestic effects.

Diazepam is irritating to veins and may cause localized thrombosis. This is a particularly important side effect in children who may have difficult venous access. Diazepam is not recommended for use in children for this reason alone.

Do not use diazepam in patients with glaucoma.

Lorazepam (0.1–0.4 mg/kg) is long-acting benzodiazepine. It is most useful for long term sedation of the intubated patient. It has no other place in RSI.

Midazolam (0.1–0.4 mg/kg IV) is a rapid onset and short-acting benzodiazepine (30–60 minutes) with potent amnestic effects. It is slower in onset than the hypnotic agents and should be administered 2 full minutes before intubation is attempted. Midazolam may require 3–5 minutes for complete effect. The typical RSI dose is much higher than a dose used for sedation and still may not be reliably effective in 0.3 mg/kg dose.

Midazolam is faster in onset, shorter in action, and has a narrower dose range than either lorazepam or diazepam.

Midazolam causes respiratory and cardiovascular depression. It does not increase ICP and may provide some small decrease in cerebral blood flow.

The effects of the benzodiazepines are generally not as reliable for RSI as the hypnotic agents. Benzodiazepines are most useful as an adjunct to provide retrograde amnesia of the procedure or as agents in the patient with ongoing seizures. Benzodiazepines have little effect on the intracerebral pressure.

All of the benzodiazepines are reversible with flumazenil. All of the benzodiazepines are suitable for use in the patient with status epilepticus.

Neuroleptic Agents

The only neuroleptic agent that is useful in intubation is ketamine. Ketamine is often described as a dissociative anesthetic, where the patient may appear to be awake, but is amnestic and unresponsive to pain. In contrast to the other sedative agents, ketamine increases the cardiac output, pulse rate, blood pressure, myocardial oxygen consumption, cerebral blood flow, intracranial pressure, and intraocular pressure.[19] Although ketamine has direct negative inotropic properties, it causes a release of endogenous catecholamines resulting in the positive overall effects. Ketamine also increases salivary and bronchial secretions.[20] Secretions can be decreased with atropine 0.01 mg/kg or glycopyrrolate 0.005 mg/kg.

Ketamine causes awakening hallucinations that many adults find unpleasant. These emergence reactions occur in up to 50 percent of adults but are rare in children under 10 years of age.[21]

Ketamine is particularly useful in the asthmatic patient as it is a bronchodilator. It is the sedative of choice in the asthmatic child with respiratory failure.[22][23]

It is contraindicated in head injury (due to both increased oxygen consumption and increased intracranial pressure associated with ketamine). It should be used with extreme caution in hypertensive patients (increases blood pressure) and those with open eye injuries and glaucoma (due to increased intraocular pressure). Ketamine may be the drug of choice in the hypotensive unstable patient, however.

The dose of ketamine for RSI in children is 2 mg/kg. At this dose, anesthesia occurs within 1 minute and lasts about 5 to 10 minutes. Some authorities feel that children who are sedated with ketamine should be also treated with atropine to reduce the secretions, but this opinion is not universal.

Neuromuscular Blocking Agents

The perfect paralytic agent for the child would have an extremely rapid onset; a duration that is proportional to the dose used; have sedative, analgesic, and amnestic properties; be safe from age 1 hour to over 100 years; have minimal side effects; and not require any special storage. This agent also does not yet exist. Current neuromuscular blocking agents may be either a depolarizing agent such as succinylcholine or a nondepolarizing agent such as pancuronium or curare. None of these have sedative properties.

Use of neuromuscular blocking agents is controversial, with anesthesiologists fearing increased morbidity and mortality when nonanesthesiologists use these agents. The largest study to date in a community hospital with emergency physician intubation with these agents has not validated these concerns.[24] The only absolute contraindication to the use of a neuromuscular blocking agent would be inability to manage the airway after making the patient apneic.

Succinylcholine Succinylcholine is considered an ideal paralytic agent because of the rapid onset of action (within 45 seconds) and the short duration of the drug (4–5 minutes). Unfortunately, succinylcholine has significant side effects, largely related to the depolarization of the muscle cell. These side effects limit the use of succinylcholine in children.

Hyperkalemia Perhaps the most clinically significant complication of succinylcholine is hyperkalemia. Although the effect has been documented for over 30 years, the precise mechanism of hyperkalemia is not yet known. It is currently thought to be due to an increased number of acetylcholine receptors in these patients. The acetylcholine receptors are found within the muscle membrane, not just at the neuromuscular junction. The increase in acetylcholine receptor sites occurs within 5 to 20 days after the development of the disease or injury. Succinylcholine can cause lethal hyperkalemia in patients with burns, crush injuries, abdominal infections, tetanus, muscle disorders, and denervating disorders.[25][26][27] Succinylcholine can be safely used in massive trauma, burns, spinal cord injuries, etc., if used within this five-day grace period. Obviously, patients with underlying hyperkalemia, such as patients with renal failure, should not be given succinylcholine.

Prolonged Paralysis Succinylcholine can cause prolonged paralysis in those children who have a deficiency of pseudocholinesterase or an atypical pseudocholinesterase.[28] Several drugs have also been associated with prolonged paralysis including magnesium, lithium, and quinidine.[29] Patients who are intoxicated with cocaine may have prolonged paralysis when given succinylcholine because cocaine is competitively metabolized by cholinesterase. The net effect of any disturbance in metabolism of succinylcholine is to prolong paralysis from 5–10 minutes to several hours. Although known pseudocholinesterase deficiency is a contraindication, the only complication would be prolongation of the paralysis.

Malignant Hyperthermia Malignant hyperthermia is thought to occur from excessive calcium influx through open channels.[30] It is associated with markedly increased temperatures, metabolic acidosis, rhabdomyolysis, and disseminated intravascular coagulopathy. It is thought to occur once in every 15,000 patients given succinylcholine.[31] This problem has prompted the FDA to ban the use of succinylcholine in infants and children except in emergency situations.[32]

Increased Intraocular Pressure Succinylcholine causes a transient rise in intraocular pressure. Theoretically, this increased intraocular pressure could cause expulsion of the vitreous in an open eye injury. There has never been a documented case of this complication despite a widespread use in open eye surgery.[33] The prudent practitioner will use a nondepolarizing agent in penetrating eye injuries if readily available.

Increased Intracranial Pressure The significance of the rise in intracranial pressure that accompanies succinylcholine is controversial. The drug has been used widely and successfully in this setting.

The transient rise in pressure may be due to a direct effect of fasciculations, increased cerebral blood flow, or sympathetic stimulation. Pretreatment with a nondepolarizing agent will blunt this response.[34] Pretreatment may not be practical when intubation is urgent.

Muscle Fasciculations Fasciculations are asynchronous contractions of every muscle fiber. These fasciculations occur until paralysis occurs. Diffuse muscle pain is a common complaint after the use of succinylcholine. During fasciculations, gastric pressure increases, enhancing the risk of aspiration.[35]

Fasciculations can be prevented by pretreatment with a small dose of a non-depolarizing agent such as vecuronium prior to the administration of succinylcholine.[36] Many physicians do not use a pretreatment dose.

If intubation is not successful during the initial paralysis, a second dose of succinylcholine can be used in adolescents. A repeated dose of succinylcholine in infants and small children may cause bradycardia and even asystole.[37] Repeated doses of succinylcholine in children should not be used.

Nondepolarizing Agents The nondepolarizing neuromuscular blocking agents bind in a competitive nonstimulatory fashion to the α-subunit of the acetylcholine receptor. Because there is no muscle stimulation prior to paralysis, these agents do not produce fasciculations. Three types of nondepolarizing drugs are available: benzylisoquinoliniums, aminosteroids, and quaternary amines. Of these, only the benzylisoquinoliniums and aminosteroids are used in RSI.

Although usually not needed in the emergency department, nondepolarizing agents can be reversed by use of an anticholinesterase agent such as edrophonium or neostigmine. Reversal may take several minutes and cannot be used as a "safety net" for a failed intubation.

The newer nondepolarizing agents (vecuronium, rocuronium, and mivacurium) can induce intubating paralysis in a time frame comparable with succinylcholine. Unfortunately, the shortest duration nondepolarizing agent has a duration of twice that of succinylcholine. Onset time of paralysis of the nondepolarizing agents is inversely related to the potency of the agent.

Some patients have significant release of histamine associated with use of the nondepolarizing muscle relaxants.[38] These symptoms can be avoided with slower infusion of the agent, but this may not be an option during intubation. None of the nondepolarizing agents should be used in patients with myasthenia gravis.

Vecuronium Vecuronium is an aminosteroid nondepolarizing agent. It has an intermediate duration of action of 30–60 minutes with an initial dose of about 0.1 mg/kg. It produces clinical effects in 30 seconds and intubation paralysis in 1–4 minutes. A priming dose of 0.01 mg/kg given 2 minutes before intubation will shorten the onset of vecuronium to about 30 seconds. Concerns of arrhythmias in children associated with succinylcholine use have made high dose vecuronium (0.28 mg/kg) a popular choice for emergent pediatric airways.[39]

Vercuronium has been associated with a myopathy of critical illness in children who have concomitantly received high doses of steroids. The exact mechanism of the myopathy is not known. It is associated with use of other aminosteroid neuromuscular blocking agents. It is unlikely that single use of these agents will be associated with this myopathy, but caution should be used in children receiving high doses of steroids.

Rocuronium Rocuronium is an aminosteroid nondepolarizing agent similar to vecuronium with a very rapid onset of action. A dose of 0.8 mg/kg will produce paralysis in infants and children in 30 seconds or less. Recovery time from paralysis is between 30 and 45 minutes. This agent may be used quite successfully as a replacement for succinylcholine, if the extended recovery time is tolerable.

Mivacurium Mivacurium is a short-acting nondepolarizing benzylisoquino-linium muscle relaxant. It has a short onset of action (30–60 seconds) with intubation conditions within 75–120 seconds. It lasts only about 15–20 minutes. The typical RSI dose is about 0.15 to 0.3 mg/kg. Mivacurium is metabolized by plasma cholinesterase, and children recover from blockade much quicker than adults do.[40] This effect may make mivacurium more useful in pediatric intubation.

Pancuronium Pancuronium is another aminosteroid neuromuscular blocking agent that will provide acceptable conditions for intubation in 90–120 seconds with paralysis that lasts from 45 to 90 minutes. It is classified as a long-acting agent with a slow onset. The slow onset limits usefulness in the ED setting.

Pancuronium is primarily excreted in the urine, so reduced renal function or urinary output will increase the duration of effect. Pancuronium can cause severe histamine reactions.

Sellick's Maneuver

Sellick's maneuver or cricoid pressure will decrease the chances of regurgitation by pressing the cricoid cartilage firmly against the esophagus.[41] The relatively soft yielding esophagus will be compressed between the cricoid cartilage and the vertebral column. Don't release cricoid cartilage pressure until you are certain that the tube is in the trachea. Since Sellick's maneuver is not certain protection against regurgitation, inflate the cuff of the tube as soon as possible.

Sellick's maneuver should always be used when the patient is ventilated with a bag-valve-mask prior to intubation. An alternative to Sellick's maneuver is BURP maneuver as previously described.

Intubate the Patient

Intubation is performed after there is full relaxation of the airway muscles. This usually occurs about 45 seconds after the administration of succinylcholine. Cricoid pressure should be maintained until the cuff is inflated and the tube position verified.

The usual caveat is that the most experienced person at intubation should be the one doing the intubation because the patient is paralyzed and sedated. This is an unacceptable policy in a training institution. If this caveat is always followed, newer physicians will remain untrained. Until the resident is completely comfortable, in the eyes of the attending physician, then the attending emergency physician should be within arm's reach of the patient until the patient is successfully intubated.

If intubation fails, cricoid pressure should be maintained and the patient ventilated with a bag-valve mask. After the patient is reoxygenated, then either another intubation should be attempted or an alternative airway technique employed.

Verify Placement

After intubation, the tube must be confirmed to be in the trachea. This verification is more important than the intubation itself. There is no sin in an esophageal intubation but there is much sin in not recognizing such a placement. The bedside clinical assessment consists of visualizing the endo-tracheal tube as it passes through the vocal cords. This is followed by listening over the epigastrium for bowel sounds and listening over each lung field for the presence and equality of breath sounds. Looking for condensation on the endotracheal tube with exhalation and watching for the chest to rise and fall with inspiration completes the clinical assessment.

The process of verification of tube placement is controversial. Each and every one of the clinical indicators of proper placement has failed. The sequence of events that precipitates intubation in the child is often accompanied by one or more conditions that can cause these failures of verification. Unrecognized esophageal intubation is catastrophic for the patient. Further confirmation of tube placement can be by documentation of carbon dioxide from the lungs, documentation of stable or increasing oxygen saturation, and by x-ray of the chest for tube placement. The astute emergency physician will always use a combination of these methods and will verify the tube placement by at least one of the other techniques. The astute clinician will always re-verify tube placement in children when clinical conditions deteriorate.

Inspection

In the perfect intubation, the tube will be seen to pass through the child's cords. Unfortunately, in the stress of an emergency intubation, with vomitus or blood, and with difficult anatomy or cervical immobilization, visualization of the tube's passage through the cords is all too often a fond aspiration.[42]

Likewise, it is difficult to look for even expansion of the chest without any gastric distention in the immobilized patient with potential chest trauma. It is nice to see, but can't be depended on as the only sign of a good intubation.

Auscultation

In the perfect patient, the breath sounds will be heard equally when the tube is in appropriate position in the trachea. Air meeting water (fluid) causes bubbling, which implies the tube is in the esophagus or stomach. In the small child, normal breath sounds may be heard when listening over the stomach. If breath sounds, but no bubbling is heard over the stomach, do not pull the tube but complete the rest of the assessment. Listen to two breaths on the right third intercostal space in the midaxillary line and compare to two breaths on the left side in the third interspace.

Pulse Oximetry

Pulse oximetry has long been a standard method of monitoring the patient with respiratory difficulties. If the oxygen saturation is rising or stays at an acceptable level in a paralyzed patient, then the endotracheal tube is certainly in the appropriate place. Unfortunately, the pulse is not particularly useful in the patient with profound shock or cardiac arrest.

Carbon Dioxide Detectors

End tidal carbon dioxide measurements or a disposable colorimetric device (CO_2 detector) can be used.[43] These devices work by measurement (colorimetric or direct measurement) of the carbon dioxide produced by the body and eliminated by the lungs. If the ET tube is placed in the esophagus, there should be no carbon dioxide in the exhaled gas. The end-tidal CO_2 detector works so well in the operating room that its use there is considered standard of care by anesthesiologists.[44] All CO_2 detectors have been shown to fail in the patient who has had a cardiac arrest and in the patient who has recently consumed a carbonated beverage.[45] These conditions occur far more frequently in emergency medicine practice than in the operating room.

Esophageal Detector Devices
Syringe aspiration esophageal detector devices have recently been used to confirm tube placement.[46 47] These devices use the rapid refill of a bulb syringe or equivalent through the endotracheal tube as proof that the tube is in the airway, rather than the esophagus. In adults, there is virtually 100 percent assurance that the EDD is *not* in the esophagus, but the EDD may misidentify endobronchial or mainstem intubation as esophageal. Marley and his colleagues showed that the esophageal detection device correctly identified 100 percent of esophageal intubation (but only 35 of 40 ED intubation).[48] There is no study that assures that these devices will be effective in the deliberate air leak associated with uncuffed tubes used in a pediatric airway. They are currently approved only for children greater than 20 kg body weight or older than five years.

Chest X-Ray
Following confirmation by auscultation, inspection, esophageal detector devices, and/or CO_2 measurement, a chest x-ray should always be obtained. A chest x-ray can also help with depth and placement of the tube. Ideally, the tip of the endotracheal tube should be in the middle third of the trachea, just proximal to the carina.

It is impractical to get a radiograph confirming tube placement in every elective intubation in the operating room or in the field, but this is not true in emergency medicine. Although the radiograph will be the gold standard by which the legal field judges our performance, a radiograph takes several minutes to obtain and process and the patient needs appropriate and adequate ventilation while the radiograph is processed. The clinician must confirm tube placement prior to obtaining a radiograph and ensure that the tube does not move during this radiograph.

Secure the Tube
The risk of inadvertent dislodgment of the ETT or mainstem bronchus intubation is much higher in the small child due to the shorter trachea and bronchus. The trachea is about 12–15 cm long in the adult and only 4 cm long in the newborn. The endotracheal tube must protrude only 3–4 cm past the cords in order to avoid a right mainstem bronchus intubation. Since the child's neck is much more flexible than the adult's is, motion of the neck can dislodge an ETT in a child.

Security of the tube includes sedation so that the child will not move and ensures that the child's head does not move during radiographs and other procedures after intubation. After each such procedure, the oxygen saturation should be carefully monitored. A falling saturation should prompt the astute clinician to reassess the placement of the endotracheal tube.

Surgical Airway in Children

If the child cannot be adequately ventilated by bag-valve-mask, and endotracheal intubation is unsuccessful, then a surgical airway is indicated.

Cricothyrotomy

Cricothyrotomy should be reserved for the child over 8 years old. The technique is as described in chapter 8.

Needle Cricothyrotomy

The equipment needed for this procedure in a child should be readily available in the resuscitation area. In infants and young children, this procedure may be quite difficult because of the short neck, floppy and redundant soft tissues, and the small diameter of the trachea. Nevertheless, it may be the only available surgical airway in the field.

A 15 mm endotracheal tube connector (fitting all resuscitation equipment) from a 3 mm endotracheal tube will fit into the large bore (12–14–16 gauge) intravenous catheter hub used for needle tracheostomy. The airway resistance will be great because of the resistance to flow in the small piping. With 100 percent oxygen source, adequate oxygen saturation can be maintained even with slower rates of ventilation. Unfortunately, hypercapnia will result in almost all of these patients. Transtracheal (needle cricothyrotomy) should be considered as a temporizing airway only.

Use of a Cook Critical Care "Melker Emergency Cricothyrotomy Catheter Set" may provide a wider bore tube with less airway resistance. This device may be used as a needle tracheostomy in larger children.

Alternative Airways

Blind Nasal Intubation

BNI should not be used on any pediatric patient who needs an airway rapidly. Despite claims to the contrary, it often requires minutes to complete. As experienced physicians can readily attest, it is more difficult in the child than in the adult. It is a poor choice for the asthmatic patient in extremis and for children in respiratory failure. The far anterior airway anatomy of the child makes BNI much more difficult than in adults.

In the child, increased size of the adenoids makes nasal intubation fraught with hazards not seen in the adult. The adenoids can make passage more difficult, bleed, or even shear off and plug the endotracheal tube.

If a nasal intubation is desired, a proper sized set of Magill forceps must be available. Vasoconstricting agents should be applied to both nostrils. After insertion of the tube into the child's nostril, the tube is observed with direct laryngoscopy. The Magill forceps are used to lift the tube into the proper position to be advanced straight into the glottis. They should not be used to push the endotracheal tube. Insertion of a nasal tube into the patient with a basilar skull fracture, a deviated nasal septum, a nasal fracture, enlarged adenoids, or a bleeding diathesis is ill-advised.

LMA in Children

The size 1 LMA has been used for neonatal resuscitation with over 94 percent success rate.[49] In the smaller device used for infants and small children, there will be leaks with positive pressure ventilation. This device has no route for suctioning or for delivering medications. It does not protect against aspiration and does have some associated gastric distention from incomplete fit of the mask. Even with appropriate position of the cuff, if airway pressure is greater than 20 cm of water, then the child's stomach may be inflated.

Manual Intubation

Manual intubation, or more correctly digital tactile intubation, has been used for centuries.[50] It fell into disfavor when Chevalier Jackson introduced laryngoscopy and direct vision of the vocal cords.[51] It may have a limited place in the field when equipment is not available or where equipment has broken during the procedure.[52 53] It is not advised for use in very small children due to the relatively large size of the adult's hand and the smaller size of the child's airway.

Indications
- Cramped quarters
- Copious oral secretions or vomitus
- Inability to visualize the vocal cords
- Suspected cervical spine trauma
- Equipment failure or lack of laryngoscope

Technique
The index and long fingers are inserted into the patient's mouth past the base of the tongue until the epiglottis is palpated. An endotracheal tube is passed between the fingers over the epiglottis and into the trachea. If the patient is breathing, air movement may further guide placement (Figure 9-1).

The patient's neck may remain in neutral position and the patient may remain in a cervical collar. The patient must be unresponsive, since the presence of a gag reflex will pose danger to the operator.

Complications
The most feared complication of this procedure in pediatric patients is the same as in adults—being bitten by the patient. This can be prevented by use of a bite block or oral airway inserted laterally along the molars. Digital intubation of conscious patients and seizing patients should be avoided.

As in all blind intubation techniques, esophageal intubation is a real possibility. This is an innocuous complication if it is promptly recognized by the standard techniques for checking tube placement.

Stylet-Guided Intubation
Lighted Stylet
Intubation with a lighted stylet depends upon transillumination of the soft tissue of the neck with a light placed in the larynx.[54] It requires neither flexion nor extension of the neck in order to insert an endotracheal tube. It is suitable for the larger child. Equipment is not available for infants and smaller children.

Method There is no specific lighted stylet that is designed for children. Orotracheal intubation is performed with a standard endotracheal tube that has been shortened to 25 cm. This tube is placed over a lubricated surgical flex-light (Concept Corporation, Clearwater, Florida-Tubestat).[55] The light extends to the end of the shortened endotracheal tube.

The method is the same as for the adult patient.

Complications and Precautions

Inability to visualize the light If the ambient lighting is extreme—as in direct sunlight—this method becomes difficult. In the original paper describing the technique, two of the three unsuccessful attempts were in sunlight. In an emergency department, simply extinguishing the overhead lights for a few seconds may solve this problem.

Blood and vomitus may further obscure the light at the end of the tube.

Esophageal intubation In very thin children, visualization of a midline glow may be found in esophageal intubation. Since this is a blind technique, the operator must ensure that the tube placement is correct. Although this complication has not been reported in children, the smaller size, lesser neck mass, and smaller body weight of most children would make esophageal visualization more likely.

Loss of the light bulb In one case in the original paper, the light bulb at the end of the flexible stylet was dislodged. This required bronchoscopy for retrieval. Newer lights from the manufacturer have a shrink-fit plastic that improves strength and reduces this risk. A fiberoptic light source and stylet has been developed that eliminates the problem of bulb loss. The original lighted stylet is quite inexpensive and may be readily supplied to EMS field agencies while the newer fiberoptic version is much more costly.

NG Tube/Suction Catheter as a Stylet

A helpful technique that is infrequently used is the use of a NG or suction tube as a guide through the cords.[56] This is most helpful where the nasotracheal tube has been passed up to the cords but can't be passed through them. A NG tube or suction tube can then be slipped through the ET tube and passed through the cords. Using the smaller tube as a guide the ET tube is then re-advanced in the proper position.

The suction catheter could also be used to provide low frequency, high-flow ventilation in a manner similar to the more invasive jet ventilation techniques described following.[57] The suction or even just oxygen tubing may be more easily passed than a larger caliber endotracheal tube.

Fiberoptic-Guided Intubation

The advantages of fiberoptic intubation in the child are the same as in the adult. Unfortunately, the fiberoptic scope is an expensive and relatively delicate instrument. Very small pediatric fiberoptic devices are correspondingly much more expensive and less likely to be readily available except in specialty pediatric emergency departments.

The primary advantage of the flexible fiberoptic technique is in negotiation of difficult anatomy. The fiberoptic laryngoscopes allow the operator to orally or nasally intubate the patient without flexion of the neck and without the disadvantages of the blind techniques. A secondary advantage is in the ready diagnosis of the patient with an inhalation injury or with epiglottic disease.

Method

The basics of the technique are the same as adults. Prepare the laryngoscope with a tube over it. 3.6 mm laryngoscopes (Olympus) have recently been developed with both suction and oxygen delivery ports. This will fit snugly through a 4.5 mm ID endotracheal tube. A 2.2mm OD fiberoptic scope is available, but this instrument is difficult to use with an endotracheal tube. With smaller adults and children, use of a pediatric bronchoscope may allow placement of a smaller diameter tube. This is a significant limiting factor in pediatric patients.

Complications

By far the most major complication of use of a fiberoptic laryngoscope in the pediatric patient is delay in oxygenation caused by an inexperienced operator. Skill with the fiberoptic laryngoscope should be gained during elective or semielective intubation rather than during an emergency. Attempting to view landmarks from a new perspective with a new instrument, in the small size of the child, while dodging bits of debris, secretions, and blood, is not calculated to be either quick or elegant.

Retrograde Intubation

A variant of the aforementioned technique is retrograde-guided intubation as described by Waters in 1963 for use in patients with drastically altered anatomy.[58] It is particularly useful in the patient with facial trauma and a suspected neck injury—in whom a blind nasotracheal intubation is unfeasible. In this technique, a transtracheal needle or a needle passed through the cricothyroid membrane is used to thread a long wire stylet cephalad through the cords. The guide wire is retrieved in the oropharynx and a tube threaded over it. The tube is then passed into the trachea past the vocal cords. Conceivably, the guide wire could be passed through a nostril and the entire process used to pass a nasotracheal tube. Successful pediatric use in a 14-month-old infant has been described.[59] This technique is no different in the child than in the adult and has been previously described.

The technique may be valuable where vomitus or bloody drainage obstructs the view or obscures the light in standard intubation. Retrograde guide wire intubation does take time to perform but is far more useful than repeated unsuccessful attempts at standard or blind nasal intubation in the difficult patient.

Both Intracath central venous pressure catheters and Seldinger guide wires have been used for this technique. The smaller Seldinger wire is more appropriate for infants and children.

Complications appear to be related to the needle stick required and are usually minor. No significant contraindications are known.[60] Ensure that both ends of the guide wire are secured while trying to pass the tube so that the guide wire will not be pulled free from the neck.

Tables

Common Pitfalls in RSI

- Lack of preparation of equipment and drugs prior to starting the procedure
- Failure to preoxygenate the patient
- Using a bag-valve-mask in the spontaneously ventilating patient
- Failing to use Sellick's maneuver or BURP maneuver
- Attempting intubation before paralysis is complete
- Failure to secure the airway after intubation
- Failure to continue sedation after intubation
- Failure to continue paralysis after intubation

Contraindications to Rapid Sequence Intubation

- Spontaneous breathing with adequate ventilation
- Operator concern that both intubation and mask ventilation may not be successful
- Major laryngeal trauma
- Upper airway obstruction
- Distorted facial or airway anatomy

Signs of Respiratory Distress in the Child

- Tachypnea
- Use of accessory muscles
- Nasal flaring
- Position of comfort
- Tripod position
- Grunting respirations
- Cyanosis

Signs of Respiratory Failure in the Child

- Decreased level of consciousness
- Grunting respirations and increased work of breathing
- Poor air entry and decreased breath sounds
- Bradycardia
- Apnea/slowed respirations

SUGGESTED PEDIATRIC EQUIPMENT SIZES

Age and Weight (kg)	Laryngoscope Blade	Endotracheal Tube Size	Suction Catheter	IV Catheter	NG Tube Size	Chest Tube Size	Urinary Catheter Size
Newborn 0–6 months (3–5 kilo)	Size 1 straight	3.0–3.5 uncuffed tube	6–8 Fr	22 gauge	12 Fr	12–18 Fr	5–8 Fr feeding tube
6–12 months (5–7 kilo)	Size 1 straight	3.5–4.5 uncuffed	8–10 Fr	22 gauge	12 Fr	14–20 Fr	8 Fr
1–3 years (10–12 kilo)	Size 1 straight	4.0–4.5 uncuffed	10 Fr	20–22 gauge	12 Fr	14–24 Fr	10 Fr
4–7 years (16–18 kilo)	Size 2 straight or curved	5.0–5.5 uncuffed	14 Fr	20 gauge	12 Fr	20–32 Fr	10–12 Fr
8–10 years (24–30 kilo)	Size 2–3 straight or curved	5.5–6.5 cuffed	14 Fr	18–20 gauge	14 Fr	28–38 Fr	12 Fr

END NOTES

[1] American Academy of Pediatrics. *Emergency Medical Services for Children: The role of the primary care provider.* Elk Grove Village, IL: American Academy of Pediatrics, 1992.

[2] Nakayma, D. K., Gardner, M. J., and Rowe, M. I. "Emergency Endotracheal Intubation in Pediatric Trauma," in *Arch Surg* 1990;211:218–223.

[3] Dickison, A. E. "The Normal and Abnormal Pediatric Upper Airway," in *Clin Chest Med* Oct 8(4):583,1987.

[4] Okhuysen, R. S., Bristow, F., Burkhead, S., et al. "Evaluation of a New Thin-Walled Endotracheal Tube for Use in Children," *Chest* 1996;109:1335–1338.

[5] Ibid.

[6] Ibid.

[7] American Heart Association. *Textbook of Pediatric Advanced Life Support*. Dallas: The Association, 1994.

[8] Todres, I. D. "Pediatric Airway Control and Ventilation," in *Ann Emerg Med* 1993;22:440–444.

[9] Rosen, M., and Laurence, K. M. "Expansion Pressure and Rupture Pressures in the Newborn Lungs," in *Lancet* 1965;2:721–722.

[10] Hirschman, A. M., and Kravath, R. E. "Venting vs. Ventilating: A danger of Manual Resuscitation Bags," in *Chest* 1982;82:369–370.

[11] Nakayama, D. K., Waggoner, T., and Venkataraman, S. T. "The Use of Drugs in Emergency Airway Management in Pediatric Trauma," in *Ann Surg* 1992;216:205–211.

[12] Sing, R. F., Reilly, P. M., Rotondo, M. F., et al. "Out of Hospital Rapid Sequence Induction for Intubation of the Pediatric Patient," in *Acad Emerg Med* 1996;3:41–45.

[13] Yamamoto, L. G. "Rapid Sequence Anesthesia Induction and Advanced Airway Management in Pediatric Patients," in *Emerg Clin N America* 1991;9:611–638.

[14] Yamamoto, L. G., Yim, G. K., and Britten, A. G. "Rapid Sequence Anesthesia Induction for Emergency Intubation," in *Ped Emerg Care* 1990; 6:200–213.

[15] Ibid.

[16] Morris, I. "Pharmacologic Aids to Intubation and the Rapid Sequence Induction," in *Emerg Med Clin North America* 1998;6:753–768.

[17] Giese, J. L., and Stanley, T. H. "Etomidate: A New Intravenous Anesthetic Induction Agent," in *Pharmacotherapy* 1983;3:251–258.

[18] Plewa, M. C., King, R., Johnson, D., et al. "Etomidate Used During Emergency Intubation of Trauma Patients," in *Am J Emerg Med.* 1997;15: 98–100.

[19] Green, L. M., Nakamura, R., and Johnson, N. E. "Ketamine Sedation for Pediatric Procedures: Parts I and II," in *Ann Emerg Med* 1990;19: 1024–1046.

[20] Epstein, F. B. "Ketamine Dissociative Sedation in Pediatric Emergency Medical Practice," in *Am J Emerg Med* 1993;11:180–182.

[21] Jankiewizc, A. M., and Nowakowski, P. "Ketamine and Succinylcholine for Emergency Intubation of Pediatric Patients," in *DICP* 1991;25: 475–476.

[22] Tobias, J. D. "Airway Management for Pediatric Emergencies," in *Pediatric Ann* 1996;25:317–328.

[23] Nichols, D. G. "Emergency Management of Status Asthmaticus in Children," in *Ped Annals* 1996;25:394–403.

[24] Dufour, D. G., Larose, D. L., and Clement S. C. "Rapid Sequence Intubation in the Emergency Department," in *J Emerg Med* 1995;13:705–710.

[25] Zink, B. J., Snyder H. S., and Raccio-Robak, N. "Lack of a Hyperkalemic Response in Emergency Department Patients Receiving Succinylcholine," in *Acad Emerg Med* 1995;2:974.

[26] Smith, R. B., and Grenvik, A. "Cardiac Arrest Following Succinylcholine Use in Patients with Central Nervous System Injuries," in *Anesthesiology* 1970;33:558.

[27] Tomie, J. D., Joyce, T. H., and Mitchell, G. D. "Succinylcholine Danger in the Burned Patient," in *Anesthesiology* 1969;31:540.

[28] McStravog, L. J. "Dangers of Succinylcholine in Anesthesia," in *Laryngoscope* 1974;84:929.

[29] Morris, I. R. "Pharmacologic Aids to Intubation and the Rapid Sequence Induction," in *Emerg Med Clin North Amer* 1988;6:753–768.

[30] Gronert, G. A., and Antognini, J. F. "Malignant hyperthermia," in Miller, R. D., ed., *Anesthesia,* 4th ed., Vol. 1. New York: Churchill Livingstone, 1994,1075–1093.

[31] Ording, H. "Incidence of Malignant Hyperthermia in Denmark," in *Anesth Analg* 1985;64:700–704.

[32] *Physician's Desk Reference,* 50th ed. Montvale, NJ: Medical Economics, 1996, pp. 1073–1075.

[33] Libonati, M. M., Leahy, J. J., and Ellison, N. "The Use of Succinylcholine in Open Eye Surgery," in *Anesthesiology* 1985;63:727.

[34] Savarese, J. J., Miller, R. D., Lien, C. A., et al. "Pharmacology of Muscle Relaxants and Their Antagonists," in Miller, R. D., ed., *Anesthesia* 4th ed., vol 1. New York: Churchill Livingstone, 1994;417–487.

[35] Kharasch, M., and Graff, J. "Emergency Management of the Airway," in *Crit Care Clinics N Amer* 1995;11:53–66.

[36] Saverese, J. J., Miller, R. D., Lien, C. A., et al. "Pharmacology of Muscle Relaxants and Their Antagonists," in Miller, R. D., ed., *Anesthesia,* 4th ed., vol. 1. New York: Churchill Livingstone, 1994;417–487.

[37] Rosenburg, H., and Gronert, G. A. "Intractable Cardiac Arrest in Children Given Succinylcholine [letter]," in *Anesthesiology* 1992;77:1054.

[38] Sarner, J. B., Brandom, D. W., Woelfel, S. K., et al. "Clinical Pharmacology of Mivacurium Chloride in Children during Nitrous Oxide-Halothane and Nitrous Oxide-Narcotic Anesthesia," in *Anesth Analg* 1989;68:116–121.

[39] Wright, J. L., and Patterson, M. D. "Resuscitating the Pediatric Patient," in *Emerg Clin N Amer* 1996;4:219–231.

[40] Goudsouzian, N. G., Denman, W., Schwartz, A., et al. "Pharmacodynamic and Hemodynamic Effects of Mivacurium in Infants Anesthetized with Halothane and Nitrous Oxide," in *Anesthesiology* 1993;79:919–925.

[41] Sellick, B. A. "Cricoid Pressure to Control Regurgitation of Stomach Contents during Induction of Anesthesia," in *Lancet* 1961;2:404–406.

[42] White, S. J., and Slovis, C. M. "Inadvertent Esophageal Intubation in the Field: Reliance on a Fool's "Gold Standard," in *Academic Emerg Med* 97; 4:89–91.

[43] Macleod, B. A., Heller, M. B., and Gerard J., et al. "Verification of Endotracheal Tube Placement with Colorimetric End-Tidal CO_2 Detection," *Ann Emerg Med* 1991;20:267–270.

[44] Ginsburg, W. H. "When Does a Guideline Become a Standard? The New American Society of Anesthesiologists Guidelines Give Us a Clue," in *Academic Emerg Med* 1993;21:1891–1896.

[45] Garza, M. "End Tidal CO_2 Detector Questions Arise," in *J Emerg Medical Services* 1991;16:22–23.

[46] Zaleski, L., Abello, D., and Gold, M. I. "The Esophageal Detector Device, Does It Work," in *Anesthesiology* 1993;79:244–247.

[47] Marley, C. D. Jr., Eitel, D. R., Anderson, T. E., et al. "Evaluation of a Prototype Esophageal Detection Device," in *Acad Emerg Med* 1995; 2:503–507.

[48] Ibid.

[49] Mitzushima, A. "The Laryngeal Mask Airway in Infants," in *Anesthesia* 1992;47:349–351.

[50] Stewart, R. D. "Tactile Orotracheal Intubation," in *Ann Emerg Med* 1984; 13:175–178.

[51] Collins, V. J. *Principles and Practice of Anesthesiology.* Philadelphia, PA: Lea & Febiger, 1952, p. 288.

[52] Hudon, F. "Intubation without Laryngoscopy," in *Anesthesiology* 1945; 6:476–482.

[53] Hardwick, W. C., and Bluhm, D. "Digital Intubation," in *J Emerg Med* 1984;1:317–320

[54] Vollmer, T. P., Stewart, R. D., Paris, P. M., et al. "Use of a Lighted Stylet for Guided Orotracheal Intubation in the Prehospital Setting," in *Ann Emerg Med* 1985;14:324–328.

[55] Ellis, D. G., Stewart, R. D., Kaplan, R. M., et al. "Success Rates of Blind Orotracheal Intubation Using a Transillumination Technique with a Lighted Stylet," in *Ann Emerg Med* 1986;15:138–142.

[56] Dryden, G. E. "Use of a Suction Catheter to Assist Blind Nasal Intubation," in *Anesthesiology* 1976;45:260.

[57] Down, M. P. "Emergency Transtracheal Ventilation," *Anesthesia* 1997;52: 84–95.

[58] Waters, D. J. "Guided Blind Endotracheal Intubation," in *Anesthesia* 1963; 18:158–162.

[59] McNamera, R. M. "Retrograde Intubation of the Trachea," in *Ann Emerg Med* 1987;16:680–682.

[60] Akinyemi, O. O. "Complications of Guided Blind Endotracheal Intubation," in *Anesthesia* 1979;34:590–592.

Chapter **Eleven**

Special Situations

Complications in Intubated and Ventilated Patients

When the intubated patient has difficulty breathing, the clinician has little time to analyze the situation. The patient is often paralyzed and usually heavily sedated to tolerate the intubation. When asked to reevaluate the patient who has been intubated, the patient's general condition and the intubation must be reassessed. Always assume that an agitated intubated patient is not getting enough oxygen and reevaluate the entire system (Figure 11-1).

Always consider that the patient may have had an esophageal intubation. At least look for moisture in the tube with every breath and consider checking the tube placement with a capnometer or direct visualization of the tube with a laryngoscope.

Ensure that the tube has not been partially dislodged by looking at the depth of the tube placement and auscultating the breath sounds. Is there an air leak? Has the cuff been overinflated or has it ruptured? Is the patient biting on the tube? Is the tube plugged by mucus?

Generally an intubated patient who has an acute difficulty will have a tension pneumothorax, a mucus plug, a fault in the ventilator or the oxygen delivery tubing, inadvertent extubation, or will have a bite obstruction of the tube. Occasionally, the patient may be fighting the ventilator and simply require more sedation or pain control.

First, take the patient off of the ventilator and attempt to ventilate the patient with a bag-valve-mask system connected to 100 percent oxygen by a transport bottle. This will eliminate all mechanical failures and most failures of oxygen delivery.

Inspect the patient and reverify the tube placement to ensure that extubation has not occurred and that the patient is not biting the tube. Carefully listen to breath sounds in both sides and evaluate the patient for retractions and abnormal breathing. If the patient is awake, then ask them to speak. (The intubated patient can't answer. If the patient can speak, then the patient has been inadvertently extubated.)

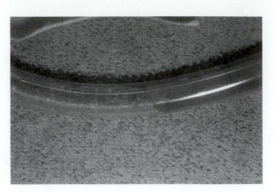

Figure 11-1 Plugged endotracheal tube.
Source: Photo by Charles Stewart and Associates; www.storysmith.net.

Rocking breathing motions, retractions, and tracheal tug argue for a plugged endotracheal tube and rapid replacement of the endotracheal tube. Suction catheters simply won't work well with mucus plugging. This is particularly true when the patient has had chemical lung injuries or inhalation injuries.

Tympany on percussion, engorged neck veins, and decreased breath sounds on one side argue for a tension pneumothorax. Although a chest x-ray may be diagnostic, there often isn't time to obtain one. Needle aspiration of the suspected pneumothorax is both diagnostic and therapeutic. A chest tube can be placed at leisure, after the immediate crisis has been managed.

If all else fails, reintubate the patient with appropriate paralysis and sedation.

Clinical Airway Crises

Laryngospasm

Acute laryngospasm may be caused by inadequate sedation, trauma to the vocal cords (such as from intubation), foreign matter on the vocal cords, effects of some drugs, idiosyncratic, or an anaphylactoid reaction. It can also be precipitated by paroxysmal coughing and emergence from general anesthesia.

Laryngospasm is generally self-limiting but can be quite frustrating and harrowing for the emergency provider. In many of the patients who develop laryngospasm in emergency practice, the trauma of an attempted intubation may be a precipitating factor. When the provider, already having difficulty

TABLE 11-1   REASONS FOR ACUTE PROBLEMS IN THE INTUBATED PATIENT

Think DOPE

• **D**isplacement of the tube (it isn't where it should be!)

• **O**bstruction of the tube (mucous plug, biting)

• **P**neumothorax, PE, pulselessness (cardiac arrest)

• **E**quipment failure (no oxygen, failure of the ventilator, disconnected tubing) with an intubation, now finds the patient has developed laryngospasm, the situation may provoke an unneeded panic. Emergent airway maneuvers are rarely required.

When faced with this situation, the provider should fall back on well-grounded basics of airway management. The initial treatment of laryngospasm is to ventilate the patient with high-pressure manual ventilation with a bag-valve-mask system. Many times, the laryngospasm will abate with hypoxia or hypercarbia.

If the provider has difficulty with this, then he or she should re-examine the patient's vocal cords with a laryngoscope. If the cords are still in spasm, a spray of lidocaine on the cords may resolve the problem.

If the provider is qualified, then paralysis with rapid sequence intubation agents will certainly resolve the laryngospasm. The vocal cords do respond well to neuromuscular blockade.

Finally, if all of these measures fail, then the patient's airway should be restored with surgical cricothyrotomy, or transtracheal jet ventilation. Laryngospasm is more of an obstruction to inhalation rather than expiration, so transtracheal jet ventilation is appropriate.

Wired Jaw

Patients with mandibular fractures or mandibular surgery will often have the fracture or surgery splinted by wiring the jaws together. The patient who has intraoral fixation (a 'wired' jaw) may be a special problem in airway management. While maintaining the structural relationship of the bones in these patients is good, the resultant access to the airway becomes quite "entertaining." The fixation devices, wires or rubber bands prevent the patient from opening his or her mouth. There are two components to this problem: airway access and management of vomiting.

There are three ways to handle this problem: open the mouth, use nasal intubation, or use a surgical airway. If the mouth cannot be rapidly opened or nasal intubation is not rapidly successful, then a surgical airway is the only option. Good mask ventilation may temporize for a short while, but is no substitute for a definitive airway procedure.

1. Nasal intubation is possible with a wired jaw. Nasal intubation is performed in the standard fashion as previously described. It may be somewhat more difficult and always may provoke vomiting. Use of a trigger control tube is strongly recommended. Successful use of this technique will preserve the patient's fracture healing or surgery. Unfortunately, this technique is often slow and may be unsuccessful. It is contraindicated if the patient has had facial trauma.

2. A cricothyrotomy can be performed in an emergent situation. This will be with standard techniques as previously described. During the attempt to open the mouth or to nasally intubate the patient, start preparing for a surgical airway.

3. Opening the mouth means removing the wires or other fixation devices used to hold the jaw together. The wiring may be done with rubber bands or with stainless steel wires. The rubber bands are easily severed with a pair of sharp scissors or a knife. The wires present more of an obstacle. This

patient should have a pair of wire cutters with them. (Well-grounded maxillofacial surgeons will often give them a pair of wire-cutters on a length of umbilical tape to hang around their neck.) Since not all patients want scissors as jewelry and not all maxillo-facial surgeons consider the future problem of airway management, the paramedic or emergency department should have a pair of wire cutters in the intubation kit.

There are no contraindications to opening the airway, but the surgical repair of the jaw may be disrupted during the intubation. Even with the proper equipment, multiple ties may be present, any one of which can prevent opening of the jaw. This should be reserved for the patient in extremis or the patient who has started to vomit.

Vomiting in the Patient with a Wired Jaw

Vomiting in the presence of a wired jaw is a disaster. Even in the awake patient, aspiration may occur. Immediately place the patient in a dependent position—either head down or on the side. A suction hose passed along the gum and posterior to the last molar may be useful. A tonsil suction tip may be used. Unless this patient is completely awake and alert, the operator needs to either open the mouth and pass an airway or perform a surgical airway procedure immediately. The wires should be rapidly cut and the patient intubated with rapid sequence intubation. Induction agents should not be given until the wires have been cut and the jaw controlled.

Total Orthopnea or The Patient Is Upright and Can't Be Moved

The patient may be trapped in a vehicle, requiring lengthy extrication and airway support. The patient may also simply not tolerate the recumbent position.

Preoxygenate the patient for 3–5 minutes with 100 percent oxygen.

If the patient is trapped, it may be quite difficult to recognize esophageal intubation. The usual field clues for appropriate intubation may not be available if you can't listen to the patient's chest. This is a good reason to routinely use CO_2 detectors in the field.

If the patient is a good candidate for rapid sequence intubation and is not predicted to be a difficult intubation, consider RSI. The patient can be sedated and the paralytic agent given while in the seated position and the patient moved to recumbent for the intubation. This is obviously not applicable to the patient who is trapped in the upright position. The blood pressure must be carefully monitored during this procedure because of many of the sedating agents cause postural hypotension.

If the patient is at risk for a difficult intubation, then consider an awake nasal intubation. This preserves the patient's spontaneous ability to breath and decreases the risk of supine position.

Depending on the circumstances, if the intubator can get into a position above the patient, a direct visualization and oral intubation may be appropriate. This may be the best solution if the patient is trapped in grain, dirt, or other bulk materials and the rescuer can get into an appropriate position.

If the patient is trapped, consider use of manual intubation or a lighted stylet for intubation. These methods can be used only in the obtunded patient. If the patient is awake but can have local anesthesia of the airway, the patient may be intubated with a lighted stylet or with a laryngeal mask airway. Fiberoptic intubation would be ideal but is seldom available in the field. A Combitube may be appropriate to get temporary airway control until the patient can be intubated under better conditions.

Intubation from the front has been described. The author describes using a Macintosh blade and "just hook into the mouth and pull straight forward."[1] He then describes the technique as "Look in and intubate." There has been no controlled series on use of this technique and both complications and success rate is unknown. If the patient requires cervical immobilization during the procedure, an assistant must stabilize the head and neck.

Finally, a surgical airway can be performed in the upright patient under local anesthesia. The patient has the same risks and complications as when it is performed in the supine position, but the procedure may be technically easier than some of the alternatives listed. The operator must be well grounded in the anatomy and landmarks in order to perform this procedure in an unusual position.

The Massively Obese Patient

The massively obese patient (weight > 200 percent of "ideal" body weight) has airway problems before they even get sick. In these patients, the weight of the abdominal viscera and the panniculus will interfere with motion of the diaphragm in the recumbent position (Figure 11-2). (This is much like the weight of the fetus pressing on the vena cava and interfering with diaphragmatic motion in the pregnant patient.)

Since these patients always have some degree of respiratory embarrassment, always give supplemental oxygen, regardless of the patient's saturation.

Most of the time the patient will be better in an upright position on the bed. Occasionally this will force the diaphragm upwards and limit respiratory excursion.

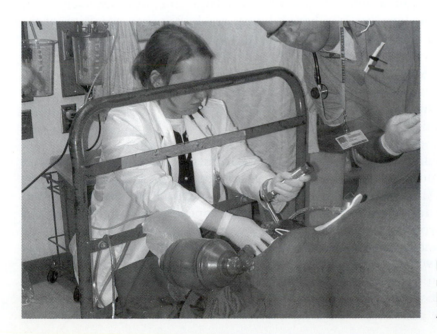

Figure 11-2 Intubating of a massively obese patient. *Source:* Photo by Charles Stewart and Associates; www.storysmith.net.

If the patient must be recumbent, then put them in left lateral recumbent position or "coma" position. This will minimize the pressure from the fat on the diaphragm and the inferior vena cava. It will also decrease esophageal reflux. The right lung will be uppermost, which decreases the chance of aspiration through the right mainstem bronchus.

Mask ventilation of the massively obese patient requires either two person technique or mouth to mask technique. One person should position the patient for airway control and seal the mask. The other person should ventilate the patient with a bag-valve-mask system. The "Seal-Easy" mask is particularly useful in these patients because it readily conforms to the obese face.

Avoid rapid sequence intubation in these patients if there is any doubt about ability to ventilate the patient. It is difficult to palpate structures in the massively obese patient's neck and difficult to perform surgical airways. Likewise, retrograde intubation may not be either easy or possible. Loss of respiratory effort and muscle tone from paralysis may convert the marginal airway into a completely irretrievable tragedy.

Consider use of ketamine for sedation. This agent preserves airway reflexes and respiratory effort in the sedated patient.

Consider intubation of this patient in the seated position with awake nasal intubation if this is clinically appropriate. Careful positioning in the sniffing position may be needed with assistants, towels, and pillows may be needed to line up the axes of the trachea, pharynx, and mouth. It may be necessary to stand above the gurney on a high step-stool in order to visualize the glottis if direct laryngoscopy or use of Magill's forceps is necessary.

An alternative is digital intubation in the seated patient from the front. The smaller intubator may have to stand on a step stool in order to intubate the massively obese patient. Other indirect methods such as a fiber-optic laryngoscope may be appropriate, but not necessarily available in field situations. These patients may be candidates for use of a LMA, Combitube, or the PTL.

When intubating this patient in the recumbent position, be sure to have extra help and equipment available. While a large curved blade may help to shove the tongue to one side, use of a very large straight blade such as the Miller or Wis-Forreger may have a longer reach, better compression of the tongue, and hold the epiglottis out of the way.

Acute Epiglottitis

Epiglottitis was classically a disease of both children and adults. The smaller airway of the child and the higher percentage of airway obstruction focused much attention on pediatric epiglottitis for the past 30 years. This has led to a supposition by unwary emergency providers that epiglottitis is only a disease of children. In fact, most cases of epiglottitis for the past few years have been in adults. The increased incidence of immunization for the most common organism, Hemophilus influenzae type B, has markedly decreased the incidence of pediatric epiglottitis in all countries supporting these immunizations.

The typical clinical scenario is that of an adult with a history of a sore throat that is getting much worse. The patient is often speaking in a hoarse or muffled voice. In children, the voice is described as speaking with a mouthful of potatoes. The patient will often be sitting up, resist lying down, and be drooling or spitting up oral secretions. The pediatric patient may be toxic in appearance with a high fever, but many adults have little fever.

The pediatric form of the disease is most treacherous, because the child's airway is so easily compromised. If the child has any retractions, then everybody should be quite careful not to alarm the child. The child may panic when examined or when an intravenous line is started. The child may remain calmer if allowed to sit on the parent's lap during the examination or transport (Figure 11-3). An oxygen mask or large bore tubing held by the parent in front of the child and blowing on the face can provide supplemental oxygen.

When the diagnosis of epiglottitis is suspected, then the prehospital providers should ensure that supplemental oxygen is provided. An intravenous line may be started in the calm older child and the adult. As long as the patient has spontaneous respirations, do not attempt to intubate the patient.

If the patient ceases to breathe or lapses into a coma, the first step should be to use a bag-valve-mask or mouth to mask respiration to push air past the obstructing epiglottis. Since the obstruction is simply edema, sometimes positive pressure ventilation will provide adequate ventilation.

If this technique is unsuccessful, then oral intubation is indicated. This will not be an easy intubation! A normal larynx will not be visible because of the edema. Indeed, often only a slit like opening remains to mark the supraglottic airway. An assistant can compress the chest and bubbles will be forced through this slit, so that the operator can identify the airway. A small tube can be inserted through this opening.

If the intubation is not rapidly successful, then proceed directly to transtracheal intubation. The obstruction of the epiglottis is often like a flap valve, so expiration will usually occur with jet ventilation. Transtracheal ventilation can also force air through the swollen glottis so that the airway can be identified and intubation facilitated.

Orotracheal intubation in the adult with epiglottitis is not nearly as difficult as in the pediatric patient. Indeed, looking at the epiglottis with indirect laryngoscopy or a fiberoptic laryngoscope is one of the better diagnostic techniques in the adult.

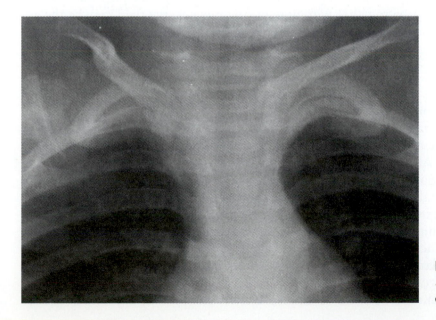

Figure 11-3 X-ray of croup.
Source: Photo by Charles Stewart and Associates; www.storysmith.net.

In the hospital setting, the intubation should be done by the person with the most experience with pediatric intubation. This person needs to stay by the bedside at all times until the patient is completely stable.

The Ear, Nose, and Throat physician should be consulted rapidly for both children and adults. Tracheostomy is indicated when the physician is unable to intubate this patient rapidly. Jet ventilation may provide some temporary relief but is not a permanent solution to the patient.

The Agitated Patient

The agitated or combative patient is a special danger for the emergency provider. Not only does this patient have a potential for hypoxia, he or she has the potential to hurt the providers. In addition, the patient may have serious internal injuries that can't be evaluated while the patient is combative.

The patient who presents with an altered mental status and no history of trauma requires a thorough diagnostic evaluation, appropriate therapeutic interventions and serial neurologic evaluations. The trauma patient who presents with a history that involves a significant mechanism of injury and an altered level of consciousness will require rapid assessment, evaluation, and intervention. If the patient is agitated and has multiple injuries, emergency paralysis with subsequent intubation will prevent the patient from further injury and will allow the managing physician to adequately examine and treat this patient.[2]

There are a number of agents that can be used to sedate the agitated patient including diazepam, fentanyl, haloperidol, or morphine. Each of these may cause airway compromise or respiratory depression in the trauma patient. Quite a few agents will cause hypotension, particularly in the traumatized patient. Obviously, airway control is essential if safe sedation is considered.

Emergent intubation and paralysis will provide patient restraint and sedation, maintain effective spinal immobilization, and provide safe airway control. Ideally, this should occur where the emergency physician has had a chance to assess the neurologic status. In cases of long transport times or significant agitation together with noteworthy injuries, the field may be the appropriate location for sedation and paralysis. These patients deserve the profound sedation of rapid sequence intubation, together with the protective effects of paralysis.

Head Trauma

Head trauma patients will pose significant problems for airway management. This is not an uncommon problem for both field and hospital emergency providers. About 120,000 severe head injuries occur each year in the United States. About 50 percent will die before reaching the hospital.[3] Severe head injuries are the most common conditions that lead to emergency endotracheal intubation in pediatric patients.[4] Multiple trauma, including potential cervical spine injuries, are the rule rather than the exception in head injured patients. Intracranial hypertension in head injury is a major concern.

The damage from a head injury results from direct forces applied to the head and from secondary damage from anoxia and brain swelling. The direct injuries include blunt trauma at the site of the injury, blunt trauma at the opposite side of the head (contrecoup injuries), and penetrating injuries such as gunshot wounds.

The primary injury to the central nervous system may be amplified by anoxia. Anoxia may result from decreased respiratory effort, from additional damage such as facial or airway damage, or from aspiration of stomach contents. Given the high rate of oxygen consumption and the unavailability of energy reserves in the brain, after only a few minutes of anaerobic metabolism, energy failure of the cells occurs.[5][6][7]

Secondary damage may also result from cerebral edema, which can lead to intracranial hypertension and the resultant herniation of brain tissue.

The clinician can do little to affect the direct damage but has substantial control over the effects of secondary damage. The progressive nature of head injuries makes resuscitation by the early providers a major factor in reducing the degree of secondary damage. Initial management includes securing the airway to protect against aspiration of secretions, blood and vomitus; maintain oxygenation; and prevent hypercarbia.

Under normal circumstances, cerebral perfusion pressure is the mean arterial pressure minus the jugular venous pressure. When the intracranial pressure exceeds the cerebral perfusion pressure, then portions of the brain get no blood flow. This situation also happens when the blood pressure falls. The precipitating factors of increased intracranial pressure are hypotension, hypoxia, hypercarbia, venous distention, and airway obstruction. Increases in intracranial pressure also occur when the patient coughs, strains, or has difficulty breathing. When these factors are controlled, secondary brain damage is minimized. Hypoxemia and hypotension on the scene in head injury are frequent and considered deleterious. Intubation and ventilation are effective for controlling this hypoxemia.[8]

In the field, the airway should always be secured in the unconscious and unresponsive patient, the patient with obstruction, the patient with altered sensorium who is vomiting, and the patient who is no longer breathing. If the patient has a Glasgow coma scale of less than 8, then immediate intubation is indicated to ensure that the patient does not deteriorate during further evaluation. Rapid intubation of all of these patients in the field is associated with improved survival and outcome.[9]

Patients with severe head trauma and a low Glasgow score (5 or less) are similar to patients in cardiac arrest. These patients can often be intubated without any adjunctive medications. Interestingly enough, many of these patients are not intubated in the field, despite significant improvement in outcome after field intubation.[10]

Securing an airway in the head injured patient can be difficult and have significant adverse effects. The patient is frequently uncooperative and may be frankly combative. This may be due to fear, anoxia, the head injury itself, or concomitant use of drugs and/or alcohol.

There is a high association of cervical injuries and head injuries, so the cervical spine injury must be assumed.[11] In most of these patients, the cervical spine must be immobilized until it is cleared by x-ray. Unfortunately, these patients often require management of the airway before the radiographs can be obtained.

The laryngeal stimulation that occurs during intubation can cause cough and reflex elevations in intracranial pressure, blood pressure, and heart rate.

These reflexes may be blunted by topical anesthesia applied to the oropharynx and nasopharynx, translaryngeal anesthesia, intravenous lidocaine, and RSI.

There is no totally safe method to intubate the patient with a head injury in the field. Direct laryngoscopy under RSI is probably the safest technique. As noted, the patient may have concomitant neck injuries, so inline fixation of the neck is essential. Movement of the mandible can also cause movement of the neck. Blind nasal intubation is dangerous, particularly when the patient has coexisting facial injuries. Cricothyrotomy in a patient without anesthesia may cause motion or straining. Cricothyrotomy or percutaneous jet ventilation may be useful when the patient has facial injuries.

In the emergency department, a more controlled environment exists. Rapid sequence intubation may be planned, alternatives considered, and the patient prepared with appropriate pharmacology to ensure that the rise in intracranial pressure is minimized. Simultaneously, the emergency physician can prepare for a surgical airway. Concomitant injuries can be assessed and treated to ensure that the patient does not develop hypotension.

The possible inability to adequately ventilate a paralyzed patient has made the use of paralytic agents somewhat controversial in management of the airway in head injuries.[12] The increase in survival associated with early intubation has swung opinion towards RSI in field operations.[13]

The semi-elective intubation in the emergency department is a planned process to avoid (as best as possible) increases in intracranial pressure. The patient should be adequately oxygenated prior to the procedure. If the patient is conscious, then adequate anesthesia for all procedures should be provided to avoid straining or release of catecholamines with stress. Ketamine should be avoided since it will precipitate release of catecholamines.

Lidocaine (1.5 mg/kg) has been given to reduce the rise in ICP associated with putting a laryngoscope into the posterior pharynx. A low dose of narcotic may accomplish the same purpose. Higher doses of narcotics may decrease the cerebral perfusion pressure. If available, thiopental (5 mg/kg) will be protective to intracranial pressure. Unfortunately, thiopental may cause counterproductive hypotension in trauma patients.

The operator must ensure that the duration of apnea during laryngoscopy is minimized. If the intubation is not successful rapidly, then the patient should be re-oxygenated before any second attempt. Prolonged attempts at intubation are inappropriate. If the clinician cannot rapidly intubate the patient with a head injury, appropriate help should be sought. After a successful intubation, the patient should be ventilated carefully to minimize the inspiratory pressure.

Hypovolemia will decrease perfusion to the brain. The clinician must tread the firm ground between adequate fluid replacement and fluid overload, since either situation can exacerbate existing brain damage.

Cervical Spine Injury

In the prehospital or emergency department setting, the trauma patient with a possible cervical spine injury and respiratory compromise also represents a very difficult situation.

There are three fundamental questions that must be answered in these patients.[14]

- What are the chances that the patient has a cervical spine injury?
- If a cervical spine injury is present, what is the risk to the patient of the airway maneuver?
- What is the "standard of care"?

What Are the Chances of a Cervical Spine Injury in the Traumatized Patient?

The cervical spine is the most mobile portion of the vertebral column and the least supported (Figure 11-4). It is therefore the most susceptible to injury and excessive movement.[15] Unstable cervical spine injuries include damage to the anterior support elements or the posterior support elements. The anterior support elements of the cervical spine are the anterior and posterior longitudinal ligaments and the vertebral bodies and discs. The posterior support elements include the capsular ligaments, the intraspinous ligaments, the interspinous ligaments, and the facet joints.

The likelihood of an unstable neck injury increases with more forceful accidents, those with a rotary component and those with linear displacement and hyperextension or hyperextension of the neck. Possible mechanisms for hyperextension include falls and blows to the face and head. The incidence may be as high as 6 percent to 10 percent in head-first falls and 3 percent or less in other accidents. The usual mechanism of hyperflexion injuries is acute deceleration in motor vehicle accidents.

In the field, it is not possible to adequately clear the cervical spine in the critically injured patient. The potential for cervical spine injury exists in almost all cases of blunt head, maxillofacial, and multiple trauma. In the most urgent situations, it is not possible to adequately diagnose a cervical injury before airway management must be started. Multiple studies have demonstrated that there is no aspect of the physical examination that reliably predicts the presence of c-spine injury in these patients. All of the manual techniques for clearing the cervical spine depend on an awake patient without other significant distracting injuries.

During airway management, the field provider must simply presume that the patient has an unstable cervical spine injury (Figure 11-5). Penetrating trauma is far less likely to cause an unstable neck injury but is possible with high energy ballistic injuries.

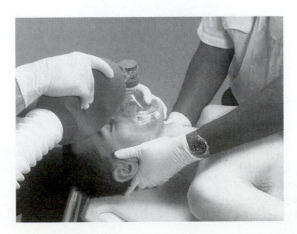

Figure 11-4 Neck immobilization. *Source:* Photo by Charles Stewart and Associates; www.storysmith.net.

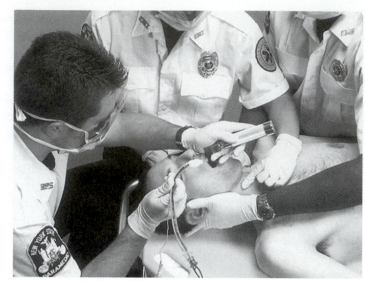

Figure 11-5 Intubation with assistance for neck immobilization. *Source:* Photo by Charles Stewart and Associates; www.storysmith.net.

In the emergency department, the role of c-spine radiography before intubation remains controversial. If the patient condition permits the time, a lateral c-spine radiograph may be obtained. The emergency provider should be well aware that lateral c-spine radiography can miss up to 20 percent to 30 percent of cervical spine injuries. Special attention must be made to the C-7/T-1 interface, since 20 percent of all cervical injuries are at C7.[16] Even a complete plain film c-spine series cannot totally exclude injury, especially if a concomitant neurologic examination cannot be performed (Figure 11-6). In some patients, the diagnosis of neurologic trauma requires both CT scan and MRI.

In a cogent analysis, Walls has estimated that a small but significant percentage (1.2 percent) of all blunt trauma victims will have an occult c-spine injury, given a 6 percent total incidence of injury and a 20 percent miss rate on lateral c-spine radiography. Based on a lateral spine film that reveals an unstable injury, the operator may decide to use a particular intubation technique.

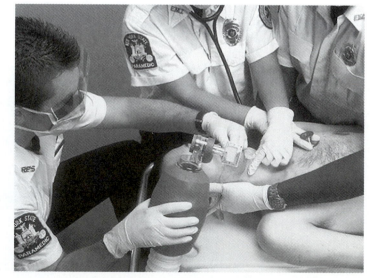

Figure 11-6 Checking tube position in potential neck trauma. *Source:* Photo by Charles Stewart and Associates; www.storysmith.net.

What Will the Airway Maneuver Do to the Cervical Spine?

Initially the airway must be cleared of blood, debris, and secretions. The chin-lift or the jaw-thrust maneuvers are appropriate to open the airway. The sniffing position will flex the lower cervical spine and extend the occiput on the atlas. Manual stabilization will decrease movement.

An oral airway may be inserted if it is needed to maintain the airway. Insertion of an oral airway produces little disturbance to the cervical spine. Bag-valve-mask ventilation produces a significant degree of movement in the unstable cervical injury.[17]

The safest method of intubation is also quite controversial. In general, the technique the operator is most comfortable with is the one that should be employed. The method is generally less important than realizing that the patient may have a cervical injury and taking reasonable care to prevent further damage. The possibility of cervical spine injury requires extreme caution in any technique of airway management that may move the neck. Regardless of which technique is used, careful control of the c-spine with in-line immobilization is essential. Traction should not be used (Figure 11-7).[18]

Until recently, oral intubation was contraindicated when a suspected c-spine injury existed. In the presence of a suspected cervical injury, blind nasal intubation or cricothyrotomy was advocated. The belief was that these maneuvers create less cervical movement. This assumption was never proven and some authorities feel quite strongly that hypoxia from failure to rapidly place an appropriate airway has caused far more damage than the manipulation of the patient during the airway insertion. With the advent of emergent use of RSI, many argue that oral intubation with meticulous attention to c-spine control is preferred in the patient at risk for c-spine injury. Oral intubation is surely the fastest and most certain method of intubating the trachea. Likewise, rapid sequence intubation is generally the safest technique that may be used to intubate the traumatized and combative patient. This technique will also decrease the possibility that the patient's own movements can precipitate spinal cord trauma.

Airway control in this setting is best performed with three people: one is the intubator, one provides in-line immobilization of the c-spine, and one applies cricoid pressure (Sellick's maneuver). This control of the cervical spine and the prevention of aspiration is important, even in the field intubation.

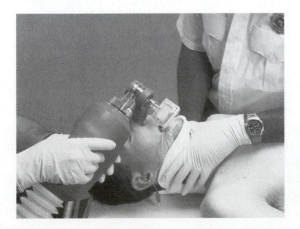

Figure 11-7 Neck immobilization after intubation. *Source:* Photo by Charles Stewart and Associates; www.storysmith.net.

Oral Intubation with Cervical Immobilization

Direct laryngoscopy with oral intubation is the fastest and surest way of intubating the trachea. The airway is completely controlled without surgical intervention and scars. The patient with head injury who is combative can be paralyzed for the procedure.

Orotracheal intubation with cervical immobilization and rapid sequence intubation technique is now considered the most appropriate intubation technique for the patient with either an actual or a potential cervical injury.[19 20 21 22 23 24 25] At "Shock-Trauma" in Baltimore, Maryland, more than 3,000 patients were intubated with RSI with no deterioration of neurologic status following intubation.[26]

Patients with an unstable C1 or C2 injury may be at more risk with oral intubation since extension of the atlantis on the occiput is needed to bring the vocal cords into alignment with the mouth.[27] Manual in-line stabilization reduces this movement by 60 percent.

Nasotracheal Intubation

Blind nasal intubation has been successful in as many as 90 percent of patients but often requires multiple attempts in up to 90 percent of successful intubations. Nasal intubation is contraindicated in the patient with unstable midface injuries (LaForte fractures) and with a basilar skull fracture. Hemorrhage produced by failed nasal intubation may make other techniques quite difficult or simply impossible.

In the nontrauma patient, nasal intubation is facilitated by rotating or flexing the neck. This is not appropriate for the trauma patient and may substantially increase the failure rate or the time to intubate as the procedure becomes more difficult.

Awake Intubation

Awake intubation is a feasible option in many trauma patients. It has been shown to be safe in the patient with cervical spine injury.[28] It may be performed by fiberoptics or direct visualization.

Awake intubation may not be an appropriate maneuver when rapid intubation is needed. Coughing may both increase intracranial pressure, threaten an unstable cervical spine, and result in failure of the procedure. Use of topical anesthesia to prevent cough may risk increases in aspiration.

Neurologic outcome with awake tracheal intubation compares favorably to the outcome seen with oral intubation. There are no prospective studies that compare the two techniques, however.

Surgical Airway

Cricothyroidotomy is a rapid but invasive method of controlling the patient's airway. The need for a surgical airway should be rapidly recognized and the procedure performed by an experienced person without delay. In injuries to the pharynx, it may be appropriate as a primary airway. It is also useful after a failed intubation attempt.

The surgical airway can be either the full surgical cricothyrotomy or a percutaneous needle cricothyrotomy with high-flow oxygen.

Jet ventilation may temporize until the trachea is intubated using another method such as fiberoptics or RSI. Although jet ventilation will provide oxygenation and ventilation for a patient, it does not protect the airway.

There are no studies that describe neurological outcome after a cricothyrotomy in the patient with known or proven cervical injury, so the advantage may be completely theoretical.

Fiberoptic Laryngoscopy

This may be the ideal intubation technique for the patient with a documented cervical spine injury. Certainly, in the hands of an experienced operator, there is no motion of the head during intubation. Unfortunately, as covered in the section on fiberoptic intubation tools, these tools are expensive, fragile, and require experience to use quickly and properly. This device is not a field tool.

Successful fiberoptic intubation requires a cooperative or comatose patient, a secretion, vomitus, and blood-free airway, no edema of the pharynx, and adequate local anesthesia. Secretions and blood can pool in the throat and gag the patient. Use of local anesthetics in the airway can consume critical time and may increase the risk of aspiration.

Fiberoptic intubation may be more difficult in the patient who is in spinal immobilization restraints. The tongue will fall backwards and obstruct the passage of the fiberoptic scope.

What Is the Standard of Care?

It has not been well substantiated that significant injury has occurred from the flexion required to intubate the patient. Unfortunately, it is all too easy for the malpractice lawyer to find abundant "authorities" who can describe in lurid details the "dangers" of intubating the patient with a cervical spine injury.

Many authors have attempted to editorialize on the impact of airway management on the unstable cervical spine. A few central principles stand out.

There is no solid support for any one approach over another. The patient's condition and the comfort of the operator with the technique employed appears to be the most significant factor. For the patient who needs the airway right now, oral intubation is significantly quicker than any other technique. Cricothyrotomy or transtracheal ventilation may be indicated in patients with anatomic features that argue for a difficult intubation.

Although the cervical spine injury must be considered and the possibility of cervical injury documented, management of the airway is the single most important task for both field medic and emergency physician alike. Failure to obtain a viable airway because the "cervical spine might be injured" is simply unacceptable medical care. The operator must ensure that cervical spine stabilization is present during any and all airway manipulations.

Axial traction is a poor technique for stabilization of the cervical spine in the emergent patient. Sudden worsening of neurologic deficits has been reported when traction is applied for spine stabilization or to expose C7 on an x-ray.[29]

A more appropriate technique is to immobilize the cervical spine to maintain the existing relationships among the head, neck, and body without traction. This will always require the operator to have an assistant who has the sole function of immobilization of the neck.

Trauma to the Airways

Blunt trauma to the major airways (larynx, trachea, and major bronchi) is an unusual event. The exact incidence of trauma to the airways is not readily available. The criticality of this event is out of proportion to the incidence, however. Up to 75 percent of the patients will die at the scene. The mortality is still between 30 percent and 60 percent when the patient makes it to the hospital and about 15 percent will die within the first hour.[30][31] Trauma to the airway presents a unique challenge to emergency providers.

The mechanisms of injury can be easily divided into two categories: the cervical portion of the larynx and trachea and the intrathoracic portion of the tracheobronchial tree. Distal tracheal and bronchial injuries are more likely to be lethal either on scene or arrival in the emergency department than the cervical airway injuries.[32] Many of these patients will have multiple injuries.

Laryngeal-Tracheal Trauma

Diagnosis Laryngotracheal trauma is fortunately uncommon. Both blunt and penetrating trauma can damage the larynx or trachea, but blunt trauma is more common (Figure 11-8). The most common etiology is from a wire or cable stretched across a path. The cyclist or snowmobiler does not notice the cable and it strikes the anterior neck. This is often called a "clothesline" type injury. Similar injuries can occur when a driver strikes the steering wheel or a cyclist strikes the handlebars of a motorcycle or bicycle.

The most common injury to the larynx is a fracture of the glottis from a direct blow. Laryngotracheal separation most frequently occurs when the patient sustains a "clothesline" type injury. When the trachea is completely transected, the lower portion of the trachea may retract into the chest. Tracheal fractures in the neck will usually be transverse and through a tracheal ring (Figure 11-9). In a complete transection of the airway, the distal segment of the trachea may retract into the chest.

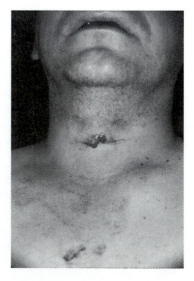

Figure 11-8 Puncture wound in neck. *Source:* Photo by Charles Stewart and Associates; www. storysmith.net.

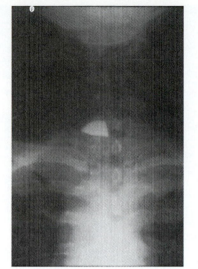

Figure 11-9 Puncture wound in neck x-ray. *Source:* Photo by Charles Stewart and Associates; www.storysmith.net.

An uncommon but important mechanism is rupture of the posterior wall of the trachea or bronchus from insertion of an endotracheal tube or overinflation of a cuffed endotracheal tube. Changing an endotracheal tube over a stylet or "tube changer" may also result in damage. These patients will initially have a good airway but will develop subcutaneous emphysema from an air leak at the site of the trauma.

The symptoms can be subtle and the emergency provider can overlook significant injuries. The most common signs and symptoms include a bruise or hematoma on the anterior neck, cervical subcutaneous emphysema, dyspnea, hoarseness, and hemoptysis. This is more common when the patient has multisystem trauma. These patients may appear stable for hours and then suddenly deteriorate. If laryngotracheal trauma is suspected, the patient needs careful evaluation and monitoring.

Important clues to the diagnosis include a high index of suspicion for this injury in all patients who have a bruise to the front of the neck. The presence of cervical subcutaneous emphysema should always suggest an injury to the major airway. Hoarseness or voice changes imply either laryngeal damage or damage to the recurrent laryngeal nerve. Persistent pneumothorax after insertion of a chest tube and worsening subcutaneous emphysema may indicate major airway trauma.

In the hospital, additional diagnostic techniques are available. On a chest or neck x-ray, the subcutaneous emphysema is obvious. The patient may also have pneumothorax, pneumomediastinum, or even pneumopericardium.

The most reliable diagnostic technique is direct visualization of the injury. The injury may be seen during surgical management of the airway or during a thoracostomy. Flexible fiberoptic laryngoscopy may visualize the higher injuries in the emergency department but injury to the bronchi require bronchoscopy.

Management Many of these patients will have already optimized their airway by assuming a sniffing position. Forcing the patient to get on a gurney and applying a cervical collar may further injure the patient or compromise the

Suspicion of an Airway Injury	
Symptoms	History of direct blow
	Motor vehicle accident
	Crush injury to chest or neck
	Dyspnea
	Hoarseness
	Voice change
	Subcutaneous emphysema/crepitus
	Hemoptysis
	Tachpnea
	Persistent pneumothorax despite a chest tube
	Worsening subcutaneous emphysema

airway. The field provider may be torn between management of the potential cervical injury and management of the airway. The airway management should always take priority.

If there is significant laryngeal trauma, then tracheostomy is the airway of choice. This should be done under local anesthesia with an awake patient if possible. (In patients with coexisting critical illness or pediatric patients, this may not be possible.)

A controversy exists about whether to intubate the patient initially or whether a tracheostomy is the first airway procedure to be performed. Proponents of initial (emergent) tracheostomy argue that intubation can cause further damage and may cause separation of the distal trachea with retraction into the chest.[33][34][35] Proponents of initial intubation feel that intubation secures the airway and allows for a less hurried and more careful urgent rather than emergent tracheostomy.

These patients have increased airway resistance and may be quite sensitive to respiratory depressant medications. The patient may already be in the optimum position for airway flow, so repositioning the patient may precipitate an airway crisis. Likewise, use of paralytic agents may be life threatening. Use of Sellick's cricoid pressure may cause obstruction if the patient's airway disruption is near the pressure point.

In the field, if the patient has a totally obstructed airway, then an attempt at intubation is appropriate. There are case reports where patients have been successfully intubated with adequate airway control. Passage of an endotracheal tube may create a false passage or the tube may not pass through the lesion. If intubation is attempted, then a smaller tube (such as 6.0 or 6.5) may be appropriate. If available, a fiberoptic laryngoscope is useful since the airway can be assessed and then intubated during the same procedure.

A Combitube or laryngeal mask is not helpful in the patient with laryngeal trauma. Both attempt to ventilate the patient above the site of injury.

Cricothyrotomy, cricothyroid puncture, and transtracheal jet ventilation are also contraindicated. The trachea may not be in the midline or may be obscured by severe subcutaneous emphysema or gross swelling of the neck. Subcutaneous emphysema may allow suction of air into the syringe used for location of the trachea. Transtracheal jet ventilation may make the subcutaneous emphysema markedly worse (even when the needle is in the proper location.) Cricothyrotomy may insert a tube above the site of injury and further damage the trachea when passage is attempted.

Vascular Neck Trauma A vascular injury in the neck can cause an expanding hematoma or vigorous external bleeding. A hematoma may compress the airway and displace it to one side. The trauma, increasing hematoma, altered anatomy, and often emergent need for an airway makes for a technically difficult intubation. Cricothyrotomy may not be possible or may be quite difficult.

Appropriate management of these patients includes early intubation. These patients are at great risk if they are paralyzed. Only if there is a surgeon standing by who feels comfortable with an emergency tracheostomy can this patient be safely paralyzed. This patient will require the most experienced available person for the intubation.

When the patient has expanding subcutaneous emphysema, the situation is not as grave, but the patient's airway access may be quite difficult. Paralysis in these patients may also be fraught with hazard.

Intrathoracic Tracheo-Bronchial Injuries

Intrathoracic airway injuries may be seen with high speed motor vehicle accidents. The patients are frequently young, male, unrestrained front seat drivers or passengers. The patient will strike the steering wheel or dashboard of the car. Rarely, industrial accidents and sporting injuries can cause this injury.

Penetrating chest trauma may injure or even sever the trachea or major bronchi. Rapid deceleration may result in shearing forces at the carina. Crush injuries when the patient has a closed glottis may produce an increase in intrabronchial pressure and rupture the large bronchi. The pathology of the injuries may range from a partial airway tear and subsequent air leak to complete transection of the airway with dislocation of the two ends. These patients often develop a massive pneumothorax or tension pneumothorax. Insertion of a chest tube is essential, and the patient will demonstrate a massive air leak from the tube.

Proximal (cervical) injuries generally have a better outcome than tracheobronchial injuries. Unfortunately, 80 percent of intrathoracic injuries occur within 2.5 cm of the carina. Field management of a patient with distal tracheal or large bronchial injury is problematic, since thoracostomy is required for management of the injury. Transport of the patient in a position of comfort is essential.

Airway Foreign Bodies

The inhalation, or more properly, aspiration, of a foreign object into the airway causes symptoms that extend from a minimal cough to death. In children under the age of four, aspiration of a foreign body is a major cause of mortality—with about 2,000 deaths per year.[36] Aspiration of foreign bodies is much more common in children than in adults—the majority of patients presenting with aspiration of a foreign body are less than three years old.[37] [38] Male children aspirate foreign bodies about twice as frequently as females.[39] [40] There have been no reports of large series of adults with nonasphyxiating foreign bodies within the airway, but anecdotal reports abound of various objects.[41]

The diagnosis of bronchial foreign body aspiration is often difficult. In several large studies, the interval from suspected aspiration to hospitalization is greater than 24 hours in over half of the patients. Delays in diagnosis can range from months to years in some isolated cases. Often the symptoms are incorrectly attributed to a diagnosis other than aspiration despite chest x-ray abnormalities. Equally often, the chest x-ray is normal, incorrectly allaying the fears and suspicions of the physician and parents.

A high degree of suspicion is necessary on the part of the provider in order to expeditiously diagnose and treat this problem. Anytime a young child presents with a new respiratory problem, the provider should be wary that this problem is caused by a new foreign body.

The changes produced by the foreign body depend on the nature, location, and the degree of obstruction of the air passages. A foreign body that occludes the upper airway completely is an immediate threat to life. Smaller objects that lodge in lobar bronchi cause more chronic and usually less severe symptoms.

Classic History

The mother that brings a blue and apneic child to the emergency department is fortunately rare. A more classic case is the ambulance call for a child with respiratory distress that was noted and has either resolved or is still ongoing. These respiratory complaints may range from persistent coughing to an episode of cyanosis or apnea.

A witnessed episode of choking is the single most important part of the history. Unfortunately, this often appears to be trivial to the parents or playmates and may be completely forgotten. It is imperative to question the family specifically about a choking episode any time that a child presents with a new respiratory symptom!

Unfortunately, the "classic history" is probably more classic in its absence. In several reviews, the history of aspiration was not found in anywhere from 6 percent to 62 percent of the cases. Since most of these children are under four years old, if the parents did observe the episode, then it is likely that the child would be unable to contribute to the history. Furthermore, as many as a quarter of patients will be completely asymptomatic at the time of presentation. Indeed, the ambulance may have not transported the child because both mother and EMS providers feel that the child is now better.

The emergency provider should be suspicious of the possibility of aspiration of a foreign body in any child who has a history of respiratory distress.

It should make no difference to the extent of evaluation if the patient's respiratory distress has resolved or is ongoing.

Why Do Children Aspirate Objects?

There is no question that curiosity and the explorations of the young are a major reason for aspiration of all objects. Young children explore tastes and shapes with their mouths. If it will fit, it will be put into the mouth.

Immature Dentition

Children do not have molars for grinding and crushing food until they are about 4 years old. Without molars, food is imperfectly chewed and may not be chewed at all. The child can inhale this food if the normal swallowing mechanism is disrupted in any way.

Physical Activity

When children are carrying food or other objects in their mouth, this food may be aspirated if the child is jostled or disturbed while playing. The child who is playing or running while eating may also inhale vigorously with food in the mouth. If the child is reclining, then the food may fall directly into the airway.

Uncoordinated Swallowing Mechanisms

In addition to all of the other problems, young children must learn to swallow and hold their breath at the same time. If the child has not mastered this skill or is disturbed during swallowing, then the food may be aspirated.

Poor Control of Chewed Food Sizes

Children will often put more food in their mouths than they can safely swallow or chew. Since the presence of food in the mouth stimulates the swallowing reflex, the child may attempt to both breathe and swallow at the same time.

Startle Reflex

Children also have a startle response that includes a gasp reflex. This permits solids in the pharynx to go through the open larynx.[42]

The Aspirated Foreign Bodies—What Are They?

Almost any object that can be inserted into the mouth or nose can be aspirated into the airway.

Toys

"Toys" ingested include coins, buttons, ballpoint pen springs, bullets, chalk crayons, plastic toys and parts of toys, safety pins, screws, tops from aluminum soda cans, cigarette filters, washers, teeth, pencil leads, pieces of Styrofoam, and beads.[43] (Remember that the three-year-old's definition of a toy is not the same as the adult parent's.) These toys may be either radiopaque or radiolucent depending upon the composition of the article—unfortunately, most are radiolucent.

Legislation has specified minimum dimensions for the components of toys intended for children under three years of age in order to further protect them from aspiration.[44] A review by the U.S. Consumer Product Safety

Commission noted that 70 percent of objects that caused death were 19 mm or less. No round object greater than 32 mm caused death.[45] The resultant laws only cover commercial manufactured toys, not everyday objects that children may play with or handmade toys. Balloons are commonly associated with asphyxiation.[46] Other round and pliable objects were noted as being easy to aspirate and difficult to extract because they impacted. This may include portions of pacifiers and formula bottle nipples used to pacify a child between feedings.

Food

Children aspirate food more frequently than objects that they are playing with. Small hard foods seem more likely to be inhaled. This may include nuts, grapes, or hard candies. Hot dogs are also likely to be aspirated. Fortunately, the majority of foreign bodies enter the esophagus rather than the respiratory tract.[47]

Peanuts are notorious as aspirated foreign bodies in the United States. In a recent large study of children with aspiration of foreign objects, one-half of aspirated food foreign bodies were peanuts and one-fifth were other nuts or seeds.[48] Because of the size, shape, and smooth surface, the peanut is readily aspirated into the mainstem bronchus. Smaller fragments of peanut may move more distally into the bronchial tree. The peanut oils, proteins, and fatty acids act as chemical irritants.[49] The resulting inflammation leads to mucosal edema and irritation that further traps the peanut fragments. As the peanut absorbs water, it swells. The result is a soft, friable particle that is trapped within an inflamed bronchus and is quite difficult to remove.[50] In other countries, other seeds are more frequent culprits.

Peanut kernels cause local granulation and may cause generalized tracheobronchitis due to the peanut oils. This can start within hours of the aspiration.

Beans, dried peas, and other dried grains can swell and cause increased obstruction as they absorb water. Removal of the object is made more difficult by this swelling. If they have been in place for a long time, they may "sprout."

Cafe Coronary

The problem of aspiration of food is not confined to children, but is much less common in adults. Acute food asphyxiation (the "cafe coronary") occurred only 141 times in 1982.[51] Indeed, only 60 adult cases were found in a 33-year survey at the Mayo clinic. In adults we are taught that the patient will have the "universal" sign of grabbing at the throat to indicate an obstructed airway. Unfortunately, this universal sign is less universal to patients who may not have read the right literature or who have forgotten the "sign" during their asphyxia. This "cafe coronary" occurs when the adult patient attempts to swallow a bolus of food that is aspirated instead.

Ingestion of alcohol, presence of dentures, and incomplete chewing of food all contribute to the problem. Indeed, the most difficult choking obstruction is not the partially chewed piece of meat that responds to the Heimlich maneuver. A bolus of chewed peanuts or similar sticky matter can be quite difficult to remove and does not respond to the usual maneuvers.

Signs and Symptoms

Immediate symptoms are usually gagging, choking, coughing, wheezing, aphonia, or dysphagia. Stridor from a foreign body implies a location in the larynx, trachea, or mainstem bronchus. Other signs that specifically suggest a location of the foreign body include

Larynx

Hoarseness, cough, dyspnea, stridor, crowing respirations, croupy cough, and respiratory obstruction, with death are signs that suggest a foreign body in the larynx. If the object lodges in the glottis or mainstem bronchus, the patient may die before medical aid is available. Fortunately, aspirated foreign bodies are more likely to pass through into the bronchi and lodge there. If the foreign body does impact in the subglottic area, the patient often has stridor that mimics croup.[52] If the patient has had prior episodes of croup and the child's aspiration is not known, then both examiner and parent may be deceived. The patient may also gag, drool, or have a muffled voice, similar to patients with epiglottitis. One should be particularly careful to obtain a cogent history in the patient suspected of epiglottitis or croup since these may produce similar clinical presentations. In rare cases, loss of voice may be the only symptom of subglottic aspiration.[53]

Trachea

Signs that a foreign body may be in the trachea include wheezes, dyspnea, stridor, crowing respirations, croupy cough, bilateral chest findings, and an "audible slap" sound heard at the patient's open mouth. A "thud" may be heard or palpated as the patient breathes. Complete respiratory obstruction may also be found at this level—and lead inexorably to death.

Bronchus

Wheezes, hyperinflation, hypoinflation, and atelectasis are common signs of bronchial foreign bodies. Partial bypass obstructions may allow air to either leave or enter with a wheeze or whistle. Ball-valve obstructions may completely block movement of airway. Entry of air into a ball-valve obstruction can cause hyperinflation of the affected area. A ball-valve obstruction that allows movement out but prohibits entry of air produces atelectasis (hypoinflation). Total obstruction will produce gradual atelectasis as the air is absorbed. Physical signs that are characteristics of partial or incomplete bronchial obstruction include limited expansion of the chest, decreased vocal fremitus, dullness to percussion, and diminished breath sounds distal to the obstruction. Children with foreign bodies lodged in bronchi for longer than 24 to 48 hours may have fever, hemoptysis, and pneumonia.

In adult patients, the foreign body is more likely to be lodged in the right mainstem bronchus. In children, the foreign body may land in either right or left side with equally facility. Careful auscultation may reveal a unilateral lung abnormality.

Symptom-Free Interval

After the initial signs and symptoms, there is often a relatively symptom-free interval that may last for hours, days, or occasionally weeks. This symptom-free interval is also when the unsuspecting practitioner evaluates a now-asymptomatic patient and does not consider the patient to be "serious" at the time of examination. This triphasic course of acute symptoms, latent asymptomatic period, and subsequent increasing symptoms is classic for mainstem bronchial foreign bodies.

Treatment

Acute Airway Obstruction

The American Heart Association recommends the Heimlich maneuver if complete airway obstruction is present. This procedure is modified for infants under one year to include four back blows and four abdominal thrusts in each attempt to dislodge the foreign object. Using the Heimlich maneuver on a child less than a year of age may cause liver damage.

The emergency provider should perform these measures once and then attempt to directly visualize the foreign body. If it is visible above the cords, it may be directly grasped and removed with Magill forceps. Sticky masses may not be able to be removed easily, even when well visualized. Be prepared for vomiting following the removal of the object. The patient may need to be intubated following removal of the mass if there has been any lengthy airway compromise.

If a partial airway obstruction is present, the patient should be constantly observed while preparations are made for removal of the object. Avoid agitating the patient and allow the child to sit in the position of comfort. Allow the parents to provide supplemental oxygen with either an oxygen tube or mask held near the patient's face or a mask. If the patient does not tolerate the mask, then holding oxygen tubing next to the patient's face will increase the inspired oxygen concentration. The child should remain under direct observation with emergency equipment at the bedside.

If there is no response to the Heimlich maneuver and the patient is not able to be intubated, then immediately perform a cricothyrotomy or needle tracheostomy. If the mass is in the trachea or in the major bronchi and you are unable to ventilate the patient, the situation is grave. At this point, some authorities recommend attempting to forcibly intubate the patient and "push the mass into the right mainstem bronchus." This is supposed to allow the patient to ventilate with the other lung and support life. In many cases, of course, it impacts the foreign body further into the trachea and makes it more difficult for the next provider to remove the foreign body.

If there is any partial airway present, use high concentration of oxygen and gently support ventilation until the patient can be bronchoscoped.

Prevention

The highest risk of aspiration by food products occurs about the end of the first year of life, although the risk continues until the child is about three.

Since this problem occurs primarily in children, prevention is an adult responsibility. Many parents have not heard of the risks of giving children inappropriate foods for their age. Others simply aren't attuned to the dangers. Parents should be warned about the dangers that common foods such as peanuts, beans, and popcorn present to their small children. Parents should carefully regulate the types and sizes of foods offered to children and left where children can get them. Young children should not be allowed to engage in activities at the same time that they eat. Access to toys and objects that serve as toys should be carefully controlled when toddlers are about.

In 1984, Mattell Corporation developed and made public a process that makes plastic parts radiopaque. This was done at no cost to other manufacturers. Emergency physicians who have patients who ingest radiolucent plastic parts are encouraged to notify the manufacturers that their product CAN be made radiopaque and request that this be done!

Other Techniques

Various authors have advocated numerous other techniques. These have included physiotherapy, postural drainage, and back slaps. These techniques have little control and may be quite dangerous. Older treatments included the use of bronchodilators and pulmonary toilet. These are so ineffective that they may be considered as simply delaying appropriate therapy.

Do not attempt to remove a foreign body by inserting a finger blindly into the oropharynx. This may force the object into the larynx and cause a complete obstruction of the airway. If a child is turned upside down, the object may be dislodged from the carina or mainstem bronchus only to impact in the subglottic area—the narrowest point in a child's airway.

Summary

The behavior of the child is well known. They explore objects by putting them in their mouth. When this happens, and they are startled, fall, or are distracted, they may aspirate these objects.

The diagnosis of aspiration of foreign bodies in the airway is difficult and requires constant suspicion on the part of the medical team. Anytime that a young child has a history of sudden onset of cough, choking, or respiratory embarrassment, an aspiration should be suspected. These children need to be completely evaluated for a foreign body. If the foreign body ingestion is not considered, the child might be discharged with a potentially life-threatening illness.

Even though the aspiration is considered, the diagnosis is not made in some cases because of the difficulties in visualizing the foreign body or its effects.

Airway Burns and Inhalation Injuries

Introduction

One of the most challenging problems the EMS provider (from EMT to physician) faces is the treatment of a victim with an inhalation injury (Figure 11-10). Four out of five deaths resulting from fires occur following smoke inhalation (not flames). Thermal injuries mainly involve the upper airway.

EMS personnel must be alert to environmental clues that suggest inhalation injury. Anticipation of pulmonary complications and problems will enable the rescuers to start necessary treatment before the insult becomes life threatening.

Smoke inhalation is an unfortunately vague term that encompasses a number of injuries from a variety of mechanisms. Smoke inhalation is also known as thermal pulmonary injury, pulmonary burn, or inhalation injury.

The lung surface is necessary for life. Other organs can suffer substantial damage, but they are able to function until healed. If the lung is unable

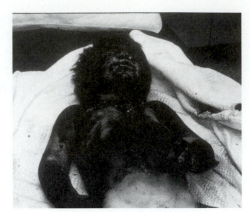

Figure 11-10 Airway burn in child. *Source:* Photo by Charles Stewart and Associates; www.storysmith.net.

to function, the remaining life span is measured in moments, and treatment options are limited. In addition, the lungs represent such a large surface area that they readily absorb toxic materials into the systemic circulation.

The importance of these toxic inhalations cannot be overstated. Between 8,000 and 12,000 people die from fires in the United States each year. Over 60 percent of these victims have no burns and are thus presumed to have died from toxic gas inhalation alone. These toxic exposures rank high in both quality and quantity. They not only do a lot of harm to a single individual, they can simultaneously affect a large number of individuals.

> **People Who Breathe Fire Tend to Die . . . A Lot.**

Over 280 chemical compounds have been identified when common household materials burn. It is impossible to catalog every toxin that is produced. Instead, a general approach to the inhalation of toxic material is more appropriate for the EMS provider. Multiple handbooks, computer catalogs, and other references exist that document inhalation agents, specific tests to identify them, treatment, and, most importantly, proper protective gear to avoid them.

The airway and pulmonary problems that can occur from the inhalation of noxious agents can be broadly classified into four groups

1. Displacement for consumption of the available oxygen—Anoxia.
2. Thermal injury.
3. Pulmonary damage from noxious fumes or particulates—Irritant Gases and Particles.
4. Inhalation of cellular toxins such as carbon monoxide or cyanide—Asphyxiant Gases.

Multiple mechanisms may have caused the inhalation injuries. It is common, for example, for the fire to partly consume oxygen, produce carbon dioxide and monoxide, cyanide, and soot and to produce superheated air. Needless to say, the injury resulting from breathing such a mixture will be multifaceted.

Types of Injury

Anoxia

When a fire consumes oxygen, ambient oxygen concentrations may drop from 21 percent to 10 percent or lower. This decrease results in simple hypoxia, aggravated by the impaired oxygen-carrying capacity and tissue injury caused by other facets of the inhalation injury. Simply, there isn't enough oxygen left to support life. Ambient oxygen concentrations of 2 percent may lead to severe anoxic injury or even death in as little as 1 minute.

Although carbon dioxide is not noxious or irritating, it will not support life. Fires produce immense quantities of carbon dioxide because carbon is a major component of most burning material.

In general, symptoms of hypoxia are produced when the oxygen content falls to below 15 percent in an enclosed space. Unfortunately, if the oxygen is less than 6 percent to 8 percent, the first symptom of hypoxia may be collapse. Self-contained breathing apparatus should be worn while entering any suspected area until the oxygen content can be verified.

Thermal Upper Respiratory Injury

As noted, most thermal injuries are in the upper airway. Thermal injury of the upper respiratory tract often causes laryngeal and supraglottic edema. Marked edema may form within minutes to hours and may be exacerbated by overzealous fluid administration. Upper airway obstruction may develop from this laryngeal edema, laryngospasm, accumulation of secretions, or extrinsic obstruction due to neck or facial burns. Injury below the vocal cords is seen in less than 5 percent of patients who present with moderate or severe surface burns.

It should be emphasized that the most common cause of death in the early phases of burn treatment is this upper respiratory tract injury. The extent of this injury and the level of respiratory tract involvement depend upon the specific inhaled gases, the length of exposure, and the environment of the exposure. Emergency intubation or tracheostomy may be required to prevent rapid airway obstruction due to edema.

Thermal Pulmonary Injury

Thermal injury of the lung itself is rare. Gases have a relatively low specific heat and, therefore, transfer of heat from the gas to the tissues occurs rapidly. As a hot gas passes through the respiratory tract, it loses most of its heat energy when it converts the liquid water normally found in the oropharynx and upper respiratory tract into water vapor. This heat transfer, even of superheated gases, usually occurs in the supraglottic and laryngeal areas, hence the propensity of burns in this area. Inhalation of superheated steam is capable of producing a direct mucosal injury as far distal as the major bronchioles. The superheated water vapor has 4,000 times the specific heat of hot air and is able to transfer more thermal energy to the distal lung. It also loses little of its energy when respiratory tract liquids are vaporized. Inhalation of steam may produce a true pulmonary parenchymal injury.

Toxic Airway Injury

Pulmonary parenchymal and tracheobronchial injuries may also result from toxic products of combustion or from inhalation of toxins. There are several variables to be considered when a victim is exposed to toxic agents.

1. The type or types of gases (or particulates) involved.

   Most fires release a large number of toxic gases including acids, aldehydes, phosgene, chlorine, ammonia, hydrogen chloride, acroleins, nitrogen oxides, and cyanides. While these products may irritate the upper airway, they can also injure the lung. This lung damage may be manifested by mucosal and pulmonary edema, increased capillary permeability, and sloughing of the mucosal lining. Since these alveolar irritants may cause little irritation to the eyes, nose, or upper airway, the internal effects of these substances may not be felt until hours after initial exposure.

2. The duration of exposure.

3. The concentration of the gas.

   Needless to say, if the toxin is present in high concentration, it will act much more quickly than a more dilute agent will. If the patient is exposed to a similar concentration for a longer duration, the effects will be more profound.

4. The water solubility of the material.

   If the agent is water soluble, it may be absorbed more easily in the oral cavity and cause less life-threatening damage. Less soluble and particulate materials tend to pass into the lower airways and alveoli.

5. The time lapse from exposure to proper treatment.

   Usually, the diagnosis of a toxic inhalation is obvious. Occasionally, the emergency provider must have a high index of suspicion in order to make the diagnosis.

6. The underlying health of the subject.

   Cardiovascular and respiratory illnesses may increase the lethality of a specific toxin. Other toxins may affect those who are very young or old or pregnant. Use of cigarettes, industrial exposures, and licit or illicit drugs may alter the effects of a toxin.

Other major complications from inhaling these toxic products include bronchospasm, chemical pneumonitis, and the adult respiratory distress syndrome (ARDS). Late deaths may be due to pneumonia in damaged lung tissue.

Particulate Matter

Besides heat and irritating gases, smoke contains suspended particulates and liquid products of combustion. These aerosolized particles are often saturated with other products of combustion. The magnitude of the injury is dependent upon the size of the particles or drops, the degree and type of contamination with other toxins, and the extent of exposure. The extent of exposure depends upon the patient's minute volume at the time of exposure, the concentration of the agents, and duration of exposure to the smoke.

These superheated particles may also cause thermal injury in distant airways. As particle size increases, the heat carrying capacity also increase, but the particle settles out in the upper airway. As particle size decreases, the particles travel into the lower airway better. About 0.06 micron appears to be deposited best in the lower respiratory tract.

Inhalation of Toxic Gases

Some toxic gases are clinically undetectable because they may be both colorless and odorless. Tests to detect many gases can be difficult to perform, whether at site or in the hospital. The result of inhalation of most gases is poorly studied, and there are few diagnostic studies that confirm an exposure after the gas has been eliminated from the body. There are, of course, exceptions to this, such as carbon monoxide.

Diagnosis of the Inhalation Injury

Diagnosis of the inhalation injury is of paramount importance. Effective early therapy is often lifesaving. Often, the injury is obvious with clinical signs including pharyngeal or laryngeal edema, wheezing, stridor, hoarseness, respiratory distress, and cough yielding carbonaceous sputum. Unfortunately, these signs often herald a fatal course. More often, the clinician makes the diagnosis from the history and physical examination.

In the absence of obvious injury, the clinician must have a high index of suspicion and respond accordingly. Certain mechanisms of injury place the victim in an extremely high-risk category.

1. History of a fire in an enclosed area
2. Exposure to the smoke of synthetic materials, particularly the plastics
3. Loss of consciousness at any time during the fire
4. Inhalation of steam

These individuals should be hospitalized and observed for at least 24 hours for the possible development of delayed symptoms. The on-scene emergency providers will often give the best information available about the mechanism of injury in these cases and should be questioned carefully.

Physical Findings

Once thought to be a clear-cut decision based upon common physical findings and historical data, the diagnosis of inhalation injuries is somewhat more complicated than previously presented. Facial burns, carbonaceous sputum, wheezing, and singed nasal hairs are often cited as classic hallmarks of inhalation injury.

1. Facial burns
2. Carbonacious sputum
3. Wheezing
4. Singed facial hair
5. Alteration of consciousness

Signs of Inhalation Injury Unfortunately, these signs are not diagnostic. Facial burns portend a possible inhalation injury, but 86 percent of patients without an inhalation injury have some degree of facial burns (Figure 11-11). Flash fires or explosions can cause facial burns or singed facial and/or nasal hair without any oropharyngeal or tracheal burns. Also, the converse appears

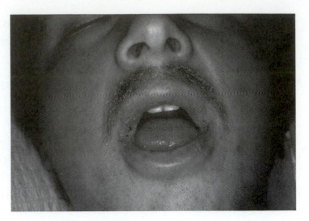

Figure 11-11 Cardinal signs of inhalation injury. *Source:* Photo by Charles Stewart and Associates; www.storysmith.net.

to be false, with only 50 percent of victims of inhalation injuries having facial burns. Singed nasal hairs are an accurate indicator of pulmonary injury in only 13 percent of patients. Only 50 percent of burn victims with a proven inhalation injury had carbonaceous sputum or wheezing.

Unfortunately, since at least 50 percent of patients with a pulmonary injury do have these facial signs, the need for possible airway intervention is not easily dismissed by examination of the patient.

Victims of a fire that have angina or syncope with normal oxygen saturation should also be suspected of having an inhalation injury. Any alteration of consciousness at the scene of the fire should be treated as an inhalation injury until proven otherwise.

Diagnostic Tests

Diagnostic tests that may yield better results than history and physical examination include flexible fiberoptic bronchoscopy, pulmonary function testing, and xenon lung scans.

Pulmonary Function Testing Pulmonary function testing will show increased work of breathing, increased airway resistance, decreased lung compliance, and decreased flow rates in the presence of a pulmonary injury. The presence of normal spirometry values probably excludes a significant injury to the lower respiratory tract. Unfortunately, pulmonary function tests are often not obtainable if the patient is unconscious or not cooperative. Arterial blood gases often show a normal pH and PCO_2 or a mild hypoxemia. An increased arterial-alveolar oxygen gradient may also be found. Measurement of carboxyhemoglobin is an important and useful screening test for inhalation injuries.

Fiberoptic Bronchoscopy Fiberoptic bronchoscopy is easily performed in the emergency department and will readily detect edema, swelling, and obstruction. Endoscopic criteria used to diagnose an inhalation injury include mucosal erythema, hemorrhage, necrosis, ulcerations, and the presence of carbonaceous deposits. Fiberoptic bronchoscopy will not help in the diagnosis of the injury that is limited to the lung parenchyma.

If upper airway burns are observed by fiberoptic bronchoscopy or laryngoscopy, the patient needs to be intubated immediately. If a fiberoptic laryngoscope is used for this examination, an appropriate endotracheal tube should be positioned over it for rapid intubation. A fiberoptic laryngoscope is useful in diagnosis of the pulmonary injury but its field of view is limited to the mainstem bronchi and trachea.

Xenon Lung Scan Another test for diagnosis of an inhalation injury is a xenon lung scan. Xenon 133 is an inert, insoluble gas that is injected intravenously. After injection, the blood carries the xenon to the lungs where it is cleared by exhalation within 90 to 180 seconds. Normally, if xenon is retained or unequal clearing of the radioactive tracer is found, an inhalation injury is suspected. Unfortunately, prior lung disease such as asthma or bronchitis may cause a false positive result. Even more problematic is the ability to obtain a xenon lung scan in a reasonable amount of time to make a clinical difference.

Other Lab Tests

Arterial Blood Gases Arterial blood gas values may increase suspicion of an inhalation injury, but they do not provide a diagnosis. A distinct advantage in obtaining arterial blood gases is that they frequently return before other laboratory tests! If good paO_2, $paCO_2$, and O_2 saturation are found in the presence of an obviously dyspneic or apneic patient, the clinician should consider that the patient might have inhaled toxins such as carbon monoxide or cyanide.

Unfortunately, the oxygen saturation is calculated from a measured oxygen tension, in most laboratories. Since the oxygen tension of arterial blood is unchanged by carbon monoxide, calculated results will be higher than if it was actually measured. For best results, the laboratory should measure the saturation and not calculate it.

Carboxyhemoglobin Level An immediate concern about any victim of suspected smoke inhalation is whether they have suffered from carbon monoxide poisoning. Carbon monoxide levels will rapidly rise to lethal levels if the fire was in an enclosed area. Measuring the carboxyhemoglobin level makes the definitive diagnosis of carbon monoxide poisoning.

As noted in the lecture on carbon monoxide (CO) poisoning, the CO level may correlate with symptoms, but absence of CO in the blood does not rule out carbon monoxide poisoning or effects. Since nearly all fires produce carbon monoxide, carbon monoxide blood levels may also be used as a screening test to increase suspicion of other inhaled toxins.

Think of CO poisoning in ALL FIRES!

Pulse oximetry is totally inadequate in judging whether a patient has carbon monoxide poisoning! A pulse oximeter measures the light absorbed at 660 and 940 nm. These values correspond to the reduced hemoglobin and oxygenated hemoglobin levels, respectively. The maximum and minimum absorption of light at these wavelengths generates the pulse signal. The ratio of the absorbed light is then used to determine the oxygen saturation. The oxygen saturation calculated by the pulse oximeter simply wouldn't change with increased carboxyhemoglobin levels because the CO molecule has a different maximum absorption wavelength.

> Pulse oximeters should not be used to monitor patients
> with suspected CO poisoning!

A co-oximeter or transcutaneous PO_2 meter is accurate in detecting a decreased oxyhemoglobin level in the presence of an increase in carboxyhemoglobin. Co-oximeters measure absorption of light on at least six frequencies, including those for reduced hemoglobin, carboxyhemoglobin, methemoglobin, sulfhemoglobin, and oxyhemoglobin. Transcutaneous oxygen monitors measure diffusion of oxygen through the skin. Since only oxygen that is available to tissues can diffuse through the skin, tissue hypoxia will be accurately measured in CO poisoning.

Chest X-ray A chest x-ray should be obtained on all patients with a suspected inhalation injury. The chest x-ray may be normal for nearly 24 hours after the injury, and, as such, is an unreliable screening tool. It will serve as a good baseline for future changes. If positive, the pattern may be mixed, show an alveolar infiltrate, an interstitial infiltrate, or congestive heart failure. Infiltrates are more common in the upper lung fields. X-rays may show concomitant injuries such as fractured ribs or pneumothorax.

> A NORMAL Chest x-ray DOES NOT RULE OUT Inhalation Injury!

The burned patient with a potential inhalation injury should *never* be sent to x-ray without a qualified attendant. Likewise, intubation should not be delayed to take an x-ray that is performed merely to confirm the obvious.

Soft Tissues of the Neck X-ray views of the soft tissues of the neck will either rule out or document any suspected obstruction of the upper airway. The epiglottis and trachea should be visible on the lateral and anterior-posterior views, respectively.

Electrocardiogram Since hypoxia is such frequent concomitant of most inhalation injuries, an electrocardiogram (ECG) is indicated both as a baseline and to assess hypoxic insults to the myocardium. If the ECG is abnormal, the patient should be monitored for any dysrhythmias. As always, if old records are available, previous ECGs should be obtained for comparison.

Urinalysis Although urinalysis may not seem like a test of the respiratory tree, the inhaled toxic gas may have systemic effects. The urine should be checked for hematuria and proteinuria. Proteinuria could suggest exposure to carbon monoxide, hydrogen sulfide, halogens, or carbon disulfide, for example. Hematuria may suggest hydrogen sulfide, halogens, or carbon disulfide inhalation.

Miscellaneous Laboratory Tests Ethanol levels should be determined, particularly if the patient has any altered mental status. Cigarette smoking and alcohol consumption is commonly and tragically associated with bed fires.

Cyanide levels are often unavailable or greatly delayed. Suspicion must guide the practitioner who does not have this laboratory exam readily available.

Clinical Course

The progression of the inhalation injury is related to the extent and intensity of both the chemical and thermal components. In severe inhalation injuries, respiratory distress may begin within minutes to hours. In these cases, the problem is likely to be multifaceted. Expect a complex injury.

Airway

Hypoxia and anoxia or direct toxic effects of rapidly acting toxins may incapacitate the patient within moments. Bronchospasm and alveolar damage may cause rapid deterioration and high mortalities in these patients. Irritant effects may cause edema of the airway that may lead to respiratory obstruction. Absorbed acids, toxins, and irritants may cause an inflammatory response with release of histamine and other vasoactive substances or smooth muscle spasm.

Although concerns about the upper airway have focused on the first few hours after the burn, the maximum edema may peak 36 to 48 hours later. The patient may have no respiratory difficulties on admission, and gradually develop stridor, hoarseness, labored breathing, and retractions. Particularly in young patients, the arterial blood gases may reflect only the tachypnea until the patient tires. This is often about the time that the patient is being transferred to a burn unit. Unfortunately, this is also the time when intubation requires maximum expertise.

Inhalation Injury = Low threshold for Intubation

Airway Plugs About days 3 to 4, soot, tars, resins, epithelial debris, and necrotic tissue may act as a physical plug to small airways. Plugging from debris and spasm may lead to atelectasis, air trapping, or emphysematous areas. This plugging may also set the stage for recurrent pneumonia, empyema, abscesses, and all of the myriad complications of the aspirated foreign body.

Look for a sudden deterioration in the PO_2 or the PCO_2 in a patient who has previously done well. These patients may have only nonspecific findings on chest x-ray, including both areas of hyperinflation and atelectasis. Increased secretions, wheezing, and increased difficulty ventilating the patient may also be found. These plugs are often easily removed with a fiberoptic bronchoscope.

Pulmonary Edema and ARDS Likewise, pulmonary edema develops between 8 and 36 hours, with some inhaled toxins. It occurs somewhat earlier in patients with underlying pulmonary disease, congestive heart failure, or past history of myocardial ischemia. An iatrogenic fluid load may also precipitate pulmonary edema. This pulmonary edema is not uncommon about the third day after the injury as the tissue edema is reabsorbed into the circulation. Sepsis may also trigger ARDS.

Pulmonary edema due to inhaled toxins responds poorly to the diuretic therapy. Early use of positive end expiratory pressure (PEEP) should be considered in these cases. If the patient develops pulmonary edema after an inhalation injury, pulmonary artery pressures should guide the administration of fluids.

ARDS may also develop as a delayed complication. It may be a challenging diagnostic exercise to differentiate between the early appearance of ARDS and pulmonary edema. A normal or low pulmonary artery occlusion pressure "wedge" in the face of pulmonary edema will suggest the diagnosis of ARDS.

Pneumonia The most delayed pulmonary complication to develop is often a bacterial bronchopneumonia. This pneumonia develops after the toxin has destroyed the lung's defenses. This complication may also be partly due to the impaired clearance of secretions, plugging, and atelectasis. Ciliary impairment due to the toxins decreases the clearance of secretions and debris. Immunosuppression from the burn decreases the patient's ability to resist the infections.

Cardiovascular Cardiovascular collapse may result from the hypoxia or from the direct action of such toxins as Freon. These toxins may precipitate arrhythmias, cardiac arrest, hypotension, conduction blocks, or pulmonary edema. The hypoxia may cause infarcts or ischemic ECG changes.

Central Nervous System Early general symptoms of toxic gas inhalation include restlessness, "intoxication," headache, dizziness, confusion, seizures, or coma. One question needs to be answered immediately: Are the symptoms due to the toxin or merely hypoxia? This question is best answered by removal of the person from the offending agent and applying 100 percent oxygen. Always remember to include trauma, alcohol, and drugs (licit and illicit) in the differential.

Hepatic and Renal Systems It is difficult to separate hepatic or renal failure due to toxic damage from hypoxic injury. The inhaled toxin may cause hepatic necrosis, such as is found with the hydrocarbons. Acute tubular necrosis may result from toxic effects elsewhere such as from the rhabdomyolysis or hemolysis that may be found with carbon monoxide and other inhaled toxins.

Skin and Musculoskeletal Systems The skin should be checked for cyanosis, cherry red color, or brownish tinge. The inhaled toxin may lead to necrosis, ulcers, or frank burns on exposed skin. Bullae formation on dependent parts is particularly common in carbon monoxide poisoning.

The toxin or the hypoxic effects of the toxin may damage the musculoskeletal system. An example of this damage is rhabdomyolysis due to carbon monoxide. Unfortunately, rhabdomyolysis is also found in improper positioning during coma.

Treatment
General Effective treatment of the inhalation injury depends first upon an accurate initial diagnosis and early recognition of complications. The appro-

priate airway treatment principles for both pre-hospital and emergency department care alike are:

1. Ensure and protect an adequate airway
2. Correct hypoxia and potential CO and hydrocyanic acid (HCN) toxicity
3. Clear airway debris and secretions

Monitoring Cardiac toxicity and arrhythmias are common in the presence of hypoxia. In suspected inhalation injuries, cardiac monitoring should be instituted promptly.

Airway Management

Intubation The victim of an inhalation injury who is alert, awake, and conversant needs no airway protection but should be placed on 100 percent oxygen pending CO levels. To intubate, by rote, the patient with "classic" hallmarks of inhalation injury but who is in no respiratory distress, phonating well, and with normal pulmonary functions is inappropriate. An alert and cooperative patient with "classic" findings of an inhalation injury deserves confirmatory flexible fiberoptic bronchoscopy and pulmonary function testing.

To deny intubation because of the lack of classic symptoms and signs when signs of respiratory distress develop or when pulmonary function testing is markedly abnormal is also inappropriate. The patient with stridor or severe dyspnea should be intubated rapidly, placed on 100 percent oxygen by endotracheal tube, and considered for bedside bronchoscopy.

The patient who is unconscious following exposure to smoke should also be rapidly intubated. If the patient has an alteration of consciousness or loss of the gag reflex, intubation is indicated for airway protection and to provide 100 percent oxygen.

Some common sense must be used in the decision of whether to intubate the patient before transport. If the patient is going to be transported following a possible inhalation injury, the means of transportation and the available room and equipment in the transporting vehicle are significant considerations. Transporting the awake, alert patient without "prophylactic intubation" for 10 minutes in a roomy Type III ambulance with full RSI equipment readily available may be quite appropriate. To transport the same patient 45 minutes, over rugged terrain, in a cramped aircraft where the head of the patient is not accessible is a different matter. Obviously, if the patient has met any other criteria for intubation, the decision to intubate for transportation is moot.

Many clinicians use the "P/F" ratio as a criterion for intubation. This is the ratio of the PaO_2 divided by the fraction of inspired oxygen. Normal values are above 400. A value of 300 or less implies that there is an impairment of oxygenation.

Although the nasal route is preferred for intubation in the literature, this is not a clear-cut decision in the patient with an inhalation injury. An adult flexible fiberoptic bronchoscope requires an 8 mm tube orifice in order to pass. Mucous plugging, soot, and debris in the airway may require repeat bronchoscopy for pulmonary toilet. Re-intubation of an edematous airway is not a trivial task. The oral route may allow placement of a larger tube and subsequent bronchoscopy through the tube.

Tracheostomy Early tracheostomy was once advocated for airway control. Now that low-pressure endotracheal tubes are available, routine tracheostomy is no longer recommended. Emergent tracheostomy has no advantage over intubation and many more complications, particularly when performed through burned skin. For facial trauma, severe respiratory distress, or massive facial burns, cricothyrotomy is preferred as the emergency surgical airway of choice (Figure 11-12).

Oxygenation Once the patient has been intubated, humidified oxygen at high flows should be maintained. As noted earlier, carbon monoxide toxicity is associated with smoke inhalation and is emergently treated by administration of high-flow oxygen. Even patients with chronic lung disease should be given high flow oxygen. Although in the patient with COPD, hypoxia may provide the stimulus for respirations, the danger of inhalation injury far outweighs the danger of oxygen therapy. The clinician should be alert to the respiratory rate and status in any case.

Pulmonary Toilet Frequent postural drainage, coughing and encouragement of deep breathing all aid in clearing the airway of debris and secretions. Frequent airway suctioning is often needed to help remove this debris. Occasionally, fiberoptic or rigid bronchoscopy is effective in removal of debris. As noted previously, escharotomy of chest and abdominal burns may be required for circumferential burns.

Bronchospasm If the patient has bronchospasm or wheezing, a trial of nebulized aerosol bronchodilators such as albuterol, terbutaline, or Bronkosol is indicated. Pulmonary edema from toxic gas exposure frequently does not resolve with diuretics. Positive pressure breathing such as PEEP and intubation are often required.

Later treatment includes prompt recognition and treatment of bacterial infections and reversal of ventilation-perfusion abnormalities. In many cases, these occur during the more prolonged hospital stays and are well covered in the many definitive texts upon the management of burns.

Adjunctive Therapy
Antibiotics
Prophylactic antibiotics should not be used. Studies have shown that organisms resistant to the antibiotics used usually results when prophylactic antibiotics are given.

Steroids
Prospective studies have indicated that steroids are not beneficial. Indeed, steroids are associated with a significant increase in mortality even when used briefly.

Pitfalls
Possible suicide attempt
Not enough fluids
Too much fluids

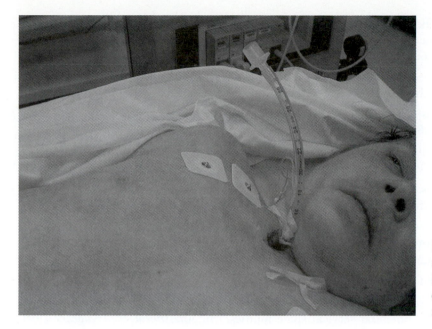

Figure 11-12 Tracheal stoma intubation. *Source:* Photo by Charles Stewart and Associates; www. storysmith.net.

<100 percent oxygen (including COPD patients)
Steroids
"Prophylactic" antibiotics
Methemoglobinemia

Managing the Patient Who Does Not Wish to Be Intubated

The patient who does not wish to be intubated should always have these wishes respected. Alternatives such as CPAP or BiPAP can bring airway relief in selected cases. The patient may be managed with bag-valve-mask techniques until the outcome is clear in other cases.

The unfortunate scenario occurs when the patient clearly expresses a wish to avoid intubation and then lapses into coma. A family member then demands that "everything must be done to save my loved one." This is, at best, an ethical dilemma. When the wishes of the patient are clear and have been set forth when the patient is not obtunded, then these wishes override the family's. If the wishes are not clear, or the circumstances are not straightforward, then an error on the side of caution would be to intubate the patient.

Notes

[1] Trimble, T. "Action-plan for Airway Problems from Hell!" http://enw. org/AirwayHell.htm (retrieved 04/10/200)

[2] Kuchinski, J., et al. "Emergency intubation for paralysis of the uncooperative trauma patient," in *J Emerg Med* 1991;9:9–12.

[3] Ampel, L., et al. "Approach to airway management in the acutely head-injured patient," in *J Emerg Med* 1988;6:1–7.

[4] Nakayama, D. K., Waggoner, T., Venkataraman, S. T. "The use of drugs in emergency airway management in pediatric trauma," in *Am Surg* 1992; 216:205–211.

[5] Stocchetti, N., Furlan, A., Volta, F. "Hypoxemia and arterial hypotension at the accident scene in head injury," in *J Trauma* 1996;40:764–767.

[6] Siesjo, B. K. "Cerebral circulation and metabolism," in *J Neurosurg* 1984; 60:883.

[7] Miller, J. D., et al. "Early Insults to the Injured Brain," in *JAMA* 1978; 240:439.

[8] Stocchetti, N., Furlan, A., Volta, F. "Hypoxemia and arterial hypotension at the accident scene in head injury," *J Trauma* 1996;40:746–767.

[9] Winchell, R. J., Hoyt, D. B. "Endotracheal intubation in the field improves survival in patients with severe head injury," *Arch Surg* 1997; 132:592–597.

[10] Ibid.

[11] Hastings, R. H., Marks, J. D. "Airway management for trauma patients with potential cervical spine injuries," in *Anesthesia & Analgesia* 1991; 73:471–482.

[12] Dufour, D. G., Larose, D. L., Clement, S. C. "Rapid sequence intubation in the emergency department," *J Emerg Med* 1995;13:705–710.

[13] Redan, J. A., et al. "The value of intubating and paralyzing patients with suspected head injury in the emergency department," *J Trauma* 1991;31: 371–375.

[14] Walls R. M. "Airway management in the blunt trauma patient: How important is the cervical spine," *Can J Surg* 1992;35:27–29.

[15] Hastings, R. H., Marks J. D. "Airway management for trauma patients with potential cervical spine injuries," *Anesthesia & Analgesia* 1991;73: 471–482.

[16] Ibid.

[17] Aphramian C., et al. "Experimental cervical spine injury model: Examination of airway management and splinting techniques," *Ann Emerg Med* 1984;13:584–587.

[18] Bivens, H., et al. "The effect of axial traction during orotracheal intubation of the trauma victim with an unstable cervical spine," *Ann Emerg Med* 1988;17:25–29.

[19] Shatney, C. H., Brunner, R. D., Nguyen, T. Q. "The safety of orotracheal intubation in patients with unstable cervical spine fracture or high spinal cord injury," *Am J Surg* 1995;170:676–680.

[20] Talucci, R. C., Shaikh, K. A., Schwab, C. W. "Rapid sequence induction with oral endotracheal intubation in the multiply injured patient," *Am Surg* 1988;54:185–187.

[21] Criswell, J. C., Parr, M. J. A. "Emergency airway management in patients with cervical spine injuries," *Anes* 1994;49:900–903.

[22] Wright, S. W., Robinson, G. G. II, Wright M. B. "Cervical spine injuries in blunt trauma patients requiring emergent endotracheal intubation," *Am J Emerg Med* 1992;10:104–109.

[23] Scannell, G., et al. "Oral intubation in trauma patients with cervical fractures," *Arch Surg* 1993;128:903–906.

[24] Norwood, S., Myers, M. B., Butler, T. J. "The safety of emergency neuromuscular blockade and orotracheal intubation in the acutely injured trauma patient," *J Am Cell Surg* 1994;179:646–652.

[25] Rhee, K. J., et al. "Oral intubation in the multiply injured patient: The risk of exacerbating spinal cord damage," *Ann Emerg Med* 1990;19:511–514.

[26] Grande, C. M., Barton, C. R., Stene, J. K. "Appropriate techniques for airway management of emergency patients with suspected cervical injuries," *Anesth Analg* 1988;67:714–715.

[27] Hastings, R. H., Marks, J. D. "Airway management for trauma patients with potential cervical spine injuries," *Anesthesia & Analgesia* 1991;73: 471–482.

[28] Ibid.

[29] Ibid.

[30] Travis, S. P. L., Layer, G. T. "Traumatic transection of the thoracic trachea," *Ann Royal Coll Surg Engl* 1983;65:240–241.

[31] Edwards, W. H., et al. "Airway injuries: The first priority in trauma," *Am Surg* 1987;53:192–197.

[32] Ecker, R. R., et al. "Injuries of the trachea and bronchi," *Ann Throracic Surg* 1971;11:289–298.

[33] Camnitz, P. S., Shepard, S. M., Henderson, R. A. "Acute blunt laryngeal and tracheal trauma," *Am J Emerg Med* 1987;5:157–162.

[34] Urschel, H. C., Razzuk, M. A. "Management of acute traumatic injuries of the tracheobronchial tree," *Surg Gynecol Obst* 1973;136:113–117.

[35] Reece, G. P., Shatney, C. H. "Blunt injuries of the cervical trachea: Review of 51 patients," *South Med J* 1988;81:1542–1548.

[36] Aytac, A., et al. "Inhalation of foreign bodies in children: Report of 500 cases," *J Thorac Cardiovasc Surg.* 1977;74:145.

[37] Rothman, B., Boeckman, C. R. "Foreign bodies in the larynx and tracheobronchial tree in children," *Ann Otol Rhinol Laryngol* 1980;89:434–436.

[38] Mu, L., Sun, D., Ping, H. "Radiological diagnosis of aspirated foreign bodies in children: Review of 343 cases," *J Laryngol Otol* 1990;104: 778–782.

[39] Wiseman, N. C., "The diagnosis of foreign body aspiration in childhood," *J Pediatr Surg* 1984, 19:531–535.

[40] Svenson, G. "Foreign bodies in the tracheobronchial tree. Special references to experience in 97 children," *J Pediatr Otorhinolaryngology* 1980;8: 243–251.

[41] Limper, A. H., Prakash, U. B. "Tracheobronchial foreign bodies in adults," *Ann Int Med* 1990;112:604–609.

[42] Rothmann, B. F., Boeckman C. R., 1980.

[43] Boothroyd, A. E., Carty, H. M. L., Robson, W. J. "'Hunt the thimble,' a study of the radiology of ingested foreign bodies," *Arch Emerge Med* 1987;4:33–38.

44 Harris, C. S., et al. "Childhood asphyxiation by food: A national analysis and overview," *JAMA* 1984;251:2231–2235.

45 Baker, S. P., Fisher, R. S. "Childhood asphyxiation by choking or suffocation," *JAMA* 1980;244:1343–1346.

46 Siwek, J. Introducing the "Henderson Maneuver." (Editorial.) AFP 1989; 40:92.

47 Ponniah, R. D., Singh, G. "Foreign bodies in the larynx in infancy," *Practitioner* 1976;217:789–791.

48 Gatch, G., Myre, L., Black, R. E. "Foreign body aspiration in children: Causes, diagnosis, and prevention," *AORN Journal* 1987;46:850–861.

49 Fries, J. H. "Peanuts: Allergic and other untoward reactions," *Ann Allergy* 1982;48:220–226.

50 Bready, L. L., et al. "Bronchoscopic administration of nebulized racemic epinephrine to facilitate removal of aspirated peanut fragments in pediatric patients," *Anesth* 1986;65:523–525.

51 Mittleman, R. E., Wetli, C. V. "The fatal cafe coronary: Foreign-body airway obstruction," *JAMA*. 1982;247:1285–1288.

52 Gay, B. B., et al. "Subglottic foreign bodies in pediatric patients," *AJDC* 1986;140:165–168.

53 Hanukoglu, A., Fried, D., Segal, S. "Loss of voice as sole symptom of subglottic foreign body aspiration. (letter)," *AJDC* 1986;140:973.

Chapter **Twelve**

Case Management Scenarios

Case 1

An 11-month-old child is brought in by a BLS unit after aspirating food at a picnic. The BLS unit is performing BVM with poor success upon arrival in the Ed. The patient has agonal respirations, a pulse of 150, and is comatose.

What is your management priority? The management priority is an open airway . . . as soon as possible.

You attempt the Heimlich maneuver as you have been taught. This yields no results. The child still has an obstructed airway. Now there is no question . . . this patient needs laryngoscopy and intubation . . . now!

How could you remove the foreign body and/or secure the airway? This calls for pediatric Magill forceps and a good look with a laryngoscope. *When you look you see a piece of hot dog. It fragments as you remove it, but you are able to get all of the hot dog out with some difficulty.*

What other methods could be used to maintain the airway? Theoretically, you could push the obstruction down the trachea and intubate one lung. I don't think that this is a good idea and there are no good series that would recommend this approach.

A better technique would be to use jet ventilation. Remember that the cricoid cartilage is the narrowest part of the upper airway in a child and that the foreign body often will hang up in this part of the anatomy. Hopefully, you will be below the piece of hot dog when you go through the cricoid membrane. If not, you could try a tracheal jet ventilation below the cricoid membrane. This may work.

In theory, you can expel the object by using pressure from the jet ventilator. In theory, you can also blow out a lung. After getting some oxygen in the lung, you can also try the Heimlich maneuver again. This has better documentation than using pressure from the jet.

This is a bad situation for the child, no matter what you do. Dealer's choice . . . and the cards are stacked against the child.

Case 2

A 43-year-old presents in status asthmaticus. The patient has a prior history of intubation and ICU time for respiratory failure. He has received SQ epinephrine 0.3 mg, IV Solu-Medrol 125 mg, and two inhalation treatments with bronchodilators. You have about 20 minutes transport time left to your medical center. The patient is obviously fatigued and failing. The patient is sitting bolt upright on the gurney with VS 165/110 140 pulse, 30 respirations per minute, and pulse oximetry of 90 percent on 100 percent NRB. After an initial improvement with oxygen, the patient becomes profoundly diaphoretic and her level of consciousness deteriorates.

What is the best approach to the airway in this patient? Obviously, this patient will require intubation. You decide to intubate the patient with Rapid Sequence Intubation.

What is your best sedative agent? This is a clear indication for ketamine (Ketalar™). The bronchodilator effect may be helpful. If ketamine is not available, this patient should be sedated with etomidate and paralyzed with succinylcholine in standard RSI fashion. Propofol would also provide some bronchodilation.

What specific problem do you face during intubation? This patient is already hypoxic and you aren't going to make her any better by preoxygenation. You simply aren't going to have the luxury of time and space for this patient. You also aren't going to have the luxury for errors during the intubation.

Case 3

A 22-year-old male was sledding and went under a fence. Unfortunately, he was struck by a wire about the face. You note an obvious unstable mandible fracture. Although the patient has limited jaw opening due to the pain, you note a large ecchymotic swelling to the floor of the mouth. The patient has a hoarse voice but appears comfortable. You have a 45 minute transport time from the scene of the accident. During the transport, you note that he develops labored respirations. Re-examination confirms a dramatic worsening of the sublingual hematoma and subcutaneous air in the neck. You decide to intubate to stave off complete airway collapse. You elect to use Rapid Sequence Intubation.

Your first intubation attempt is unsuccessful due to airway distortion by the hematoma on the floor of the mouth.

Your second attempt is likewise unsuccessful.

The patient's oxygen saturation is 85 percent and the pulse is now 120.

Thinking you might be having a bad day, you let your partner attempt to intubate the patient. She is unsuccessful in two subsequent attempts.

What is the next step in management of this difficult airway?

What other alternatives should you consider?

Should you have intubated this patient with RSI?

What other techniques could you have used in this patient?

This is a real problem. This patient has a crushed larynx, and your field solution is definitely not the recommended solution. The patient needs a low tracheostomy, not field intubation. Rapid sequence intubation is clearly *not* indicated for this patient.

Your only option now is to do a jet ventilation.

If this patient has an intact airway, the optimum field solution is to transport the patient rapidly to an emergency department and advise the emergency physician that your patient may have a crushed larynx.

If the patient starts to lose the airway en route, then tracheal jet ventilation may be an appropriate technique. Some authors recommend a single pass at awake nasal intubation, but this is going to be problematic. You can't RSI, and you shouldn't sedate.

Case 4

An 18-year-old female is status post auto versus pedestrian accident. The patient was struck by a fast-moving vehicle and thrown 25 feet. The patient is unconscious, diaphoretic, and pale at the scene. GCS = 8; HR = 120; BP = 90/50; Resp = 24. There is obvious right chest, hip, and head trauma. There is clear fluid leaking from the right ear. You are with the responding ambulance service.

What are your management priorities?
What medication choices would you make for RSI in this patient?

You need the usual field survey in this patient. Clearly, the patient has significant internal injuries, a head injury, and depressed level of consciousness. The patient should be intubated rapidly to protect the airway. A nasal intubation is contraindicated by the suspicion of a basilar skull fracture.

Cervical spine precautions are in order before, during, and after your intubation.

You need an agent that will not lower the blood pressure and will not cause increased intracranial pressure. My choice would be etomidate, although propofol would also be appropriate. Benzodiazepines, sodium thiopental, and narcotics are poor choices.

Case 5

A three-year-old immigrant child is brought in to the emergency department by his worried mother. The mother notes that the child was well until just a few hours ago, when he started to complain of a sore throat. He has developed a fever of 102 and is drooling and having difficulty swallowing. As you examine the child, you note that he is sitting upright with chin thrust forward and his neck slightly extended. He is supporting his upper body weight on his arms. You notice that the child is anxious, apprehensive, and toxic appearing. He has a slight stridor on inspiration.

Does this child need emergent intubation?
If you transport this child, what precautions should you take?
What can you do to prevent further respiratory distress in this child?

This is epiglottitis. We don't see it as much in children as we used to, because they are getting anti-H-flu vaccines, but it is still out there.

This child DOES need emergent intubation, but I wouldn't want to do it in the field. In fact, I'd only do it in the emergency department if I was absolutely forced to. The child needs to be admitted to the OR and intubated with an ENT surgeon standing by in case a tracheostomy is urgently needed.

Transport the child in the position of comfort, mother holding the child, and using "blow-by" oxygen held by mother. No needle sticks, no oxygen masks, no fuss if you can help it.

Slick technique . . . use Heliox™ to give the little tyke a bit more oxygen. The helium-oxygen mixture is less dense than the normal oxygen-nitrogen mixture of air. It goes through the narrowed airway more easily. This can buy you time to get to that OR.

Case 6

A four-and-a-half year old child was running with a Superball™ in his mouth. Mother calls 911 and an ALS unit is dispatched. Upon arrival, the child is in respiratory arrest. A pulse is still present.

What options does the paramedic have to manage this airway problem?
What method would the emergency physician use to control the airway
once the child arrives in the emergency department?

This is Case 1 all over again without the ability to grab the foreign body. This is truly a lethal event.

Case 7

Your ambulance is called to transport a 13-year-old obese child with asthma. As you get the history from her stepfather, you find that the child has been admitted to the hospital three times in the last month for asthma, and once was to the intensive care unit. The child ran out of her nebulizers today after using them extensively all night and day. The child was treated with prednisone upon the last discharge, but the prescription ran out two days ago and the stepfather has not yet gotten a refill.

The respiratory rate is 42, the pulse ox is 85 percent, the patient's pulse is 140, and the blood pressure is 105/65. When you examine the child, you find her sitting in a tripod position. There are extensive retractions about the neck. You are unable to appreciate any wheezes and note the air movement is inadequate. The nail beds are slightly blue.

What should you do to help this child's respiratory distress? First, let's try the standard techniques. You need to give the child continuous nebulization treatments with Ventolin™ or equivalent bronchodilator. The child may benefit from subcutaneous epinephrine or terbutaline.

If you elect to intubate this child, what technique would you use? RSI, of course. You want to control the problem not exacerbate it by using a sedative. You also don't want to wait until the patient starts to crash before you can intubate.

What agent(s) would be appropriate for sedation in RSI? This is another
   ketamine case.

Case 8

A 67-year-old man presents to the ED with COPD. He has been generally well
except for his COPD. He has been under a lot of stress with the death of his
best friend about three days ago. He has started to smoke again. The patient's
breathing has been deteriorating over the past two days, and he is much
worse today. The vital signs are 150/90, 140 pulse, 40 respiratory rate.

   You start him on a Ventolin™ nebulizer treatment with oxygen and he
starts to deteriorate. He becomes somnolent, his tidal volume starts to fall,
and his oxygen saturation starts to fall.

Should you have used oxygen for the nebulizer treatment?
What should you do now?

   The use of oxygen has not harmed the patient. He has, however, run
out of steam. He will require intubation and ventilation. Again, this patient
deserves your best efforts, and RSI is surely the proper choice. A sedative in
this patient will take away the last vestige of his respiratory drive, and you'll
need to intubate an apneic patient. With RSI, you control the timing of the
intubation.

Case 9

You get a 911 call from the wife of a 45-year-old physician for help with her
husband. The dispatcher tells you that the patient has a sore throat and can't
breathe.

   Upon arrival, you find a youthful 45-year-old who is sitting bolt upright
on the couch. He is unable to speak with a normal voice and is quite hoarse.
His wife tells you that he started himself on azithromycin (Zithromax™)
samples for a sore throat yesterday. She notes that he has gotten progressively
worse despite the antibiotics. Your vital signs include a respiratory rate of 40,
pulse of 120, and blood pressure of 140/85.

What are you going to do?
What is this patient's problem? This patient has epiglottitis. (This was an
   actual case of mine). The patient needs transport to the emergency department with high-flow oxygen. If you have Heliox, this is a good
   time to use it.

   Intubation of this patient can be fraught with hazard and quite difficult.
If you can avoid it in the field, you should do so. I did an awake nasal intubation in the emergency department with a fiberoptic laryngoscope. My ENT
doctor was standing by and ready to do a tracheostomy. The doctor spent
two days in the ICU and was discharged to home in three days.

   This is the disease that killed President Washington. By the way, this was
Hemophilus influenza. The older folks didn't get the immunization, and this
is the most common organism in this age group.

Case 10

A 24-year-old female presents to the emergency department from the scene of a fire. She is brought in by family, directly from the fire as a victim of smoke inhalation. She is very intoxicated. She responds with appropriate answers to questions but has a slurred speech with hoarseness. She coughs frequently and is expectorating carbonaceous sputum. Her eyebrows and lips are singed. Vital signs include blood pressure of 125/80, pulse of 100, and respiratory rate of 22. Oxygen saturation is 98 percent. Arterial blood gases have pH 7.44, 36 $PaCO_2$, 88 PaO_2. Her carboxyhemoglobin is 15 percent.

What is your approach to this patient's airway?

You have three problems:

Inhalation injury, carbon monoxide intoxication, and alcohol intoxication. The alcohol intoxication is probably not going to cause life threatening problems but may complicate your other treatments.

You need to have this patient on 100 percent oxygen for the carbon monoxide intoxication. You should probably intubate the patient for airway control. If you are going to transport the patient, intubation is mandatory.

Some authors would suggest that you could use fiberoptic laryngoscopy to look at the carina and see if there is soot, swelling, and burns. If there is, then the patient can be intubated at the same time. If there is not, then intubation can be approached at leisure, if needed at all. If you can't look at the carina, then intubation is mandatory.

Chapter **Thirteen**

Summary

O ne of the most frightening experiences that the emergency provider faces is the critically ill patient with a difficult airway. Knowledge of alternatives, familiarity with the instruments and anatomy, and practice with the procedures should be gained in the cool light of day rather than during the heat of the crisis. Complications are more frequent during intubation of the moribund patient when time and technique are critical.

The astute emergency provider should diligently review the immediate actions for management of the difficult airway in the same spirit that a pilot reviews emergency procedures. Both expect not to have to employ these skills on any one journey, but others stake their lives on rapid and accurate response during an urgent situation.

Appendix 1

Airway Aphorisms

- If you are properly prepared for the difficult airway, it becomes increasingly difficult to find a difficult airway.
- If the patient has an airway obstruction or a potential obstruction, it is generally safer to let them continue to breathe than to paralyze them.
- Drugs that last a long time tend to last far longer when you really want (or need) the patient to breathe on his or her own.
- Have a low threshold for calling for help. It is so much easier to apologize to a colleague for unnecessarily bothering him or her than it is to apologize to the grieving family.
- The very obese patient is always a challenge.
- If you wait until a difficult airway to learn an advanced technique for the airway . . . well, you just won't be elegant and slick when you do it.
- A surgical airway is better than a pretty neck in a corpse. (Far easier to explain, too!)
- Surgical airways are a bloody mess!
- Fiberoptic intubation requires skill, an airway free of blood and edema, and experience. Of these, the most important is probably experience. In the middle of a dire emergency is probably not the time to try to get that experience.
- Good judgment is the result of experience.
- Bad judgment will build a lot of experience quickly!

Appendix 2

Pitfalls in Intubation

- Inadequate training, experience, and practice
- Failure to properly prepare the equipment before starting
- Failure to preoxygenate the patient
- Using the laryngoscope as a pry bar
- Forcing a tube against resistance
- Pushing the tube in too far
- Prolonged attempts without oxygenation

Appendix 3
Difficult Intubation Cart/Bag

Oxygen Delivery Equipment

Laerdal bag-valve-mask (or equivalent) with multiple size masks and reservoir
Oxygen tubing extension for connection to wall outlet or tank
Suction equipment
Endotracheal suction catheters #10, #12, #14
Yankauer oral suction catheter
Suction tubing

Suction device (battery-powered, hand-powered, or wall attachment, as appropriate)

Nasal:

Nasopharyngeal airways sizes #6, #7, #8
Endotrol blind nasal trigger endotracheal tubes sizes 6.0, 7.0, and 8.0

Oral:

Guedel oropharyngeal airways #8, #9, #10, #11
Stylets/intubating guides
        Endotracheal tube stylet (satin tip) size 14 Fr.
        Eschmann gum elastic bougie sizes 10 Fr, 15 Fr.
        Trachlight (Laerdal)
Cuffed endotracheal tubes 5.0, 5.5, 6.0, 6.5, 7.0, 7.5, 8.0, 8.5

Laryngoscope Blades and Handles:

Curved: #3 and #4 Macintosh, McCoy, Left handed #3 Macintosh, Huff-man prism for Macintosh blade
Straight: #3 and #4 Miller, #2 Seward, #3 and #4 Wisconsin, #3 and #4 Wis-Forregar.
Handles: C-cell, D-Cell, AA-Cell, Short handle

Laryngeal Mask Airways:

Sizes #3, #4, #5
Fastrach intubating laryngeal masks #3, #4
Endotracheal tubes for laryngeal masks sizes 6.0, 6.5, 7.0 cuffed
Size 6.0 Sheridan LTS
Combitube

Cricothyroidotomy Tools

Transcricothyroid membrane jet ventilation
        Intravenous catheters size 12 gauge and 14 gauge (2 inch)
        Jet ventilation hose and controller handle and Luer lock connector
Retrograde transcricothyroid membrane wire
Melker percutaneous dilational cricothyrotomy set (uncuffed #6.0 tra-cheostomy tube) included in set
Surgical cricothyrotomy equipment
        #3 scalpel handle, #10 blade, #11 blade
        Tracheal retraction hook
        Size 6.0 endotracheal tube
        Shiley cuffed tracheostomy tubes #4, #6, #8, #10

Accessory Equipment

Confirming position of ET tube—Easy Cap ETCO$_2$ detector
Endotracheal tube exchange catheters
        With jet ventilation capability
                Cardiomed
                Cook catheter, small, medium, large
        Without jet ventilation capability
                Sheridan catheter, small, medium, and large

Other
    Spare batteries and bulbs for laryngoscope
    Bite blocks
    Magill forceps
    Lidocaine spray
    Cetacaine spray

Appendix 4
Adjuncts and Measures to Assist Intubation

Changing Laryngoscope Blades
Changing the size or type (curved vs. straight) of laryngoscope blade may allow for better visualization of the glottic opening. When the patient has overriding teeth or a floppy epiglottis, the straight blade may provide better visualization. Straight blades are more useful in children.

Use of a Stylet
Guiding Stylets
When the glottic opening can be seen but insertion of the endotracheal tube is difficult, a stylet may be useful. Suction catheters, tracheal tube exchangers, and gum bougie stylets have all been used successfully for this purpose.

Lighted Stylets
A lighted stylet as described earlier can be used to aid the difficult intubation.

Magill Forceps
Magill forceps can move the tip of the tube into a better location.

Use of a Directional Tip Control Endotracheal Tube
The Endotrol endotracheal tube allows the operator to control the curve of the distal part of the endotracheal tube. Although these tubes were originally developed for blind nasotracheal intubation, they are invaluable for the difficult oral intubation.

"Blind" Passage Based on Landmarks
Sometimes the only structure seen during the intubation is the epiglottis. The endotracheal tube can be passed successfully by sliding the end of the tube along the underside of the epiglottis and (hopefully) through the glottic opening. When the operator can only see the arytenoids, the tube may be directed superiorly to these structures. Needless to say, confirmation of tube placement in this occasion is essential.

Use of an Assistant
The assistant can do more than hold pressure on the cricoid. In a difficult intubation, the assistant can employ the laryngoscope with the intubator's guidance. When adequate glottic exposure is attained, the operator has both hands free to use Magill forceps.

Index

Boldface page numbers refer to figures and tables